PHARMACOLOGY IN DRUG DISCOVERY AND DEVELOPMENT

THIRD EDITION

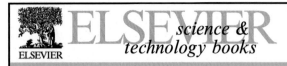

∴ *Companion Web Site:*

https://www.elsevier.com/books-and-journals/book-companion/9780443141249

Pharmacology in Drug Discovery and Development, Third edition
Terry P. Kenakin

Resources available:

• https://coursewareobjects.elsevier.com/objects/elr/ExpertConsult/Kenakin/pharmacologydiscovery3e/quizzes/

**ACADEMIC
PRESS**

PHARMACOLOGY IN DRUG DISCOVERY AND DEVELOPMENT

UNDERSTANDING DRUG RESPONSE

THIRD EDITION

TERRY P. KENAKIN

Department of Pharmacology, University of North Carolina, School of Medicine, Chapel Hill, NC, United States

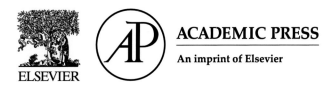

ACADEMIC PRESS
An imprint of Elsevier

ELSEVIER

For Information on all Academic Press publications
visit our website at https://www.elsevier.com/books-and-journals

Publisher: Mica H. Haley
Acquisitions Editor: Andre G. Wolff
Editorial Project Manager: Himani Dwivedi
Production Project Manager: Omer Mukthar
Cover Designer: Vicky Pearson Esser

Typeset by MPS Limited, Chennai, India

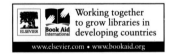

Working together
to grow libraries in
developing countries

www.elsevier.com • www.bookaid.org

Dedication

As always . . . for Debbie

Contents

Preface

Pharmacology is unique in that it is the only scientific discipline that considers the fact that drugs can demonstrate different behaviors in different organs through common mechanisms, a fact that makes the prediction of therapeutic effects sometimes very difficult. Over the past few years, a "perfect storm" has descended upon the pharmacology of drug discovery with the introduction of two important forces, namely, molecular dynamics and new assay technology. Molecular dynamics describes proteins as moving bodies with a nearly limitless capacity to change conformation. These ideas counter the previous simple models of drug action in pharmacology, which essentially described drugs as turning target proteins on and off like simple switches. Molecular dynamics allows us to describe nuanced drug activity and better define exactly what is required in the treatment of disease. The second force is the increasing availability of new assays to view the complex behaviors of drug targets as they sample these new conformations predicted through molecular dynamics. These assays redefine what is meant by "drug activity" and now allow a more informed selection of new drug candidates for human testing. The impact of these new ideas on drug discovery is prevalent in this new edition, which hopefully will bring these new ideas into focus for new drug therapy.

Terry P. Kenakin
Professor, Department of Pharmacology, University of North Carolina,
School of Medicine, Chapel Hill, NC, United States

Acknowledgments

I wish to thank Andre Wolff at Elsevier for generous support during the preparation of this edition, and I am indebted to the University of North Carolina School of Medicine for giving me the means to explore pharmacology and apply it to drug discovery. Finally, I am very grateful to my wife and family for their boundless patience during the writing of this book.

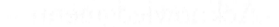

1

Pharmacology: the chemical control of physiology

By the end of this chapter, the reader should be able to understand how drug response is quantified by the use of dose-response curves, the way in which different tissues process drug stimulus to provide tissue response, and what qualifies a drug to be classified either as an agonist or antagonist.

Pharmacology and cellular drug response

Pharmacology (from the Greek φάρμακον, pharmakon, "drug" and -λογία, -logia, the study of) concerns drug action on physiological systems (physiology from the Greek φύσις, physis, "nature, origin" and -λογία, -logia is the study of the mechanical, physical, and biochemical functions of living organisms). With regard to the application of

Pharmacology in Drug Discovery and Development
DOI: https://doi.org/10.1016/B978-0-443-14124-9.00006-9

pharmacology to the discovery of drugs for therapeutic benefit, the main focus of pharmacological theories, procedures, and mechanisms relates to the *chemical control of physiological processes*. Insofar as the understanding of these physiological processes benefits the pharmacologic pursuit of drugs, pharmacology and physiology are intimately related. However, it will also be seen that complete understanding of the physiologic processes involved is *not* a prerequisite to the effective use of pharmacology in the drug discovery process. In fact, often an operational approach is utilized whereby the complexity of the physiology is represented by simple surrogate mathematical functions.

The important practical aspect of these ideas that pharmacology captures, in a unique way, the fact that drugs work in partnership with physiology and that this predicts the effect of any given drug can change depending on the physiological environment in which it is placed to produce effect. As shown in Fig. 1.1, a given drug, interacting with various setpoints of complex physiological system, can have a variety of observed effects. Within this context, an in vitro experiment revealing the activity of a drug in a system with defined sensitivity and reactivity can be considered a limited "snapshot" of the drug's activity. Once this same drug is exposed to the wide variety of tissues (with varying sensitivities), then the full range of the activities of this drug will be revealed. In this sense, the snapshot becomes the "movie" of the range of drug behaviors potentially observed. Understanding the relationship between the primary properties

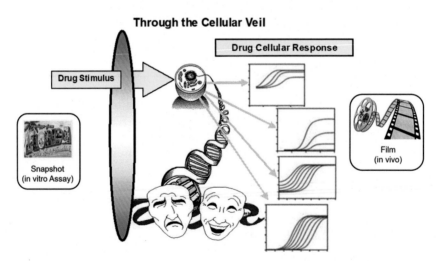

FIGURE 1.1 One view of the activity of a drug can be obtained in an in vitro experiment (the "snapshot"). However, drugs are used in vivo where they encounter a vast array of tissues of differing sensitivities and these can change the response to the drug (the "movie"). Pharmacology furnishes the tools and scales that bridge the gap between a single experiment and in vivo activity.

of the drug and the relative sensitivity and reactivity of the physiological system with which it will interact is the key to the selection of the ideal drug candidate for the modification of any defined pathophysiology. These effects demonstrate an obvious value of pharmacology in that the tools and concepts of the discipline can differentiate capricious and erroneous drug behavior from behavior correctly predicted by complex systems. For example, the b-adrenoceptor prenalterol agonist can produce a full agonist effect in the right atria, but no agonist response at all (in fact full antagonism) in skeletal muscle. Given this, it might be supposed that one of the experiments giving these two profiles is wrong but in fact, both could be correct, the difference being a complex interplay of agonist affinity, efficacy, and system sensitivity in physiology. Another example would be that a given antagonist produces decreases in agonist sensitivity with no diminution of agonist response in one system and a depression of the maximal agonist response in another. However, this would be correctly predicted in systems with differing kinetic sensitivities and would not be indicative of erroneous experimental data.

In contrast, understanding how pharmacologic behavior can change observed behavior can highlight obviously erroneous data. For example, two experimental systems indicating that a given antagonist produces steric hindrance-based orthosteric antagonism in one system and an allosteric-based (separate sites of interaction) in another highlights that one of these systems yields erroneous data. The point of this is that understanding what pharmacology predicts is the discerning factor in determining elucidation of complex activity from erroneous data.

The starting point of any pharmacologic modification of physiology is the drug target, thus it is useful to define what is meant by pharmacological target.

New terminology

The following new terms will be introduced in this chapter:

- *Affinity*: The propensity of a drug molecule to associate closely with a drug target.
- *Agonists*: Drugs that produce an observable change in the state of a physiological system.
- *Antagonists*: Drugs that may not produce a direct effect, but do interfere with the production of cellular response to an agonist.
- *Dose-response curve*: The relationship between doses (if the drug is used in vivo) or concentrations (if used in vitro) of a drug and pharmacologic effect.

- *Drug target*: The protein (or in some cases DNA, mRNA) to which a drug binds to elicit whatever pharmacologic effect it will produce. These proteins can be seven transmembrane (or one transmembrane) receptors, enzymes, nuclear receptors, ion channels, or transport proteins.
- *EC50*: Concentration of agonist producing half the maximal response to the same agonist; usually expressed for calculation and statistical manipulation as the pEC_{50}, negative logarithm of the molar concentration producing 50% response.
- *Efficacy*: The change in state of the drug target upon binding of a drug.
- *Efficiency of target coupling*: The relationship between the net quanta of activation given to a cell and the number of drug targets available for activation.
- *Full agonists*: Agonists that produce the full maximal response that the system can produce.
- *Null method*: The comparison of equiactive concentrations (or doses) of drug to cancel the cell-based processing of drug response. The assumption is that equal responses to a given agonist are processed in an identical manner by the cell.
- *Partial agonists*: Agonists that produce a maximal response that is of lower magnitude than the maximal response that the system can produce to maximal stimulation.
- *pEC50*: The negative logarithm of EC_{50} values. For arithmetic and/or statistical manipulation, numbers must be normally distributed. This is true only of pEC_{50}s, not of EC_{50}s; thus all averages, estimates, or error and statistical procedures must use pEC_{50}.
- *Potency*: The concentration (usually molar) of the drug needed to produce a defined response or effect.
- *Target density*: The concentration of drug targets at the site of activation, that is, on the cell surface for receptors.

Pharmacological targets

The term "pharmacological target" refers to the biochemical entity to which the drug first binds in the body to elicit its effect. There are a number of such entities targeted by drug molecules. In general, they can be proteins, such as receptors, enzymes, transporters, ion channels, or genetic material, such as DNA. The prerequisite for pharmacologic targets is that they have the ability to discern differences in electronic structure minute enough to be present in small drug-like molecules; in this regard, the most predominant targets for drugs are protein in nature. Proteins have the tertiary three-dimensional structure necessary for a detailed definition of the electronic forces involved in small molecule binding. Signals are initiated through complementary binding of drug molecules to protein conformations that have a physiological purpose in the cell. The act of these molecules binding to the protein will change it, and with that change, a pharmacologic effect will occur.

At this point, it is worth considering the beginning and end processes. The first process is the drug binding to the target. The result(s) of this process are totally dependent on the affinity and efficacy of the drug. These are drug parameters unique to its chemical structure. In pharmacologic terms, this is the most important effect, since it occurs in every tissue and organ possessing the target. Therefore characterization of this event enables a general quantification of drug-target activity to be made in the test system, which will also be true for all systems including the therapeutic one. Therefore *the characterization of affinity and efficacy becomes the primary aim of pharmacologic analysis.* However, it can be seen that the various (and variable) biochemical reactions linking the target to cellular response intervene, thereby causing a tissue-dependent abstraction of the link between affinity and efficacy and observed cellular potency. The magnitude of this abstraction depends upon the number of responding target units and the efficiency of target coupling.

The major protein target classes are membrane receptors, enzymes, ion channels, and transporter proteins. Of these, the most prominent drug targets are receptors. While there are a number of types of receptor, one of the most important from the standpoint of therapeutic drug targets is seven transmembrane receptors (7TMRs). These are so-called because they span the cell membrane seven times to form complex recognition domains both outside and inside the cell. These proteins are capable of recognizing chemicals, such as hormones and neurotransmitters present in the extracellular space, and transmit signals from these to the cell interior. Due to the fact that these are on the cell surface and thus exposed to the extracellular space, these entities were the subject of experiments that originally defined the receptor concept (see Box 1.1 for history).

Historically, pharmacology evolved from the medical discipline of physiology (see Box 1.1). It should be stressed that pharmacology is the study of the molecule producing the physiological change (i.e., the drug) and not the physiological change itself (although the latter is intimately involved with defining the nature of the drug). A unique feature of pharmacology is that the effect of the drug is often observed indirectly, that is, while the drug affects a select biochemical process in the cell, the outcome to an observer is an overall change in the state of the whole organism, and this is often the result of multiple interacting cellular processes. A major aim of pharmacology is to define the molecular events in initiating drug effects, since these define the action of drugs in

---

BOX 1.1

The birth of pharmacology

Pharmacology may be considered the child of Physiology, itself an offspring of medicine. Historically, Physiology as a discipline is many hundreds of years old, beginning with pioneers such as the Greek physician Galen (129–200) and the English physician William Harvey (1578–1657). In their quest to understand the workings of the human body, early physiologists would probe systems with chemicals to see what changes occurred and how the body dealt with chemically induced response. In time, a subset of these physiologists, such as Bernard (see below), became more interested in the probes than the systems and pharmacology was born.

I would in particular draw the attention to physiologists to this type of physiological analysis of organic systems which can be done with the aid of toxic agents...

Claude Bernard, Pharmacologist

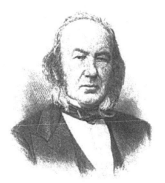

Claude Bernard
(1813–78)

The first Pharmacological Institute was created by Rudolf Buchheim (1820–79) in 1849 at the University of Dorpat in Estonia. The first Pharmacology Department in the United States was established by John Jacob Abel in 1891 at the University of Michigan School of Medicine.

---

all systems. If quantified correctly, this information can be used to predict drug effect at the pharmacological target in all systems including therapeutic one(s). While the ultimate aim of pharmacology in drug discovery is to define the therapeutic actions of drugs, the fact that drugs may have different behaviors in different organs depending on the state of the tissue means that it may not be possible to explicitly predict what a given drug will do in all tissues (since the state of these tissues in the human body may be quite heterogeneous). Moreover, physiological and pathophysiological conditions may change the state of tissues making for even more heterogeneous therapeutic conditions. Therefore the drug discovery process of characterizing drug candidate molecules is aimed at defining what a given molecule has the capability of doing in a tissue, not necessarily what it will do in all tissues. For instance, one molecular activity an excitatory drug may have is to elevate the second cellular messenger cyclic adenosine monophosphate (AMP) through activation of a signaling protein called Gs protein. If it can be shown that a given candidate molecule has no Gs protein stimulating activity, then it is known that this will not be a therapeutic outcome for the molecule. However, if the candidate does show Gs protein activating capability, this means that the molecule may elevate cyclic AMP therapeutically but only if the conditions are right to do so. The heterogeneity of tissues in the body also requires discovery efforts to utilize pharmacological concepts and procedures to convert descriptive data (what the experimenter sees in a particular experiment) into predictive data (enabling logical prediction of effects in other tissues). This is done through generic pharmacological, scales, such as affinity and efficacy (*vide infra*).

Historically, while the actual physical nature of receptors was unknown, it was realized that a distinct entity on the cell surface allows cells to recognize drugs and read the chemical information encoded in them—Box 1.2. Early concepts of receptors likened them to locks with drugs as keys (i.e., as stated by the biologist Paul Ehrlich: ... *substances can only be anchored at any particular part of the organism, if they fit into the molecule of the recipient complex like apiece of mosaic finds its place in a pattern...*). The main value of receptors is that they put order into the previously disordered world of physiology. For example, it can be observed that the hormone epinephrine produces a wealth of dissimilar physiological responses, such as bronchiole muscle relaxation, cardiac muscle positive inotropy, chronotropy and lusitropy, melatonin synthesis, pancreatic, lacrimal and salivary gland secretion, decreased stomach motility, urinary bladder muscle relaxation, skeletal muscle tremor, and vascular relaxation. The understanding of how such a vast array of biological responses could be mediated by a single hormone is difficult until it is realized that these processes are all mediated by the interaction of epinephrine with a single receptor protein, in this case, the β-adrenoceptor. Thus when this receptor is present on the surface of any given cell it will respond to epinephrine, and the nature of that response will be determined by the encoding of the receptor excitation produced by epinephrine to the cytosolic biochemical cascades controlling cellular function. This forms a unifying concept in pharmacology,

BOX 1.2

The evolution of the receptor concept in pharmacology

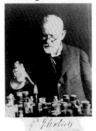

Numerous physiologists and pharmacologists contributed to the concept of "receptor" as minimal recognition units for chemicals in cells. Paul Ehrlich (1854–1915) studied dyes and bacteria and determined that there are "chemoreceptors" (he proposed a collection of "amboreceptors," "triceptors," and "polyceptors") on parasites, cancer cells, and microorganisms that could be exploited therapeutically.

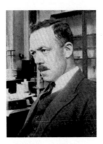

John Newport Langley (1852–1926), as Chair of the Physiology Department in Cambridge, studied the drugs jaborandi (containing the alkaloid pilocarpine) and atropine. He concluded that receptors were "switches" that received and generated signals and that these switches could be activated or blocked by specific molecules.

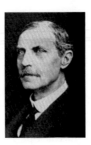

continued

BOX 1.2 *(cont'd)*

AJ Clark (1885–1941), who could be considered as the father of modern receptor pharmacology, was one of the first to suggest from studies of acetylcholine (ACh) and atropine that a unimolecular interaction occurs between a drug and a "substance on the cell." As stated by Clark: *"... it is impossible to explain the remarkable effects observed except by assuming that drugs unite with receptors of a highly specific pattern..."*

which is the melding of chemistry and physiology because the receptor becomes a focus for medicinal chemists in efforts to modify physiology, that is, a simple interaction of molecules with a single protein in simplified assay systems can be used to illuminate the structure–activity relationships that govern the complex physiology. In a conceptual sense, the term "receptor" can refer to any single biological entity that responds to drugs (i.e., enzymes, ion channels, transport proteins, DNA, and structures in the nucleus). This information is transmitted through changes in protein shape (conformation), that is, the drug does not enter the cell nor does the receptor change the nature of the drug (as an enzyme would).

Pharmacologic effects on cells can include a wide variety of outcomes, from changes in the mechanical function of cells (i.e., cardiac contractility, contraction of bronchiole smooth muscle), biochemical metabolic effects (levels of second messengers such as calcium ion or cyclic AMP) and modulation of basal activity (level of catalytic degradation of cyclic AMP by enzymes, such as phosphodiesterase, rate of uptake of neuroamines, such as norepinephrine and serotonin).

It is worth considering the process of target choice in the drug discovery process. Specifically, effective prosecution of any drug target requires a minimal effort in resources and time (perhaps 1–2 years per target), thus it can be seen how an incorrect choice of target could lead to a serious dissimulation in the drug discovery process. While there are considerations in target choice, such as target tractability (how difficult it is to produce a molecule to alter the behavior of the target), one of the most important factors is a strong association with the disease that is being treated. It has been estimated that there are approximately 600–1500 possible drug targets that may be valid to pursue for therapy. These are made up of genes that are known to be associated with diseases and that also code for a protein that may be modified through binding to a small molecule [1]. No discovery program could pursue a number of genes close to the number available, making target validation a very important step in the process. Table 1.1 shows some of the factors involved in the process of target validation, with particular reference to the problem of HIV-1 viral entry to cause Acquired Immune Deficiency Syndrome (AIDS). Data also has shown that a given target can be pleiotropic with respect to the number of signaling pathways to which it is linked in the cell; this is especially true of 7TMRs. With signaling pleiotropically it has been seen that different drugs can choose to activate different pathways (see chapter: Predicting Agonist Effect); this extends the classical concept of "target validation" as the main focus of discovery to "pathway validation," that is, it may not be enough to activate a given 7TMR, but rather it may be necessary to limit the signal that emanates from that receptor. As a preface to the discussion of cellular drug effect, it is useful to consider the major pharmacological tool used to quantify it, namely, the dose-response curve.

Pharmacologic targets can be used to modify physiological processes. Specifically, chemicals can be used to cause activation, blockade, or modulation of protein receptors and ion channel targets. For enzymes and transporter proteins, the main drug effect is the inhibition of ongoing basal activity of these targets (chapter: Enzymes as Drug Targets discusses these targets in detail). Another difference between these

TABLE 1.1   Factors relevant to target validation with reference to acquired immune deficiency syndrome (AIDS).

Factor	CCR5 in AIDS[a]	References
Target is linked to sensitivity to disease	CCR5 receptors must be present on cell surface for HIV-1 infection	[2,3]
Cell level of target alters sensitivity and course of disease	Downregulation of CCR5 leads to resistance to HIV-1 infection	[4]
	Genetically high levels of CCR5 lead to rapid progression to AIDS	[5]
Interference with target will not lead to harm	CCR5 knockout mouse lacks the receptor but is otherwise healthy	[6]
Ligands for target interfere with disease	CCR5 interaction with chemokines interfere with HIV-1 infection	[7–11]
	Patients with high circulating levels of chemokine have retarded progression to AIDS	[12,13]
Specific genetic association	Δ32 deletion in CCR5 gene leads to lack of receptor expression and complete resistance to AIDS	[14–18]

[a]*Genetically altered mouse that does not naturally express the CCR5 receptor.*
CCR5, cysteine cysteine chemokine receptor 5.

target classes is location; while receptors, ion channels, and transporter proteins are usually found on the cell surface (exposed to the extracellular space), enzymes are most often found in the cytosol of the cell (drugs must enter the cell to act on enzymes). Exceptions to this general rule are nuclear receptors which reside in the cell nucleus. Finally, it should be recognized that there are other drug targets present in the cell, such as DNA, and that chemicals can have physical effects (i.e., membrane stabilization) that can change cellular function.

Dose-response curves

A characteristic feature of drugs acting on a specific target in a physiological system is that there will be a graded increase in response with an increase in drug concentration (dose). If the drug effect can be observed directly, then the magnitude of effect can be displayed as a function of drug concentration in the form of a dose-response curve. For example, epinephrine is known to cause increased heart rate in humans; Fig. 1.2 shows

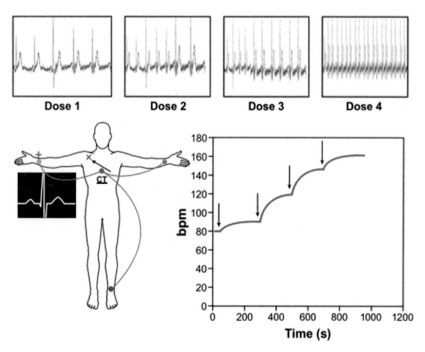

FIGURE 1.2 Dose-response curve for epinephrine given to a human at increasing doses. The heart rate is obtained from noninvasive electrocardiography (EKG) leads. It can be seen that there is a relationship between heart rate and increasing dose of epinephrine.

how increasing doses of epinephrine produce increases in heart rate. The curve-defining dose and resulting observed response can be used as short-hand to characterize the effect of the drug in the system. This relationship can then be used to predict what any dose of the drug will do in the system, in the form of an empirically derived line joining the observed data points. Fig. 1.3 shows the increased heart rate as a function of epinephrine concentration. The lines joining the data points infer that there is a continuous relationship between epinephrine dose and heart rate. Such an empirical relationship can allow interpolation of values, but the predictions must be bounded by real data to do so. Usually, the basal activity of the system is known (i.e., in the case of the example, the patient had a resting heart rate of 80 bpm). Dose-response relationships are characterized by three parameters; a threshold, slope, and maximum.

In the example shown in Fig. 1.3, the threshold can be inferred from the increase from 80 bpm and the slope from the existing real data points. The maximum response can be problematic since, unless it can be defined by real data, it must be projected from the existing data; this will be discussed in more detail in the following consideration of dose-response relationships. In this case, as in many pharmacological cases, there are safety issues for experimentally determining the maximal

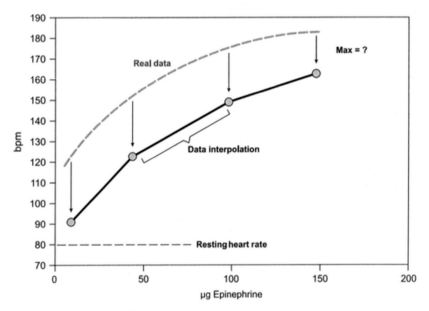

FIGURE 1.3 Empirically determined dose-response curve for data shown in Fig. 1.2. Real data points joined by straight lines enable responses to doses between 8 and 144 µg to be predicted. While the basal activity of the system is known (patient's resting heart rate = 80 bpm), the true maximum of the curve is unknown.

heart rate increase to epinephrine (i.e., a fatal arrhythmia could ensue). For this reason, dose-response data is often used to apply mathematical models that can fully define the dose-response relationship. As a preface to this discussion, it is useful to consider what a dose-response relationship represents in a physiological system.

Fig. 1.4 shows a typical dose-response curve. Considering a living cell as an idling engine, there is a basal level of activity that is an ambient baseline for the dose-response curve; an analogy could be that cellular metabolism is a faucet of water filling a container with a hole in it. If the level of the water in the container is the cellular effect, then an input can be subthreshold if the rate of exit of the water keeps the level low (see Fig. 1.4). As the stimulus to the cell increases (increased flow of water into the container), the level rises visibly, and this can be viewed as the cellular response to the drug. At some point, a maximum will be attained whereby the system can return no further response to a stimulus. These cellular maxima can be dictated by the physiological or mechanical properties of the cell (saturation of a biochemical process or attainment of a maximal mechanical contraction). This can be modeled as an overflow valve to prevent the level of water from going above a certain level

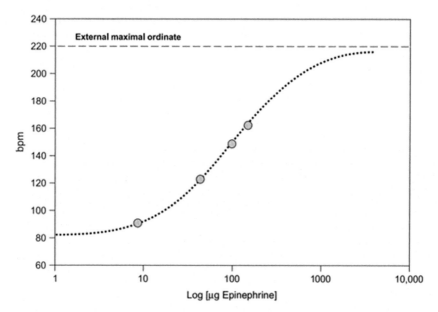

FIGURE 1.4 Shows the dose-response relationship given in Figs. 1.2 and 1.3 on a logarithmic scale fit with a mathematical function. The maximum response in this case was obtained from historical data suggesting that a maximal heart rate of 220 bpm is common for human heart muscle. The nature of various mathematical fitting functions for dose-response data will be discussed further in Chapter 2, Drug Affinity and Efficacy.

(Fig. 1.4). Thus a window of response for the cell exists between the threshold and maximum where a drug may change cellular effect, and the strength of that effect will be linked to the concentration of the drug by a quantifiable function. This function is visualized as a dose-response curve. A useful expedient is to express the dosage on a logarithmic scale. This allows a wide range of doses to be shown concisely and the maximum to be more easily observed. These details will be discussed more fully in the section on the Langmuir adsorption isotherm.

Fig. 1.5 Schematic of a cell process described by a dose-response curve. The stimulus input is the amount of fluid entering the vessel from the spigot and the level of fluid in the vessel is the cellular response. It is assumed that the cell has a basal activity, given by a low level of fluid entry into the vessel. The level of the fluid at this point describes the basal activity of the cell. As a drug increases, the stimulus to the system (increases fluid entry), the level of the fluid rises (cellular response increases). At some point, the level exceeds the limits of the vessel and escapes through the overflow; this represents the maximal capability of the cell to increase activity.

Data from Fig. 1.3 fit to a semilogarithmic sigmoidal mathematical function that covers a larger range of doses. The maximal heart rate is taken from historical data (220 bpm for normal healthy humans).

It is worth mentioning at this point how the design of pharmacologic experiments is based on an independent variable (drug concentration) being put into an organ system to yield a dependent variable (drug response); on the basis of the magnitude of the dependent variable, drugs are characterized in terms of potency and efficacy. This system is based on the tacit assumption that the value of the independent variable is accurately known. If the concentration of the drug at the target is not known accurately, then all subsequent estimates of drug activity (which go on to be ascribed to be characteristics of the drug) are also wrong. Therefore it is imperative that exemplary care be taken to accurately determine the value of the drug concentration interacting with the target. This is exceptionally difficult in vivo; hence, an entire discipline around this problem has evolved in the form of *pharmacokinetics*. This will be dealt with explicitly in Chapter 7, Pharmacokinetics I: Permeation and Metabolism, and Chapter 8, Pharmacokinetics II: Distribution and Multiple Dosing. In experiments aimed at determining drug activity, the dependent variable actually transforms into a variant of the independent variable; that is, the desired result is an identified concentration denoting a defined activity, such as an EC_{50} as the effective dose producing 50% maximal response. This makes it even more important to know the value of the independent variable (concentration) in the experiment. If this is an error, then all concentrations characterizing the activity of the drug for a defined response will also be incorrect. Pharmacology also utilizes in vitro experimentation in which tissues are incubated in media mimicking true physiology in chambers of constant volume, to obviate variance in drug concentration and thus accurately link concentration to drug activity. This technology was first introduced into pharmacology by pioneers such as Magnus at the turn of the century (see Box 1.3).

On a semilogarithmic scale, dose-response curves are characteristically sigmoidal in shape (i.e., see Fig. 1.4). The location parameters of such curves denote the *potency* of the drug. If the dose-response curve is obtained in vivo, then the EC_{50} will be a measure, such as mg/kg body weight. If the experiment is done in vitro, then a molar potency can be obtained. For in vitro experiment, a convenient parameter to numerically quantify potency is to report the pEC_{50} of the curve, literally the negative logarithm of the molar concentration of the drug that produces half the maximal response to the drug (see Fig. 1.6A). The pEC_{50} is the correct form to use for EC_{50} manipulation (arithmetic and/or statistical),

---

BOX 1.3

Isolated tissue pharmacology

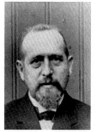

Rudolf Magnus (1873–1927) was a German pharmacologist who became the first Professor of Pharmacology at the University of Utrecht. Widely known for his work on secretions of the pituitary gland, his work on muscle tension gained such acclaim that he was nominated for the Nobel Prize in 1927. Tragically, his sudden death prevented him from receiving the award. In pharmacology, Magnus is most noted for his pioneering work in the use of isolated tissues. A basic tenet of pharmacological research is that all experimentally derived dependent variables (i.e., potency, drug activity) depend upon an accurate value for drug concentration at the target.

Magnus pioneered an apparatus that could sustain an isolated tissue physiologically for many hours, thereby allowing the quatitative measurement of drug effect. The drug was added to a chamber of constant volume ensuring that the concentration of drug acting on the tissue was constant.

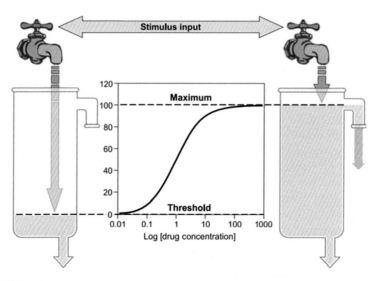

FIGURE 1.5 Dose response curve as a augmentation of an ongoing process.

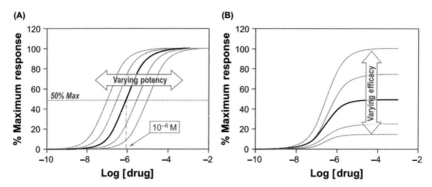

FIGURE 1.6 Two measures of drug activity in a cellular system. (A) The location parameter along the concentration axis represents the drug potency. This is usually quantified by the molar concentration that is seen to produce 50% of the maximal response. For the solid line dose-response curve the concentration producing 50% response is $10 - 6$ M; this is reported as the negative logarithm of this value (pEC$_{50}$), in this case the pEC$_{50}$ is 6.0. (B) Another measure of drug activity in a system is the maximal response. While the potency is a complex product of both the affinity and efficacy of the drug, the maximal response is solely dependent upon efficacy.

since pEC$_{50}$s (but not EC$_{50}$s) are normally distributed. In this example, 50% of the maximal effect is produced by a drug concentration of 10^{-6} M. The negative logarithm of this number is the pEC$_{50}$, in this case 6.0. The other observed effect is the maximal response. It will be seen that the potency and maximal response of a drug depends on different molecular properties, with the maximal response being primarily dependent on the drug's efficacy (Fig. 1.6B).

Fig. 1.7 Summarizes the characteristics of a semilogarithmic dose-response curve. In this example, the maximal response is expressed as a fraction (or percentage) of the maximal capability of the system (called the system maximal response). The maximal response to the drug being studied may or may not equal the system maximal response.

It is worth describing some general drug nomenclature at this point; this nomenclature is based on the behavior of a drug in a particular system which may change in different systems (tissues). In general, a drug that causes a cellular system to change its state and produces a measurable biological response is referred to as an *agonist*. A drug that produces the maximal response of the system (a maximal response equal to the maximal capability of the system to report cellular response) is termed a *full agonist* (Fig. 1.7B). It should also be noted that a drug may not produce a response equal to the maximal response capability of the system, that is, a given drug may only produce a maximal response that is below the maximal capability of the system. When this occurs, the drug is referred to as a *partial agonist*. A drug that reduces the biological effect of another drug is called an *antagonist*. An antagonist may itself produce a low level of direct response (i.e., a partial agonist can produce antagonism

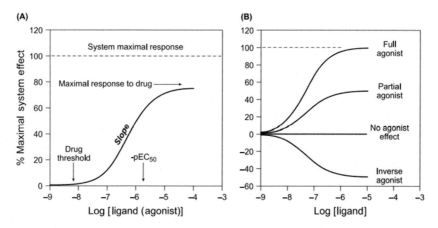

FIGURE 1.7 Features of dose-response curves and different behaviors of drugs characterized by those curves. (A) A dose-response curve is characterized by a threshold effect, a slope of the relationship between dose and response, and a maximal response. This maximal response may or may not equal the maximal response capability of the cell system. (B) The dose-response curve produces a profile of behavior of a drug in a given system. If it produces the maximal response of the system, it is a full agonist; if it produces a submaximal response it is a partial agonist. In other cases no observed response may be observed (but the drug may bind to the receptor to be an antagonist). Some systems have an elevated basal response, which can then be decreased through drug action; this behavior is inverse agonism.

in responses to full agonists). Finally, there are cases where the tissue itself possesses elevated basal activity due to a spontaneous activation of receptors. A class of drug that reverses such elevated basal effect is termed an *inverse agonist*; these will be described in later discussions of antagonists (see chapter: Drug Antagonism Orthosteric Drug Effects). It will be seen that the common currency of pharmacology in describing drug effect is the dose-response curve. As a prerequisite to a discussion of these properties, it is useful to describe the cellular target that responds to agonists to yield observable cellular response, in this case the receptor.

Linking observed pharmacology with molecular mechanism

Drug targets are coupled to the organism (cell, organ) through a myriad of biochemical reactions, and these can vary with different cell types. However, these reactions are similar in terms of how they relate input (the stimulus at the start of the process) to output (the result of activating the process). Specifically, the reactions that link cell surface signaling to cytosolic response are saturable (they reach a finite endpoint with infinite stimulation); an example of such a process is shown in Fig. 1.8. This figure shows a typical relationship between the input to a biochemical reaction (x-axis, to be referred to as the stimulus) and output (y-axis, to be referred to as the response), that is, low levels of stimulus cause the most change in output until a maximal output is attained. This is consistent with the idea that, in the absence of stimulus, the system is open to activation; therefore the first molecules interacting have the most opportunity to produce response. As the level of stimulus increases, the probability that new stimulus will encounter a part of the system already interacting with the previous stimulus increases and the new output is reduced. Finally, at very high levels of stimulus, the system is maximally engaged and no further response can be elicited.

In addition to saturability, the curved relationship between stimulus and response leads to amplification. For example, in Fig. 1.8, 20% maximal stimulus leads to 64% maximal response. This type of amplification is compounded when such saturable reactions are in series, as often occurs in cells (Fig. 1.9). The nature, capacity, and sensitivity of the biochemical reactions linking stimulus and response vary from cell to cell; in fact, this is one way that a cell can tailor its sensitivity to input to its needs. This will be referred to as the efficiency of coupling. This fact precludes the direct linking of the actual sensitivity of the organ to the effect of the drug on the biochemical process; the target-coupling process intervenes in a variable way.

There are two main cell-based control points for cellular sensitivity mediated by a pharmacological target; the number of targets available

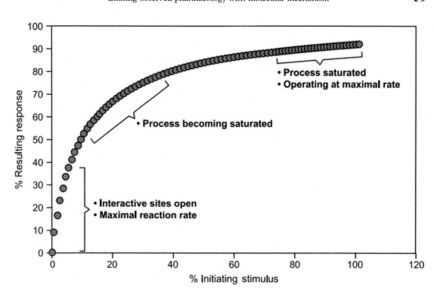

FIGURE 1.8 Depiction of a saturable biochemical process (as would be operative in working cells). The x-axis shows the incoming signal and the y-axis the resulting response. The initial steep rise reflects the fact that the system is open to stimulation; as the system becomes engaged, fewer open sites are present and the slope of the response—curve decreases. Once the interacting sites are occupied, no further stimulus can cause increased response, that is, the response is the maximal response that the process can return.

to produce stimulus and the efficiency of coupling of the target to cellular metabolism. Cells use both of these control points to maintain appropriate levels of stimulus to sustain their function. Differences in target density levels and the components of the cell that control the efficiency of coupling of the target are what cause drugs to have a wide range of potencies and activities in different cell types. It is this variation that must be dealt with and accounted for when drug activity is assessed in a test system for prediction of effect in a therapeutic one.

Agonist effect results from the interplay of four factors; two are related to the drug and two to the system. The drug effects are:

- *Affinity*: The force(s) that cause the agonist and the protein target to interact with each other, that is, what causes the drug to bind to the target.
- *Efficacy*: The property of the drug that causes the target to change its behavior toward the host cell once the drug is bound.

These drug-related properties are what can be quantified in pharmacological procedures to characterize drug activity. The result of the interaction of the drug with the target provides the cell with a stimulus, that is, each target furnishes a degree of stimulus to the cell commensurate with the drug's target occupancy (controlled by the

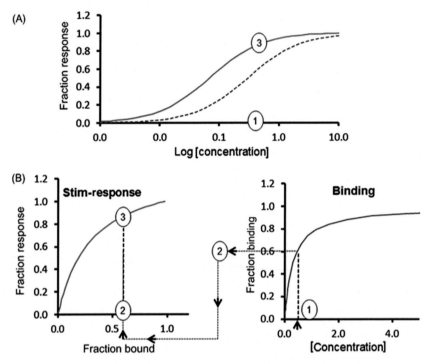

FIGURE 1.9 Amplification of cell signaling through a series arrangement of saturable functions. (A) Semilogarithmic curves showing binding (blue dotted line) and response (red solid line) as a function of concentration. (B) Right panel shows binding as a function of concentration (blue line). A concentration of 0.5 units (circle 1) yields a fractional binding value of 0.6 (circle 2). This level of binding stimulus enters a second saturable stimulus–response function (left panel, red line) to yield a value for observed response of 0.88 (circle 3).

concentration of the drug and its affinity for the target) and efficacy. Two cell-based properties control the overall stimulus received by the cell. These are:

- *Target density*: The actual number of responding target units exposed to the drug, that is, receptors on the cell surface.
- *Target coupling efficiency*: The efficiency with which each target is coupled to the cellular response machinery. The series of biochemical processes linking target activation with final cellular response is referred to as stimulus–response coupling.

Each process along the stimulus–response chain, beginning with the binding of the drug to the target, can be described with a dose-response curve. As seen in Fig. 1.9, as successive biochemical reactions feed into each other (i.e., the response of one reaction becomes the stimulus for the next), amplification occurs. Therefore the potency of the drug, as the process is viewed further down the stimulus–response chain of reactions, increases. This effect causes the potency for the final effect of the drug to be considerably higher than it is for the first initiating reaction (binding to the target).

The main pharmacological tool used to negate the variable effect of biochemical target-coupling is the null method. Through this device, drugs are compared in terms of their potency (the concentration of drug needed to produce a defined response) to produce a common effect. This imposes the condition that the stimulus of each drug to the cell is subject to the *same system-dependent modification* and, therefore this effect will cancel when two drugs are compared in the same system (see Fig. 1.10). Through the use of null methods, the relative potency of agonists can be compared in one system to yield a parameter (relative potency ratio) that may be constant for all systems. There is a major assumption required for this method, and this is that the agonists involved activate the target receptor in the same manner, that is, produce the same receptor active state. There are cases where this is true and other cases where it is *not*. In the cases where it is not true, the

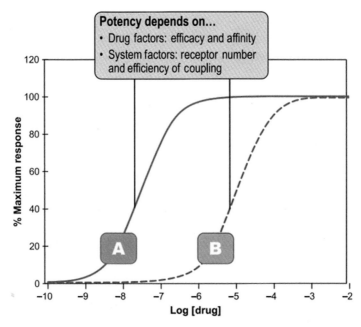

FIGURE 1.10   Dose-response curves to two agonists (A and B). Their respective potencies depend upon the two drug factors of affinity and efficacy, and two tissue factors of receptor number and efficiency of receptor coupling. The null method compares equal responses (e.g., the concentrations of each agonist producing 50% of maximal response); this ratio is still dependent upon the drug factors (the respective affinities and efficacies of the agonists), but the tissue factors are common to both and thus cancel each other. This potency ratio is a system-independent measure of the relative affinity and efficacy of the two agonists.

relative potency of agonists in whole cell systems is not constant and thus cannot be used for therapeutic predictions.

Pharmacology can identify drug mechanisms of action through the comparison of the verisimilitude of observed drug effects (i.e., effects on the dose-response curve) to mathematical models defining the interaction of the drug-bound receptor with various components of the physiological systems. This is a very powerful tool in that a mathematical model can predict the effects of the drug, not only in the given experimental system defining dose-response curves, but rather in *every* experimental system encountered by the drug. The key to this effect is the correct application of a mathematical model to describe observed effects. If this can be identified, then a wealth of predictions of the effects of a drug can be made. As stated by the astrophysicist Stephen Hawking...'what is it that breathes fire into the equations and makes a universe for them to describe?' Therefore a model can be an extremely useful tool to identify subtle effects in complex physiological systems.

Fig. 1.11 shows a model for two molecules (A,B) interacting with a receptor (R) to produce physiological response through a response element (E). This is a model for allosteric effects produced by B on the response given by

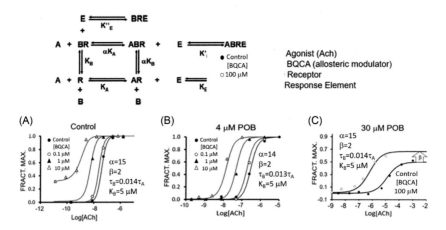

FIGURE 1.11   An example of fitting data to a mathematical model to elucidate the mechanism of action. Top panel: A model for the activation of receptors by a molecule A and the modification of the response by an allosteric modulator B. Panel A. The effects of the allosteric modulator BQCA on dose-response curves to acetylcholine are mediated by muscarinic M1 receptors expressed in CHO cells producing inositol-1-phosphate through activation of Gq protein. The parameters in the red square substituted into the model equation furnished the curves shown to fit the data. Panel B. The same experiment was done in a system of lower receptor expression (and thus lower sensitivity to Ach). It can be seen that the same parameters as those used to fit the curves in panel A were also viable to fit this different pattern of allosteric effect. Panel C. In an even less sensitive system, the same model parameters fit the experimental data. Experimental data from [3].

A. An example of an allosteric profile described by this model is the allosteric modulator BQCA acting on muscarinic ACh receptors [19]. Fig. 1.11 A shows the effect on the muscarinic activation of receptors indicating that low concentrations of BQCA produce sensitization to the muscarinic agonist ACh and higher concentrations of BQCA produce continue sensitization to ACh but with an added activity, namely a direct receptor agonism. This pattern of activity is consistent with BQCA producing an allosteric effect on the ACh receptor to produce a sensitization to ACh and a concomitant direct activation of the receptor. The functional allosteric model fits these data through allosteric parameters a, b, t_A, and K_B; the values for the data in panel A are shown in the red box. If this model is truly a valid description of the mechanism of BQCA, then it should also describe BQCA patterns in other systems of differing sensitivity (i.e., cells with different cell surface level of receptors) to ACh. In a tissue of reduced sensitivity (reduced receptor level), a different pattern of response is observed—see Fig. 1.11B. The model fits these data suggesting it can be a viable predictor of the effects of the drug in other systems. In the case shown for BQCA, it can be seen that the model fits very well with the experimental dose-response curves and moreover, the parameters of the model needed to fit the experimental data are actually the same (which is a required property of the model). A further reduction in system sensitivity produces a system where BQCA produces yet another array of effects. In this case, application of the same model, with only an adjustment for the sensitivity of the system, fits very well with the data and also does so with parameters that are consistent with previous application of the model—see Fig. 1.11C. These data, in total, indicate that the model chosen to describe the effects of BQCA is robust and able to fit experimental data in a variety of experimental conditions and thus can be thought to be a good indicator of the effects of BQCA in all systems. In this case, the model describes the mechanism of action of BQCA as allosterically increasing the affinity of Ach (a = 15), increasing the efficacy of ACh (b = 2), and having a direct positive efficacy (1.4% that of ACh) that produces cell response. Through such fitting of experimental data to mathematical models two important aims of drug discovery can be achieved:

1. Understanding of how molecules function in complex physiological systems.
2. Prediction of the effects of drugs in all systems including the therapeutic one. This latter effect can be important as drugs are seldom, if ever developed directly in human therapeutic systems but rather in surrogate system with projected activity of therapeutic value.

The process of fitting data to models can be considered to be the process of converting "descriptive" data (what we see) to "predictive" data, which can transcend the specific conditions under which the measurements were made.

Descriptive pharmacology: I

This monograph is designed to guide the reader in the application of pharmacological principles to describe the biological activity of drugs. At the end of each chapter, the specific progress toward this end will be summarized. As shown in Fig. 1.12, a new chemical entity (which may or may not be a drug) is tested in a biological preparation and one of two outcomes may result. The chemical may not produce a visible response and this may be due to the fact that it does not bind to and activate the target (inactive), or it does bind but has such a low efficacy that no change in the state of the cell can be observed. The presence of the chemical on the target may preclude further activation of the target by other molecules in which case the chemical is an antagonist; a further set of tests can then be done to define this activity (see chapters: Drug Antagonism Orthosteric Drug Effects, and Allosteric Drug Effects). If an agonist response is observed in the preparation, then this suggests that the chemical has efficacy and may be an agonist. It should be stressed that specific tests for selectivity must be carried out before this conclusion is firm; these are described in Chapter 3, Predicting Agonist Effect. The assay may also show the chemical to be a full or partial agonist; this is a general measure of the strength of efficacy of the test substance. This also

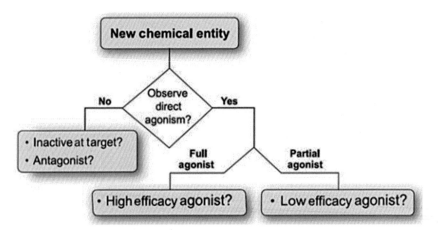

FIGURE 1.12 Schematic diagram of logical progression for determination of drug effect. The end result of this progression at this point is to determine, if the new chemical entity produces a visible effect in a pharmacologic assay and, if so, to describe some characteristics of that effect, namely a statement describing efficacy (full or partial agonism) and potency. It should be stressed that this analysis is necessarily linked to the particular assay used to make the measurements, and also that a specific target-based effect requires separate testing of selectivity before conclusions can link effect with specific target activation.

underscores a general tenet for a complete analysis at this stage of testing, namely that the classifications of the new chemical entity will still be uniquely tied to the particular biological preparation in which the testing is done. It will be seen in subsequent chapters that a different assay may show what previously appeared to be an antagonist to be an agonist, and vice versa. Also, many low-efficacy agonists can produce partial agonism in some tissues and full agonism in others. For this reason, observations made in a single test system must be considered to be system-dependent and subject to change when tests are conducted in other tissues. Procedures outlined in the next chapters will extend these approaches to obtain measures of drug activity that are independent of the test system and thus can be used to predict drug activity in all systems.

At this stage, tests done in a given system (or person) can yield general statements, such as:

- The compound produces no observed effect in the system.
- The compound produces partial or full agonism with a potency of x mg/kg (if tests done in vivo) or a pEC_{50} of x (if tests done in vitro).

Summary

- Drugs bind to and activate biochemical targets in physiological systems.
- Identification of these targets enables chemical access to modify physiology.
- Drugs that produce observed change in cellular processes are termed agonists; those that block such effects are antagonists.
- Agonist effect can concisely be described with a dose-response curve, which relates drug effect to drug concentration. The properties of potency and maximal response describe the effect of the agonist in any given system.
- Cells amplify initial chemical signals through a series of saturable biochemical processes; this produces a difference in the dose-response curves describing the initial interaction of the agonist with the receptor and the dose-response curve for cellular response.
- The observed potency of an agonist depends upon two drug-related parameters (affinity, efficacy) and two cell-dependent parameters (target density and efficiency of target coupling).
- The cell-dependent factors can be canceled when the relative potency of agonists is compared in the same system (null method). Under these circumstances, the observed relative potency reflects differences only in the drug-related parameters of affinity and efficacy (and thus is system-independent). This is true only for agonists that activate the receptor in the same manner.

References

[1] A.L. Hopkins, C.R. Groom, The druggable genome, Nat. Rev. Drug Disc. 1 (9) (2002) 727–730. Available from: https://doi.org/10.1038/nrd892.

[2] A.D. Luster, Mechanisms of disease: chemokines - chemotactic cytokines that mediate inflammation, N. Engl. J. Med. 338 (7) (1998) 436–445. Available from: https://doi.org/10.1056/NEJM199802123380706.

[3] M. Zaitseva, A. Blauvelt, S. Lee, C.K. Lapham, V. Klaus-Kovtun, H. Mostowski, et al., Expression and function of CCR5 and CXCR4 on human Langerhans cells and macrophages: implications for HIV primary infection, Nat. Med. 3 (12) (1997) 1369–1375. Available from: https://doi.org/10.1038/nm1297-1369.

[4] L. Cagnon, J.J. Rossi, Downregulation of the CCR5 β-chemokine receptor and inhibition of HIV-1 infection by stable VA1-ribozyme chimeric transcripts, Antisense Nucleic Acid Drug Dev. 10 (4) (2000) 251–261. Available from: https://doi.org/10.1089/108729000421439.

[5] M.P. Martin, Genetic acceleration of AIDS progression by a promoter variant of CCR5, Science 282 (5395) (1998) 1907–1911. Available from: https://doi.org/10.1126/science.282.5395.1907.

[6] D.N. Cook, M.A. Beck, T.M. Coffman, S.L. Kirby, J.F. Sheridan, I.B. Pragnell, et al., Requirement of MIP-1α for an inflammatory response to viral infection, Science 269 (5230) (1995) 1583–1585. Available from: https://doi.org/10.1126/science.7667639.

[7] M. Baba, O. Nishimura, N. Kanzaki, M. Okamoto, H. Sawada, Y. Iizawa, et al., A small-molecule, nonpeptide CCR5 antagonist with highly potent and selective anti-HIV-1 activity, Proc. Natl. Acad. Sci. U S Am. 96 (10) (1999) 5698–5703. Available from: https://doi.org/10.1073/pnas.96.10.5698.

[8] F. Cocchi, A.L. DeVico, A. Garzino-Demo, S.K. Arya, R.C. Gallo, P. Lusso, Identification of RANTES, MIP-1α, and MIP-1β as the major HIV-suppressive factors produced by CD8 + T cells, Science 270 (5243) (1995) 1811–1815. Available from: https://doi.org/10.1126/science.270.5243.1811.

[9] P.E. Finke, B. Oates, S.G. Mills, M. MacCoss, L. Malkowitz, M.S. Springer, et al., Antagonists of the human CCR5 receptor as anti-HIV-1 agents. Part 4: synthesis and structure-activity relationships for 1-[N-(methyl)-N-(phenylsulfonyl)amino]-2-(phenyl)-4-(4-(N-(alkyl)-N- (benzyloxycarbonyl)amino)piperidin-1-yl)butanes, Bioorg. Med. Chem. Lett. 11 (18) (2001) 2475–2479. Available from: https://doi.org/10.1016/S0960-894X(01)00492-9.

[10] M. Mack, B. Luckow, P.J. Nelson, J. Cihak, G. Simmons, P.R. Clapham, et al., Aminooxypentane-RANTES induces CCR5 internalization but inhibits recycling: a novel inhibitory mechanism of HIV infectivity, J. Exp. Med. 187 (8) (1998) 1215–1224. Available from: https://doi.org/10.1084/jem.187.8.1215.

[11] G. Simmons, P.R. Clapham, L. Picard, R.E. Offord, M.M. Rosenkilde, T.W. Schwartz, et al., Potent inhibition of HIV-1 infectivity in macrophages and lymphocytes by a novel CCR5 antagonist, Science 276 (5310) (1997) 276–279. Available from: https://doi.org/10.1126/science.276.5310.276.

[12] A. Garzino-Demo, R.B. Moss, J.B. Margolick, F. Cleghorn, A. Sill, W.A. Blattner, et al., Spontaneous and antigen-induced production of HIV-inhibitory β-chemokines are associated with AIDS-free status, Proc. Natl Acad. Sci. U S Am. 96 (21) (1999) 11986–11991. Available from: https://doi.org/10.1073/pnas.96.21.11986.

[13] H. Ullum, A.C. Lepri, J. Victor, H. Aladdin, A.N. Phillips, J. Gerstoft, Production of beta-chemokines in human immunodeficiency virus (HIV) infection: evidence that high levels of macrophage in inflammatory protein-1-beta are associated with a decreased risk of HIV progression, J. Infect. Dis. 177 (1998) 331–336.

[14] M. Dean, M. Carrington, C. Winkler, G.A. Huttley, M.W. Smith, R. Allikmets, et al., Genetic restriction of HIV-1 infection and progression to AIDS by a deletion allele of the CKR5 structural gene, Science 273 (5283) (1996) 1856−1862. Available from: https://doi.org/10.1126/science.273.5283.1856.

[15] Y. Huang, W.A. Paxton, S.M. Wolinsky, A.U. Neumann, L. Zhang, T. He, et al., The role of a mutant CCR5 allele in HIV-1 transmission and disease progression, Nat. Med. 2 (11) (1996) 1240−1243. Available from: https://doi.org/10.1038/nm1196-1240.

[16] R. Liu, W.A. Paxton, S. Choe, D. Ceradini, S.R. Martin, R. Horuk, et al., Homozygous defect in HIV-1 coreceptor accounts for resistance of some multiply-exposed individuals to HIV-1 infection, Cell 86 (3) (1996) 367−377. Available from: https://doi.org/10.1016/S0092-8674(00)80110-5.

[17] W.A. Paxton, S.R. Martin, D. Tse, T.R. O'Brien, J. Skurnick, N.L. VanDevanter, et al., Relative resistance to HIV-1 infection of CD4 lymphocytes from persons who remain uninfected despite multiple high-risk sexual exposures, Nat. Med. 2 (4) (1996) 412−417. Available from: https://doi.org/10.1038/nm0496-412.

[18] M. Samson, F. Libert, B.J. Doranz, J. Rucker, C. Liesnard, M. Farber, et al., Resistance to HIV-1 infection in caucasian individuals bearing mutant alleles of the CCR-5 chemokine receptor gene, Nature 382 (6593) (1996) 722−726. Available from: https://doi.org/10.1038/382722a0.

[19] Sara Bdioui, Julien Verdi, Nicolas Pierre, Eric Trinquet, Thomas Roux, Terry Kenakin, The pharmacologic characterization of allosHeteric molecules: Gq protein activation, J. Recept. Signal. Transduct. 39 (2) (2019) 106−113. Available from: https://doi.org/10.1080/10799893.2019.1634101.

2

Drug affinity and efficacy

By the end of this chapter, the reader should understand the concept of a molecule having an "affinity" for a protein, what the uniquely pharmacologic concept of "efficacy" means, and its mechanism. The reader should also understand how drugs can have many efficacies and how these can be expressed in either "full" or "partial" agonism. The reader will also see how particular methods to compare full and partial agonists with respect to relative activity are used in discovery.

Introduction

Up to this point, drug activity (specifically that of an agonist) is described as an observed effect quantified by a dose-response curve.

Pharmacology in Drug Discovery and Development
DOI: https://doi.org/10.1016/B978-0-443-14124-9.00018-5

Thus the maximal response and the potency of an agonist (location of the curve along the drug concentration axis) in any specific system yield the measure of activity in that system. Also, as noted in the last chapter, the magnitude of the observed organ response is controlled by four factors, two drug-related and two tissue-related. This chapter describes the two drug-related parameters of *affinity* and *efficacy*. The value in quantifying these parameters is that they are unique properties of the drug acting on the target and thus are true for that target in all tissues and organs in which it resides. Therefore if the affinity and efficacy of a given molecule can be determined in one system (referred to as the "test" system), then these parameters may be used to assess drug activity in any other system, including the therapeutic one. This is of great value since drugs are very rarely discovered and studied directly in the therapeutic system. A prerequisite to the determination of the affinity and efficacy of agonists is to know that the agonism is selective for the particular target of interest. There are two main strategies for making this determination.

New terminology

- k_1: The rate of association of a molecule as it binds to the target in units of $s^{-1}\ mol^{-1}$.
- k_2: The rate of dissociation of the molecule away from the target during the binding process in units of s^{-1}.
- K_{eq}: Equilibrium dissociation constant of the molecule—target complex in units of mole ($K_{eq} = k_2/k_1$); also equal to the concentration of drug that binds to 50% of the target population available for binding. For agonists, K_{eq} is denoted K_A; for antagonists K_B. Affinity $= K_{eq}^{-1}$.
- *Lead*: In new drug discovery, a molecule that fulfills criteria for possible activity from a screening process is termed a "hit." A hit with the added qualities of chemical tractability (opportunity to change the chemical scaffold to modify structure), selectivity, and lack of toxicity is termed a "lead."
- *Lead optimization*: The process of iterative medicinal chemistry to modify structure to enhance primary activity and selectivity.

Agonist selectivity

As discussed in the previous chapter, there are numerous potential biological targets in any given cell that a chemical could activate to cause agonism. Usually, a nonspecific activation is not therapeutically useful, as it comes with a nonspecific activation of organs, leading to unwanted side effects. By definition, the chemical control of pathology through pharmacological agonism requires a selective activation of the predetermined therapeutic biological target. There are two basic approaches for identifying the selective agonist effect.

The first is pharmacologic intervention, whereby a specific antagonist of the target is given as a pretreatment to the preparation (either in vitro or in vivo) to see if the observed agonism to the test agonist is eliminated (or ablated) (see Fig. 2.1). If the agonist action emanates from the binding of the test agonist to the same site as that utilized by the antagonist, a steric hindrance will occur and agonism will be blocked. However, it will be seen that in the case of allosteric activation of the target where the test agonist binds to a site separate from that of the antagonist, interference of the agonist response with antagonist binding may not occur. Therefore another strategy that may be employed in

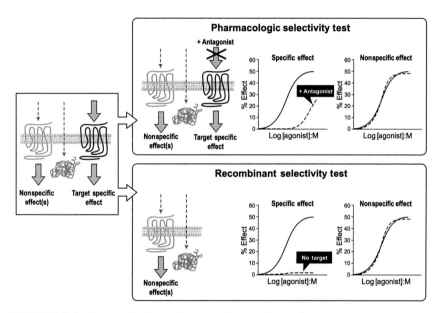

FIGURE 2.1 Two methods to determine the specificity of agonism. A given agonist may activate a specific biological target (solid arrows) or cause a response through the activation of elements within the cellular host (dashed arrows). Specific target activation can be confirmed by specific blockade of the response with a specific antagonist for the target (Pharmacologic Selectivity Test). Alternatively, if recombinant cells consisting of host cells containing and not containing the target are available, the observance of a response to the agonist only in cells containing the target provides presumptive evidence of selective agonism (Recombinant Selectivity Test).

these cases (or in general to ensure that this possibility is considered experimentally) is to use a recombinant system. In this approach, genetic material for the biological target of interest (specifically comple- mentary DNA (cDNA)) is used to transfect host cells. The test agonist is then tested in the transfected cell and the nontransfected host cell (i.e., the same cell line but with no receptor present). If the response is observed only in the transfected cell line (containing the target of inter- est), this is presumptive evidence that the agonist activates the biologi- cal target of interest (see Fig. 2.1).

Affinity

A simple model of ligand binding originally designed to describe the binding of chemicals to metal surfaces in the making of filaments for light bulbs was published by the chemist Irving Langmuir (see Box 2.1); accordingly, it is referred to as the Langmuir adsorption isotherm and it still forms the basis for the measurement and quantification of drug affinity. In Langmuir's model, a drug molecule has an intrinsic *rate of association* with the receptor (referred to as the "rate of condensation" by Langmuir).

In Langmuir's system, the target was the surface of metal, but in the context of pharmacology, the target is the binding pocket of a biologi- cally relevant protein, such as a receptor. This rate of association (denoted k_1) is driven by changes in energy, that is, the energy of the system containing the drug in the receptor-binding pocket is lower than the energy of the system with the drug not bound in the pocket. The drug also has a *rate of dissociation* from the receptor (referred to by Langmuir as a rate of "evaporation"), which describes the change in energy when the molecule diffuses away from the surface (denoted k_2). When a drug is present in the compartment containing the recep- tor, then the concentration gradient controls the movement of drug molecules. The absence of a drug in the receptor-binding pocket drives the binding reaction toward drug binding to the receptor but, as more drug binds, the bound drug will diffuse out of the binding pocket in accordance with its natural tendency to do so. This leads to an equilib- rium whereby the rate of drug leaving the binding pocket will equal the rate of drug approaching and entering the binding pocket. The ratio of k_2/k_1 determines the amount of drug bound to the receptor at any one instant and this becomes a measure of how well the drug binds to the receptor. This ratio is referred to as the equilibrium

---

BOX 2.1

Irving Langmuir and the Langmuir adsorption isotherm

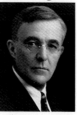

Irving Langmuir (1881–1957)

Irving Langmuir (born in Brooklyn, New York) graduated as a metallurgical engineer from the School of Mines at Columbia University in 1903. He went on to achieve a PhD in Physical Chemistry with Nernst. He returned to America to join, and eventually become director of, the Research Laboratory of the General Electric Company in Schenectady, New York. Langmuir's studies of vacuum phenomena led him to investigate the properties of adsorbed films, leading to his derivation of the adsorption isotherm. He contributed to the Lewis theory of shared electrons and his work led to the gas-filled incandescent lamp and the discovery of atomic hydrogen. Langmuir won numerous awards for his work, including the Nobel Prize for Chemistry in 1932.

---

dissociation constant of the drug–receptor complex (denoted K_{eq}). Under these circumstances, the reciprocal of K_{eq} is a measure of the affinity of the chemical for the target. The derivation of Langmuir's isotherm, in his original terminology, is given in Box 2.2; the form utilized by pharmacologists is:

When the concentration of the drug is equal to K_{eq}, then $\rho = 0.5$, that is, the K_{eq} is the concentration of drug that occupies 50% of the available receptor population. Therefore the magnitude of K_{eq} is inversely proportional to the affinity of the drug for the receptor. For example, consider two drugs one with $K_{eq} = 10^{-9}$ M and another with $K_{eq} = 10^{-7}$ M. The first drug occupies 50% of the receptors at a concentration 1/100 of

BOX 2.2

Derivation of Langmuir's isotherm

Langmuir's model was centered on the calculation of the fraction of the total area of a surface bound by a chemical (denoted by Langmuir as $\theta\mu$). The fraction of total area left free for further binding of new molecule to the surface is given by $1 - \theta\mu$. In Langmuir's terminology, the amount of chemical bound to the surface is the product of the concentration of drug available for binding (denoted as μ), the rate of "condensation" of chemical onto the surface (α), and the fraction of surface left free for further binding $(1 - \theta\mu)$ (Rate of condensation $= \mu\alpha(1 - \theta\mu)$). Similarly, the amount of drug diffusing away (denoted "evaporation" by Langmuir) from the surface is given by the amount already bound ($\theta\mu$) multiplied by a rate of evaporation (denoted V_1) (Rate of evaporation $= \theta\mu\, V_1$).

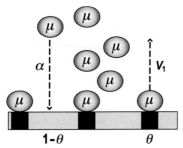

At equilibrium, the fractional amount diffusing toward the receptor is equal to the fractional amount diffusing away from the receptor:

$$\mu\alpha[1 - \theta_\mu] = \theta_\mu V_1 \tag{2.1}$$

Rearranging to isolate $\theta\mu$, the fraction of chemical bound to the surface yields:

$$\theta_\mu = \frac{\alpha\mu}{\alpha\mu + V_1} \tag{2.2}$$

Pharmacologists and biochemists define the fraction of biological target bound by a chemical (denoted A) as ρ_A and α as k_1 (a rate of association with the target), V_1 as k_2 (rate of dissociation from the target) and combine k_1 and k_2 into an equilibrium dissociation constant denoted K_{eq} ($K_{eq} = k_2/k_1$).

$$\rho_A = \frac{[A]}{[A] + K_{eq}} \tag{2.3}$$

$$\rho_A = \frac{[A]}{[A] + K_{eq}} \tag{2.1}$$

that required by the second. Clearly, the drug with $K_{eq} = 10^{-9}$ has a higher affinity for the receptor than the one with $K_{eq} = 10^{-7}$ M.

It can be seen from Eq. (2.1) that, for a ligand with K_{eq} of 10^{-7} M (100 nM), the fraction of sites bound can be calculated for any concentration (e.g., 30 nM would occupy (30 nM)/(30 nM + 100 nM) = 23% of the sites). In fact, Eq. (2.1) enables the calculation of a complete binding curve. Experimentally, if the binding of a series of concentrations can be measured, then a relationship between concentration and percent bound can be determined (Fig. 2.2). As is the case with dose-response curves, these curves are best described using a semilogarithmic format (see Fig. 2.2). Assuming that a direct measure of the amount of bound ligand can be made (for instance, if the ligand is radioactive and the quantity of radioactive–ligand complex could be quantified), then K_{eq} can be measured directly; this can be accomplished with saturation binding experiments with radioactive ligands.

Under certain circumstances, the affinity of an agonist may also be directly observed from the agonist effect. Specifically, the EC_{50} value for

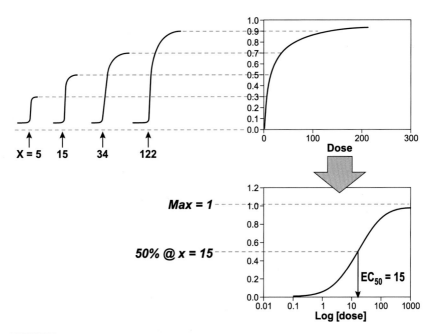

FIGURE 2.2 Binding defined by the Langmuir adsorption isotherm. Different concentrations of ligand, when added to the preparation, bind different fractions of the available binding sites according to a curve defined by the adsorption isotherm. This defines a curved relationship, which is sigmoidal when plotted on a semilogarithmic axis (Log Dose vs fraction of sites bound). The midpoint of this sigmoidal relationship is the EC_{50}, the concentration binding to 50% of the available sites.

a *partial agonist* (an agonist that does not produce the full maximal response of the assay preparation) is a good approximation of the affinity for the agonist. The reason for this effect is the fact that a partial agonist does not saturate the stimulus-response capability of the tissue; therefore the maximal receptor occupancy can be identified through observation of the functional maximal response. Under these circumstances, the response to a partial agonist is proportional to the receptor occupancy. Therefore the EC_{50} of the partial agonist becomes a reasonable approximation of the concentration of agonist occupying 50% of the available receptors; by definition the K_{eq} for receptor binding (the affinity of a partial agonist $= 1/K_{eq} = 1/EC_{50}$) can directly be obtained from the dose-response curve for a partial agonist (see Fig. 2.3).

Unfortunately, the same simple relationship does not hold for the EC_{50} of a full agonist and agonist affinity. This is because the maximal response to the full agonist cannot be reliably related to 100% receptor occupancy (in fact, the opposite is true). Due to the amplifying effect of agonist response by cells (specifically agonist efficacy coupled with the cellular effects of high target densities and efficient target-coupling mechanisms to cellular response; see chapter: Pharmacology: The Chemical Control of Physiology), the receptor binding curve is displaced to the right of the observed agonism. Because of this effect, the

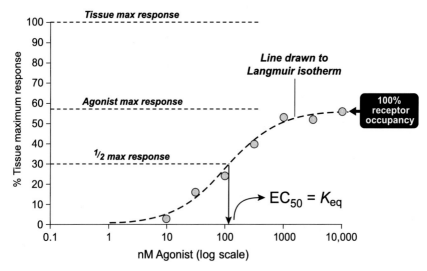

FIGURE 2.3   Dose-response curve for a partial agonist. If the maximal response to the agonist is lower than the system maximal response, then the concentration producing maximal response approximates the saturation binding concentration of the agonist (concentration binding to 100% of the available receptors). Under these circumstances, the EC_{50} of the curve also approximates the K_{eq} for binding (concentration binding to 50% of the sites).

EC_{50} of a curve to a full agonist will be lower than the concentration that occupies 50% of the target sites; that is, it is no longer an estimate for K_{eq} (1/Affinity). The magnitude of the EC_{50} for a full agonist is a complex function of the affinity and efficacy of the agonist (see Derivations and Proofs, Appendix A) and also the effect of stimulus-response amplification by the tissue (Fig. 2.4).

In many cases, agonist response can be characterized in a system-independent manner by the measurement of the affinity and efficacy of the agonist; this will be described in more detail in the following chapter. However, while both the parameters of affinity and efficacy are required to describe agonists, only affinity is required to character-ize the activity of target antagonists (molecules that block the activa-tion of the target by agonists). The various methods employed to measure the affinity of antagonists will be described in Chapter 4, Drug Antagonism Orthosteric Drug Effects and Chapter 5, Allosteric Drug Effects.

Efficacy

The property of a molecule that causes the target to change its behav-ior toward the cellular host when the molecule is bound to the target is

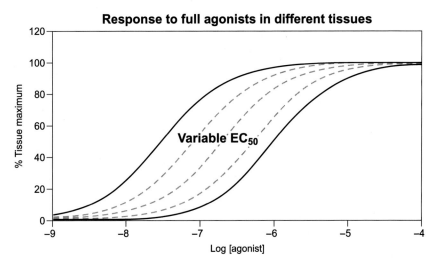

FIGURE 2.4 In contrast to curves for partial agonists (see Fig. 2.3), changes in cellular sensitivity to full agonists result in variation in the EC_{50}. However, the EC_{50} is a complex function of both the affinity and efficacy of the agonist; therefore no specific information about the affinity of the full agonist can be derived from the EC_{50}.

called *efficacy*. However, small a drug molecule may be compared to the receptor protein, the receptor with drug bound to it is a different thermodynamic species than the receptor with no drug bound. Therefore by definition, there is a property imparted to the receptor through the binding of a drug. The term *efficacy* was coined by the British pharmacologist R.P. Stephenson (see Box 2.3). The compelling observation in these studies was the fact that a collection of highly related alkyltrimethylammonium partial agonists produced contractions of the guinea pig ileum with nearly identical affinity (pEC_{50}), but with varying maximal responses (see Fig. 2.5) [1]. These data made it apparent that there must be another drug-related property causing these molecules to have differing capabilities of inducing response; this property was given the name efficacy. While Stephenson defined efficacy as both a drug-related

---

BOX 2.3

R.P. Stephenson and drug "efficacy"

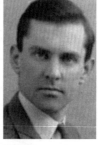

R.P. Stephenson (1925–2004)

Robert Stephenson, renowned for introducing the concept of efficacy into pharmacology, was an English pharmacologist who worked in the Pharmacology Department at Edinburgh University. He studied the activity of alkyltrimethylammonium compounds as contractile agonists in the guinea pig ileum through activation of muscarinic receptors. It was here he noted that, while the compounds had fairly uniform affinity for the receptors, they differed considerably in their ability to cause contraction. This led him to postulate that the compounds need to have another intrinsic property to differentiate one from the other; he gave this fundamental property of drugs the name efficacy. Stephenson considered both the intrinsic efficacy of the agonist and the sensitivity of the tissue to be a combined description of the efficacy of an agonist in any tissue.

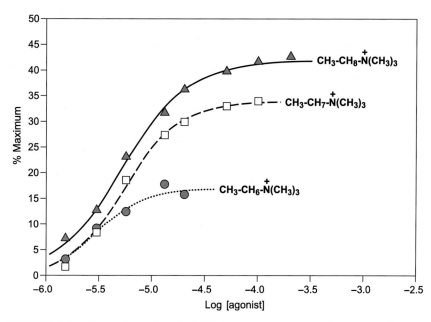

FIGURE 2.5   Data redrawn from Ref. [1] showing contractions of guinea pig ileum to three alkyltrimethylammonium partial agonists. While these molecules are of comparable affinity for the muscarinic receptors in this preparation, clearly the molecules differ in their ability to induce maximal response. Stephenson reasoned that the critical property causing these differences is efficacy.

and a tissue-related property, it will be seen that there are pharmacological procedures that allow the cancellation of the tissue-dependent aspects of efficacy to allow it to be used as a strictly drug-dependent parameter (*vide infra*).

The most common setting for observing efficacy is the effect of agonists on cellular systems. On a molecular scale, it is useful to consider how an agonist elicits a change in the receptor to cause cellular activation. Whereas enzymes bind their substrates in energetically constrained conformations to stretch bonds to a breaking point (or to create a new bond), receptors do not change their "substrates," nor are they permanently altered by their interaction with drugs. Instead, an agonist activates the receptor when it binds and the activation ceases when the agonist diffuses away. Historically, it was thought that the binding of the drug deformed the receptor and produced an activated state through drug binding (protein conformational induction). However, such a mechanism is energetically extremely unfavorable. In thermodynamic terms, a much more reasonable mechanism is through protein *conformational selection* (see Fig. 2.6). In this scheme, drugs bind to a limited number of preexisting receptor conformations and stabilize those through binding (at the expense of other conformations—Le Chatelier's principle of an equilibrium responding to perturbation—see Box 2.4). Because of the selective affinity of the ligand for receptor active states a bias in the collection of conformations results. If two conformations are interconvertible, then a ligand with a higher affinity for one of the conformations will enrich the system with this conformation at the expense of other conformations. The mathematical description of how this occurs is given in Box 2.5. This defines binding as an active process, not a passive process. Specifically, if a ligand has a selective affinity for a collection of protein conformations, it will actively change the makeup of that collection. It is this active property of ligands that can result in physiological cellular response (efficacy).

Affinity and efficacy can be dissociable properties that vary independently with changes in chemical structure (i.e., see Fig. 2.5). It is useful to note the independence of affinity and efficacy on chemical structure for drug development, as these properties can be manipulated separately en route to a defined therapeutic entity (as in the case of the discovery and synthesis of the important class of histamine receptor H_2 antagonists for

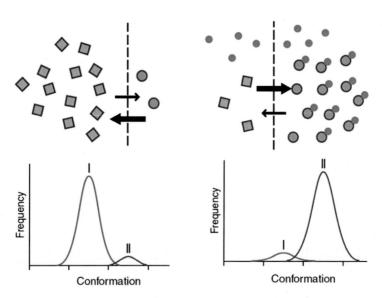

FIGURE 2.6 Conformational selection as a molecular mechanism for efficacy. The system is comprised of two protein conformations (green squares and red circles) in equilibrium with each other. A given ligand (blue filled circles) does not bind well to the inactive state of the receptor but rather selectively binds to the active state (red circles) producing a new thermodynamic species. This drives the equilibrium toward the free red circle state causing the system to be enriched in this species. If the red circles induce cellular response, then the ligand is an agonist.

BOX 2.4

Le Chatelier's principle

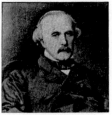

Henry Louis Le Chatelier (1850–1936)

Henry Louis Le Chatelier was a French-Italian chemist most famous for devising "Le Chatelier's principle." This idea is used by chemists to predict the effect a change in conditions has on a chemical equilibrium. Although he trained as an engineer, Le Chatelier chose chemistry as a career and went on to explore general chemical laws and principles (... all my life I maintained a respect for order ... order is one of the most perfect forms ...). His famous principle stated "... If a dynamic equilibrium is disturbed by changing the conditions, the position of equilibrium moves to counteract the change." This concept was first presented to the Academie des Sciences in Paris in 1885. This principle applies to isoenergetic interconvertible protein conformations, and dictates how ligands bias protein ensembles toward active states to produce a cellular response.

the treatment of peptic ulcer). In this instance, a chemical effort to enhance the affinity and eliminate the efficacy of the natural agonist histamine for the target H_2 receptor resulted in the synthesis of cimetidine, a potent molecule with high affinity for the H_2 receptor but no efficacy (see Box 2.6). This molecule competes with histamine to antagonize the production of stomach acid and thus promotes the healing of ulcers. Utilizing separate scales of affinity and efficacy for agonist activity is preferable to using amalgam scales, such as agonist potency. This latter value is a complex function of both affinity and efficacy thereby making potency a possibly insensitive scale to gage the pharmacological effects of changing chemical structure. For instance, a structural change that reduces affinity but increases efficacy may produce little effect on potency. Valuable data for chemical lead optimization would be lost by assuming that the change in structure produced no effect, if potency were the sole scale for activity.

BOX 2.5

Protein conformational selection

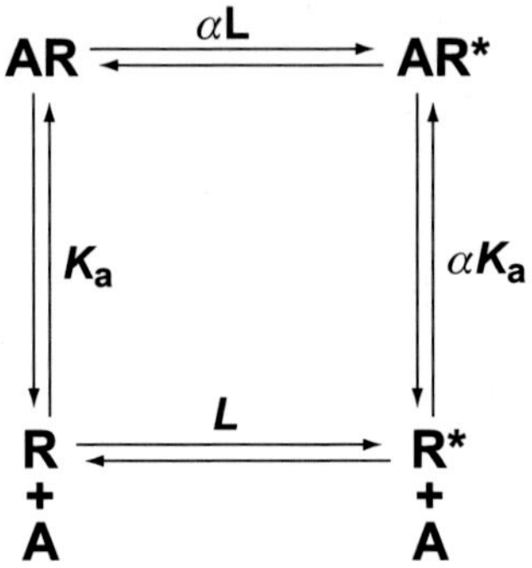

Assume two protein conformations R and R* are controlled by an equilibrium dissociation constant L, where $L = [R^*]/[R]$. Similarly, consider a ligand A with an affinity (defined as the equilibrium association constant $K_a = k_1/k_2$) of K_a for receptor state R and αK_a for receptor state R*, where the factor α denotes the differential affinity of the agonist for R*, that is, $\alpha = 10$ denotes a 10-fold greater affinity of the ligand for the R* state. The effect of α (selective affinity) on the ability of the ligand to alter the equilibrium between R and R* can be calculated by examining the amount of R* (both as R* and AR*) present in the system in the absence of A, and in the presence of A. The equilibrium expression for $([R^*] + [AR^*])/[R_t]$ where $[R_t]$ is the total receptor concentration given by the conservation equation $[R_t] = [R] + [AR] + [R^*] + [AR^*]$ is:

$$\rho = \frac{L(1 + \alpha[A]/K_A)}{[A]/K_A(1 + \alpha L) + L + 1} \tag{2.4}$$

where K_A is the equilibrium dissociation constant of the agonist–receptor complex. In the absence of agonist ($[A] = 0$), $\rho_0 = L/(1 + L)$, while in the presence of a maximal concentration of ligand (saturating the receptors; $[A] \to \infty$) $\rho_\infty = (\alpha[1 + L])/(1 + \alpha L)$. Therefore the effect of the ligand on the proportion of the R* state is given by the ratio ρ_∞/ρ_0. This ratio is given by:

$$\frac{\rho_\infty}{\rho_0} = \frac{\alpha(1 + L)}{1 + \alpha L} \tag{2.5}$$

It can be seen from this equation that if the ligand has an equal affinity for both the R and R* states ($\alpha = 1$) then ρ_∞/ρ_0 will equal unity and no change in the proportion of R* will result from maximal ligand

continued

BOX 2.5 *(cont'd)*

binding. However, if $\alpha > 1$, then the presence of the conformationally selective ligand will cause the ratio ρ_∞ / ρ_0 to be >1 and the R* state will be enriched by the presence of the ligand. If the R* state promotes physiological response, then ligand A will promote response and be an agonist. This defines binding as an active, not a passive, process. Specifically, if a ligand has a selective affinity for a collection of protein conformations, it will actively change the makeup of that collection. It is this active property of ligands that can result in physiological cellular response (efficacy).

Drugs with multiple efficacies

Up to this point, efficacy has been discussed as if it is a single drug property. In early considerations of efficacy, test systems were simple and consisted of a single index of tissue response (e.g., Stephenson used the in vitro contraction of guinea pig ileum). The assumption at that time was that efficacy was linear, meaning that it was a reflection of all the biological actions mediated by that target in the cell. Also at that time, receptors were thought to be more simple units controlling single functions (i.e., calcium entry into the cell to mediate contraction). With increasing technology, different assays have been developed that can monitor the functions of receptors and cells, and with this has come an appreciation of how receptors perform multiple tasks and have complex behaviors. Fig. 2.7 shows some prominent behaviors of seven transmembrane (7TM) receptors that have been elucidated through separate assay technologies. These proteins can process numerous signals from extracellular molecules to activate different cytosolic signaling proteins, such as G proteins and β-arrestin; these targets also have a dynamic lifetime on the cell surface as they are expressed, reside in the cell membrane, and then disappear into the cytosol again to be recycled or destroyed. Activation of these targets by agonists changes the dynamics of receptor behavior through processes, such as phosphorylation by kinases, desensitization, and internalization (Fig. 2.7). It is important to realize that different agonists can produce these effects differentially, that is, not all agonists produce a uniform set of behaviors in 7TM receptors. This being the case, it will be seen that different molecules can have more than one efficacy as they cause activation of different aspects of target behavior. For example, there are agonists that primarily

---

BOX 2.6

James Black and dissociation of affinity and efficacy

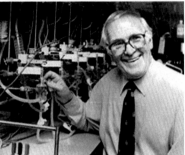

Sir James Black (1924–2010) was a Scottish pharmacologist who discovered two major classes of therapeutic drugs; beta-blockers and H_2 histamine antagonists. The discovery of this latter class was based on the principle that the structure-activity relationships governing drug affinity and efficacy could be different. His aim was to cure stomach ulcer by blocking the histamine-induced release of acid that prevented ulcers from healing. As stated by Black: "... we knew that the receptor bound histamine, so it was a matter of keeping affinity and losing efficacy ..." For his ground-breaking discoveries Black received the Nobel Prize for Medicine in 1988. Below are shown the key molecules that illustrate how efficacy can be reduced and affinity enhanced.

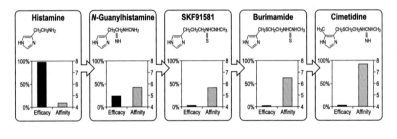

---

activate only G proteins through a receptor, while other agonists activate only β-arrestin through the same receptor. The mechanism by which this occurs is the formation of different active states of the receptor. This presents the receptor in the therapeutic role of a microprocessor able to receive different signals from the extracellular space and yield correspondingly different intracellular signals (see Box 2.7). There are two major consequences of this mechanism. First, the formation of drug-specific receptor active states allows the reduction in the breadth

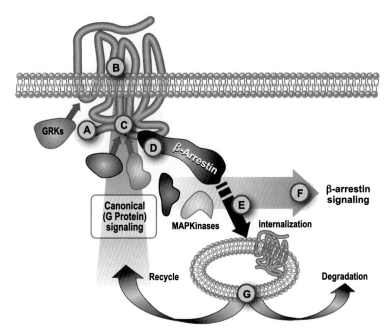

FIGURE 2.7   Seven transmembrane (7TM) receptors have complex behaviors in cells and these may be exploited therapeutically. Thus binding of ligands to these proteins can cause activation of signaling proteins called G proteins (C) and subsequent phosphorylation of receptors by G protein receptor kinases (A). These targets may also accommodate binding of allosteric ligands (B—see chapter: Allosteric Drug Effects). These targets also bind the cytosolic molecule β-arrestin (D), which can cause recycling of the receptor to the cell surface or internalization of the receptor into endosomes. Internalized receptor can be degraded (G) or form a scaffold for cytosolic MAPKinases to produce cellular signals (F).

of effect to an agonist with a resulting potential for greater selectivity. Second, this functional selectivity produces varying agonist potencies in whole cells, thereby negating characterizations of potency ratios as system-independent measures of affinity and efficacy of agonists (as was shown in chapter: Pharmacology: The Chemical Control of Physiology, Fig. 1.9). This is because the actual microscopic efficacy of functionally selective agonists is different. Therefore the relative activities of these agonists depend on the dominance of various cell types for each of the separate signaling pathways. For example, a primarily β-arrestin signaling molecule will be differentially more active in cells containing large amounts of β-arrestin than in cells that do not.

This can lead to ambiguity in classifying drugs for therapeutic purposes. Specifically, molecules with numerous efficacies can be both agonists for some cellular functions and antagonists for others. For instance, some β-blocker antagonists (antagonists of β-adrenoceptors; see chapter: Drug Antagonism Orthosteric Drug Effects) are also

BOX 2.7

Receptors as microprocessors

Receptors as Microprocessors

Angiotensin   TRV120027

With the advent of new assays to independently measure multiple agonist responses has come the realization that drugs do not need to produce all of the signaling mechanisms associated with a given receptor. Instead, some ligands may emphasize the activation of some signaling pathways at the expense of others; such agonists are said to produce "biased" signaling, an effect discussed in further detail in the next chapter. The molecular mechanism for this effect is the selective stabilization of different receptor active states [2,3]. For example, the natural hormone angiotensin produces activation of Gq protein and also β-arrestin signaling in cells. In contrast, the biased angiotensin receptor ligand TRV120027 binds to the angiotensin receptor but does not activate Gq protein, only β-arrestin [4]. Such a profile is proposed to be beneficial in heart failure [5]. Thus receptors, with the ability to form multiple active conformations, take on the role of microprocessors, which, by definition, receive varying signals and yield differential output based on those incoming signals.

activators (agonists) of extracellular receptor kinases. Similarly, two agonists could have similar primary activities but different and important secondary properties. For example, while natural hormones and neurotransmitters, such as endomorphins, produce activation of receptors leading to desensitization and receptor internalization into the cytosol with prolonged activation, there are agonists that produce activation with considerably less desensitization. This type of functional selectivity can lead to superior therapeutic agonism (i.e., sustained opioid analgesia with no tolerance). Another form of functional selectivity defines antagonists that produce no activation but nevertheless produce receptor internalization. Such drugs produce better antagonism in cases where all effect needs to be abolished (internalization of C-C chemokine receptor type 5 (CCR5) receptors for removal of HIV-1 sites of infectious binding).

These ideas have changed the way drug efficacy is regarded in pharmacology. While historically efficacy has been considered to be a homogeneous drug property differing mainly in the strength of the signal given to the cell, the realization that receptors are pleiotropically linked to multiple signaling mechanisms has led to an appreciation of the quality of efficacy inherent in any drug molecule. The key to the actual quality of efficacy is locked in the receptor conformations stabilized by the drug molecule. Thus as drug molecules create different conformations of receptors, these then go on to activate signaling mechanisms in different ways to create a "bias" in the combination of signals given to the cell—see Box 2.7. Such signaling bias can be applied to discovery to create therapeutically useful signaling profiles. For instance, the creation of analogs of parathyroid hormone that selectively activate a signaling molecule called β-arrestin-2 known to build bone may provide a superior treatment for bone wasting osteoporosis [6]. Similarly, biased molecules may de-emphasize signaling that otherwise causes harm, such as the respiratory depression produced by morphine through β-arrestin, which limits its analgesic utility. In this regard, the application of genetically engineered animals can be very useful in identifying beneficial and/or harmful signaling pathways—see Box 2.8.

An appreciation of the quality of efficacy for an agonist may be obtained from an inspection of the different signaling elements activated by the molecule upon receptor binding. Fig. 2.8 shows a radar plot of various intracellular signals produced by molecules; the overall pattern forms a geometric web, which can serve to characterize the efficacy of the molecule and hopefully, the association of such webs with in vivo phenotypic activity can be used to optimize drugs for therapeutic application.

BOX 2.8

Identifying therapeutic pathways through knock-out genes

Beneficial and harmful signaling pathways can be identified through the drug testing in genetically modified animals where specific genes have been removed. For instance, it is known that activation of μ-opioid receptors by morphine causes the therapeutically beneficial analgesia but also debilitating respiratory depression. The analgesia is mediated through activation of G protein by the receptor while the respiratory depression results from a receptor β-arrestin interaction. Such signaling can be elucidated by testing morphine in normal (wild-type; WT) mice and β-arrestin knock-out (β-arr. KO) mice where the gene responsible for β-arrestin has been removed from birth, leaving the animal bereft of the protein. It can be seen that there is significantly less morphine-induced respiratory depression in the β-arr. KO mice than in WT mice [7], supporting the assignment of the harmful μ-opioid effect to this signaling pathway and thus indicating a need for a μ-opioid analgesic that is biased toward G protein and away from β-arrestin.

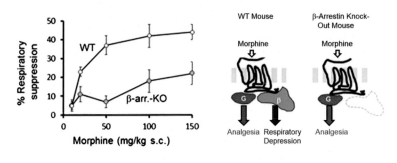

Quantifying agonist activity

Under ideal circumstances, the affinity and relative efficacy of agonists can be quantified and used in a system-independent manner to predict therapeutic agonism (see chapter: Predicting Agonist Effect). However, even when this is not the case, in some cases agonism can still be quantified to describe agonists. The methods for doing this are different for full versus partial agonists. For full agonists, equiactive potency ratios are used. Thus the ratios of EC_{50} values are used to quantify the relative potency of full agonists. If the agonists produce responses by an identical mechanism of activation of the target (i.e., stabilize the same active state

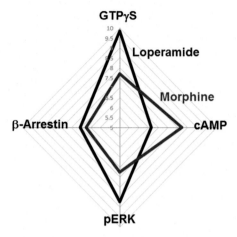

FIGURE 2.8 Radar plot showing the activation of four separate signaling pathways (interaction of the receptor with G protein (GTP-γS), generation of the second messenger cyclic AMP, phosphorylation of extracellular signal-regulated kinase 1 and 2 (pERK), and interaction of the receptor with β-arrestin-2) linked to μ-opioid receptors by two opioid agonists loperamide and morphine. The different geometric forms indicate different patterns of signal activation, which also will result in different qualities of efficacy for these two agonists when they activate the receptor. Source: Data from G.L. Thompson, J.R. Lane, T. Coudrat, P.M. Sexton, A. Christopoulos, M. Canals, Biased agonism of endogenous opioid peptides at the μ-opioid receptor. Mol. Pharmacol. 88 (2015) 335–346 [8].

of the protein), then these potency ratios are system-independent measures of relative agonist activity. For example, for two agonists of identical mechanism, one with a pEC_{50} of 8.2 and another with a pEC_{50} of 7.1, the potency ratio is $10^{(8.2-7.1)} = 12.6$. This ratio should be true of these two agonists in every tissue where they function as full agonists. An example of ranking full agonists through potency ratios is shown in Fig. 2.9.

More detailed information can be obtained for partial agonists. When the agonist does not produce the system's maximal response, as discussed earlier, the EC_{50} becomes a surrogate estimate of the K_{eq} for binding to the target (affinity = $1/K_{eq}$). Similarly, the maximal response, although not numerically equal to the efficacy of the agonist, can be used to rank agonists according to a scale of efficacy. Thus it can be assumed that if the maximal response to a given partial agonist [A] is greater than the maximal response of another partial agonist [B], the efficacy of A is greater than the efficacy of B. An example of how agonist affinity and efficacy can be estimated for partial agonists is shown in Fig. 2.10. In this figure it can be seen that there are different orders of potency for efficacy (maximal response) and affinity (potency); this is a clear indication that the structural differences in the molecules have different effects on efficacy and affinity.

2. Drug affinity and efficacy

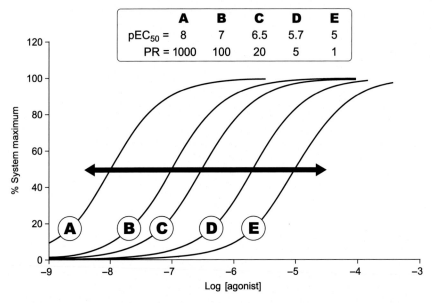

FIGURE 2.9 Quantifying full agonist effect through the measurement of potency ratios. Full agonists A–E have the potencies shown (pEC$_{50}$ values). The relative potencies (measured as the ratio of EC$_{50}$ values) should be constant for these agonists in all cell types, if they produce a response through identical mechanisms.

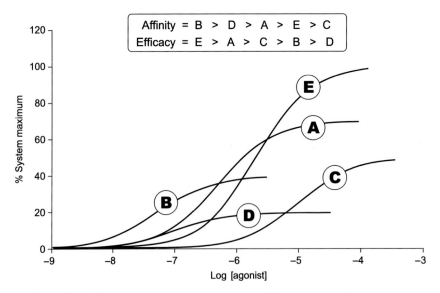

FIGURE 2.10 Characteristics of partial agonist dose-response curves. The EC$_{50}$ values of the curves to partial agonists reflect affinity, thus, for the partial agonists shown, the affinities of molecules are B = 30 nM, D = 100 nM, A = 300 nM, E = 1 μM and C = 100 μM. The rank order of efficacy of the agonists can be discerned from the relative maximal responses as shown.

The behavior of full and partial agonists in cell systems suggests ideal test systems for lead optimization and screening for new drugs. In terms of screening, the most sensitive system possible is best since this will detect weak agonists. Given the known amplification of signals, as they are measured distal to the initial point of initiation (see Derivations and Proofs, Appendix A), the end organ cellular response is optimal for new drug screening. Once a chemical scaffold is identified and medicinal chemists begin to optimize activity, a system where the effect of changing chemical structure on affinity and, separately, on efficacy, is optimal since much more information can be obtained. As noted in Fig. 2.10, this would be assays in which the agonists demonstrate partial agonist activity.

Descriptive pharmacology: II

Continuing the process of pharmacologic characterization of new molecules (from Linking Observed Pharmacology with Molecular Mechanism, chapter: Pharmacology: The Chemical Control of Physiology), this chapter discusses the characterization of agonists from the point where a cellular response to the molecule has been observed (see Fig. 2.11). The next step is to confirm that the agonism is specifically related to the biological target of interest. It is also possible to begin to characterize the agonism in more detail, either through quantifying full agonist potency ratios or, for partial agonists, estimation of agonist affinity through measurement of the pEC_{50}. Partial agonism also enables the ranking of efficacy through comparison of maximal responses.

Summary

Specific agonism can be confirmed by determining that specific antagonists of the target block response to the agonist and/or that the presence of the target is required to demonstrate a response to the agonist.

Affinity is quantified through a ratio of the rate of dissociation of the molecule from the protein (k_2) and the rate of association to the protein (k_1) in a parameter referred to as K_{eq} (where $K_{eq} = k_2/k_1$). This is the concentration of ligand that binds to 50% of the available receptors.

Efficacy is the property of a molecule that changes the behavior of the biological target toward its cellular host, when it is bound to that target.

Molecules can have multiple efficacies depending on which behavior of the biological target is considered.

Potency ratios can furnish system-independent (constant for all tissues) measures of relative agonism (providing the agonists have identical modes of action).

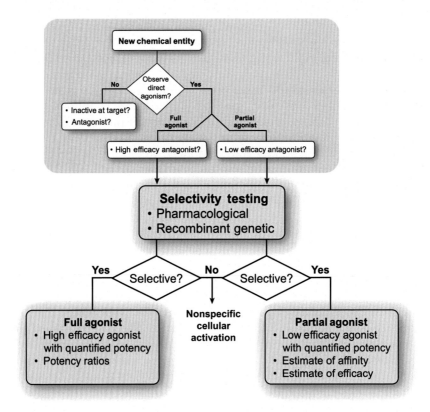

FIGURE 2.11 Continuation of logical progression for determination of new drug effect. *(From Fig. 1.10). Once agonism has been observed, it must be determined that it is selective for the biological target of interest. If the response is full agonism, then system-independent characterization of relative efficacy (that may transcend cell type) can be made through relative potency ratios (if the agonists produce a response in an identical manner). For partial agonists, the EC_{50} value is an estimate of affinity and the maximal response denotes relative efficacy.*

The pEC_{50} value for agonism is a reasonable approximation of the affinity of a partial agonist.

The maximal response of partial agonists can be used to rank order the efficacy of the partial agonists.

The ideal assay for new drug screening is a highly sensitive one (end organ response), whereas a good assay for lead optimization is where the agonists produce partial agonism.

Questions

2.1. The response to a test agonist is not blocked by conventional antagonists of the target. What could be happening?

2.2. Drug A has an equilibrium dissociation constant (K_{eq}) of 10^{-8} M while drug B has a K_{eq} of 10^{-10} M. Which drug has the higher affinity and why?

2.3. Two agonists produce responses in a system both with a pEC_{50} of 7.5. However, one produces 25% maximal response while the other produces 90% maximal response. What is the difference between these two agonists?

2.4. The potency ratio for two full agonists A and B is 15.4 in one cellular system and 2.3 in another. What does this lack of correlation of full agonist potency ratio suggest?

2.5. Why is it important to test putative agonists in as many functional assay systems as possible?

2.6. Why are the overall descriptive terms "agonist" and "antagonist" now seen to be confining in terms of characterizing new drugs?

References

[1] R.P. Stephenson, A modification of receptor theory, Br. J. Pharmacol. 11 (1956) 379–393.

[2] T. Kenakin, P.H. Morgan, The theoretical effects of single and multiple transducer receptor coupling proteins on estimates of the relative potency of agonists, Mol. Pharmacol. 35 (1989) 214–222.

[3] T. Kenakin, Agonist-receptor efficacy. II. Agonist-trafficking of receptor signals, Trends Pharmacol. Sci. 16 (1995) 232–238.

[4] J.D. Violin, S.M. DeWire, D. Yamashita, D.H. Rominger, L. Nguyen, K. Schiller, Selectively engaging β-arrestins at the angiotensin II type 1 receptor reduces blood pressure and increases cardiac performance, J. Pharmacol. Exp. Ther. 335 (2010) 572–579.

[5] G. Boerrigter, M.W. Lark, E.J. Whalen, D.G. Soergel, J.D. Violin, J.C. Burnett, Cardiorenal actions of TRV120027, a novel β-arrestinbiased ligand at the angiotensin II type I receptor, in healthy and heart failure canine: a novel therapeutic strategy for acute heart failure, Circ. Heart Fail. 4 (2011) 770–778.

[6] S.L. Ferrari, D.D. Pierroz, V. Glatt, D.S. Goddard, E.N. Bianchi, F.T. Lin, Bone response to intermittent parathyroid hormone is altered in mice null for beta-arrestin2, Endocrinology 146 (2005) 1854–1862.

[7] K.M. Raehal, J.K. Walker, L.M. Bohn, Morphine side effects in beta-arrestin2 knockout mice, J. Pharmacol. Exp. Ther. 314 (2005) 1195–1201.

[8] G.L. Thompson, J.R. Lane, T. Coudrat, P.M. Sexton, A. Christopoulos, M. Canals, Biased agonism of endogenous opioid peptides at the μ-opioid receptor, Mol. Pharmacol. 88 (2015) 335–346.

Predicting agonist effect

By the end of this chapter, readers should be able to use the Black—Leff operational model to quantify agonist affinity and efficacy. They should also be able to use ratios of these values obtained in a test system to predict agonism for the same agonists in any other system as well as quantify any biased agonism produced by a test agonist.

Agonist response in different tissues

As discussed in Chapter 1, Pharmacology: The Chemical Control of Physiology, the potency of an agonist depends on the drug-related properties of affinity and efficacy, and the cell-related properties of

Pharmacology in Drug Discovery and Development
DOI: https://doi.org/10.1016/B978-0-443-14124-9.00009-4

target density (number of responding units in the cell) and the efficiency with which these target units are coupled to the cell response producing machinery. These two latter factors vary with cell type, leading to variable potency of any given agonist in different cell types. It is useful to consider the pattern that the dose-response curves to a given agonist will assume in a range of tissues of varying target density and/or target coupling efficiency. As discussed in Chapter 2, Drug Affinity and Efficacy, the EC_{50} of the curve to a partial agonist is an approximate estimate of the binding K_{eq} (affinity^{-1}). This is a molecular property of the agonist that is constant for all tissues, so it follows that in tissues where the agonist produces partial maximal effect, the EC_{50} will be relatively constant and equal to a value near the K_{eq}. Also as noted in Chapter 2, Drug Affinity and Efficacy, in more sensitive tissues where full agonism is produced, the EC_{50} dissociates from K_{eq} and becomes a complex function of both affinity and efficacy (see Derivations and Proofs, Appendix A.2). With increasing sensitivity of the tissue, the dose-response curve to the full agonist will progressively shift to the left along the concentration axis. Fig. 3.1 shows dose-response curves to a given agonist in a range of tissues of varying sensitivity (from low to high). It can be seen from this figure that the curves showing submaximal activity have similar EC_{50} values until the tissue maximal response is produced. Then, in the more sensitive tissues where full agonism is observed, the EC_{50} values progressively diminish (i.e., the curves shift to the left along the concentration axis).

The behavior of agonist dose-response curves in different tissues is important to understand to predict agonist response in all tissues. In general, in the least sensitive tissues, the dose-response curve to any agonist emanates from concentrations around the K_{eq} for binding. At this point, this will be denoted as K_A, which is the nomenclature for the binding K_{eq} for agonists. In more sensitive tissues, the curve shifts to the left of this value. Fig. 3.2 shows the dose-response curves of two agonists (denoted A and B) in a range of tissues of varying sensitivity (numbered 1−4, with 1 being the most sensitive). In the lower panels, the curves for each agonist in tissues 1−4 are shown. It can be seen that the relative potencies of agonists A and B do not follow a uniform pattern once partial agonism is observed. This has practical ramifications for drug discovery. Specifically, consider the relative potency profiles of agonists A and B in tissue 1 and tissue 4. In efficiently coupled tissues where both are full agonists, it can be seen that agonist B is more potent than agonist A. However, in a more poorly coupled tissue (tissue 4), it can be seen that agonist A now yields a more robust response than agonist B. Such discontinuities in agonist potency can only be predicted if affinity and efficacy are known. In the

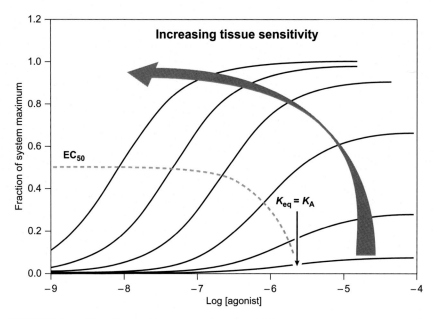

FIGURE 3.1 The effects of increasing tissue sensitivity on response to an agonist. In low sensitivity systems, the curve shows a maximum that is below the tissue maximal response and the EC_{50} can be approximated by the K_{eq} for agonist binding to the receptor (denoted as K_A). As tissue sensitivity increases, the maximal response increases until the tissue maximum is attained. Increases in sensitivity beyond this point have no further effect on the maximal response to the agonist (i.e., the agonist produces the tissue maximum), but do shift the dose-response curve to the left (increased agonist potency). At this point, the EC_{50} is $\ll$ the K_{eq} for binding.

absence of this information, the behavior of the agonists in different systems cannot be predicted accurately. The major tool to make such predictions is the Black–Leff operational model of agonism.

New terminology

The following new terms will be introduced in this chapter:

- *Michaelis–Menten kinetics*: Description of the interaction of molecules with proteins based on the enzyme catalysis of substrate molecules as first described by Michaelis and Menten. Kinetics are characterized by a maximal rate of enzyme action (denoted V_{max}) and a sensitivity to catalysis (denoted K_m, referred to as the Michaelis–Menten constant). This latter term is the concentration of substrate that causes the enzyme to function at $^1/_2\ V_{max}$.

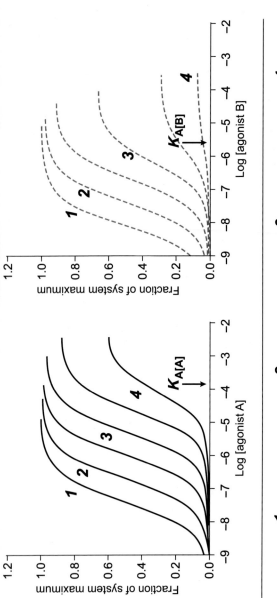
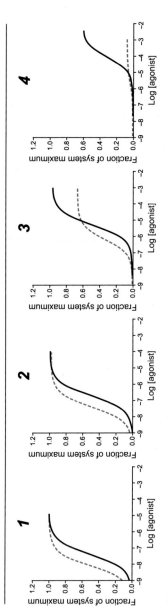

FIGURE 3.2 Dose-response curves to two agonists (agonists A and B) in a range of systems of varying sensitivity. It can be seen that in systems of low sensitivity, both are partial agonists with potencies (EC$_{50}$ values) approximating the binding constant to the receptor (K_{eq} for agonist A = $K_{A[A]}$ and for agonist B = $K_{A[B]}$). With increasing sensitivity, both become full agonists with increasing potency. Lower panels show the relative responses of each agonist in four systems ranked from most to least sensitive. It can be seen that the relative effects range from agonist B being a more potent full agonist in system 1, to agonist A being a more efficacious agonist in system 4. Thus, there is no uniform decrease and preservation of the relative activity of these agonists in the different systems due to the fact that agonist activity results from a complex interplay of affinity and efficacy.

- *Receptor reserve (spare receptors)*: This refers to the condition in a tissue whereby the agonist needs to activate only a small fraction of the existing receptor population to produce the maximal system response. The magnitude of the reserve depends on the sensitivity of the tissue *and* the efficacy of the agonist.
- τ: efficacy of an agonist (according to the Black—Leff operational model of agonism) is made up of drug-specific properties (the intrinsic efficacy of the molecule) and tissue-related factors (the K_E of the drug-bound receptor interacting with the stimulus-response biochemical reactions of the cell).
- *Biased Agonism*: If the receptor is linked to multiple signaling pathways in a cell, then agonists may differentiate these and produce emphasis of some pathways at the expense of others; this is referred to as biased signaling.

The Black—Leff operational model of agonism

The model used to link stimulus with cellular response is the operational model devised by Black and Leff [1]. The basis of this model is the experimental finding that the observed relationship between agonist-induced response and agonist concentration resembles a model of enzyme function presented in 1913 by Louis Michaelis and Maude L. Menten (see Box 3.1 and Fig. 3.3). This model accounts for the fact that the kinetics of enzyme reactions differ significantly from the kinetics of conventional chemical reactions. It describes the reaction of a substrate with an enzyme as an equation of the form: reaction velocity = (maximal velocity of the reaction × substrate concentration)/(concentration of substrate + a fitting constant K_m). The parameter K_m characterizes the tightness of the binding of the reaction between the substrate and enzyme; it is also the concentration at which the reaction rate is half the maximal value. It can be seen that the more active the substrate, the smaller is the value of K_m. Comparison of this equation with Eq. (2.1) shows that it is formally identical to the Langmuir adsorption isotherm relating binding of a chemical to a surface ($K_m = K_{eq}$). Both of these models form the basis of drug receptor interaction, thus the kinetics involved sometimes are referred to as "Langmuirian" in form.

The Black—Leff model views the cell as a virtual enzyme and the amount of agonist-target bound complexes as the substrate for that enzyme (see Box 3.2). The first step in the response chain is the transduction of the activated receptor stimulus (quantified by the number

BOX 3.1

Michaelis—Menten enzyme kinetics.

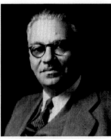

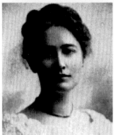

Leonor Michaelis (1875—1949) and Maude Menten (1879—1960) worked in the Berlin Municipal Hospital and together formulated one of the earliest quantitative laws of biochemistry. Specifically, their famous equation described the velocity and mechanism of the formation of the complex between an enzyme and substrate. In form, the Michaelis—Menten equation describes a relationship between input and output that is applicable to a wide variety of biochemical processes, such as enzymes, transport processes, and other saturable reactions. Black and Leff utilized the general form of this equation to define τ as a representation of agonist efficacy and the sensitivity of tissues to agonist action.

of agonist-receptor complexes denoted [AR]) into a cellular response. The number of [AR] complexes is given by the fraction of the receptor population bound by agonist (ρ_A given by the Langmuir adsorption isotherm, Eq. 2.1) multiplied by the number of receptors on the cell surface (denoted [R_t]; [AR] = $\rho_A \cdot$ [R_t]). The operational model relates tissue response to a Michaelis—Menten type of equation of the form:

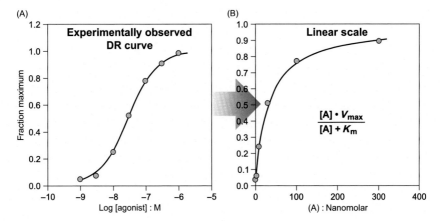

FIGURE 3.3 Similarity of cellular response to enzymatic function. Experimentally determined dose-response curve from an intact cell system (left panel, A) and the same curve plotted on a linear scale to show the similarity of the shape of this curve to a Michaelis–Menten kinetic system (right panel, B). This similarity prompted Black and Leff to use Michaelis–Menten kinetics to model cellular transduction of drug response.

$$\text{Response} = \frac{[AR]E_m}{[AR] + K_E} \tag{3.1}$$

where [AR] is the concentration of the amount of agonist-activated receptor, E_m is the maximal response that the system is able to produce under saturating stimulation (as the V_{max} in the Michaelis–Menten enzyme reaction) and K_E is the equilibrium dissociation constant of the activated receptor and response element (cellular machinery that responds to the activated receptor to generate a cellular response) complex. The similarity between a standard pharmacological dose-response curve and Michaelis–Menten kinetics is shown in Fig. 3.3. In this sense, Eq. (3.1) treats the cell as a comprehensive virtual enzyme utilizing the activated receptor as the substrate and cellular response as the product. The magnitude of the K_E reflects the activating power of the agonist, that is, high-efficacy agonists will have a lower K_E value than low-efficacy agonists. The amount of [AR] complex is given by the Langmuir adsorption isotherm for the fractional receptor occupancy of the agonist (ρ_A from Eq. 2.1) to yield [AR] from $[AR] = \rho_A \cdot [R_t]$ where $[R_t]$ is the concentration of receptors. Combining Eq. (2.1) and the Michaelis–Menten equation (see Fig. 3.4 and Derivations and Proofs, Appendix A.3):

$$\text{Response} = \frac{[A]/K_A[R_t]/K_E E_m}{[A]/K_A([R_t]/K_E + 1) + 1} \tag{3.2}$$

BOX 3.2

The operational model of drug action (shoebox model).

Stephenson's concept of efficacy was empirical in nature with no mechanistic basis. Black and Leff considered this to be a weakness in receptor theory and set out to redefine efficacy in biochemical terms as a function of a saturable transduction mechanism capable of being described with the Michaelis–Menten function for enzyme action. This model is rooted in what was observed in pharmacological experiments, namely, that there is a hyperbolic relationship between agonist-receptor occupancy and tissue response. An early version of the operational model was referred to by its creators as the "shoebox model" because of the fact that a three-dimensional rendering of the curves for agonist occupancy, signal transduction, and end-organ dose-response (as pasted on the internal faces of a shoebox) gave a concise view of the relationships between receptor occupancy and cellular response.

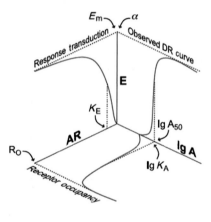

where E_m is the maximal response of the system. The model defines a parameter τ as $[R_t]/K_E$ to present the description of agonist response as:

$$\text{Response} = \frac{[A]\tau E_m}{[A](\tau + 1) + K_A} \tag{3.3}$$

An important and versatile parameter in the operational equation is τ; this constant incorporates the intrinsic efficacy of the agonist (a property of the molecule) and elements describing the efficiency of the tissue as it converts agonist-derived stimulus into tissue response

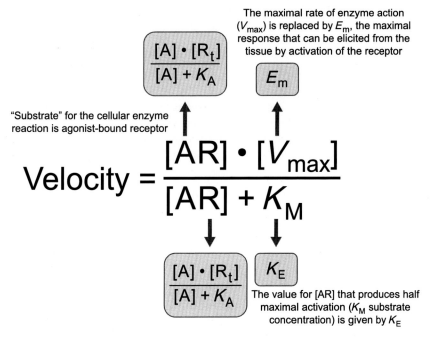

FIGURE 3.4 Operational model counterparts of the parameters of the Michaelis—Menten equation. Modeling cellular response as an enzyme velocity characterized by the Michaelis—Menten equation, the "substrate" for the cell is the agonist-receptor complex ([AR]) (given by the Langmuir adsorption isotherm). The sensitivity of the cell to agonist activation is quantified by K_E, while the maximal response of the system is denoted E_m.

(receptor density and K_E, the constant relating receptor activation and cellular response). The magnitude of K_E is unique for each tissue, since it is an amalgam of the series of biochemical reactions unique to the cell.

Applying the Black—Leff model to predict agonism

The first step in predicting agonism is to fit experimental data to the Black—Leff model; the variable slope version of the Black—Leff equation (see Derivations and Proofs, Appendix A.4) should be used to accommodate varying dose-response curve slopes observed experimentally (see Box 3.3). There are three basic steps in this process; the first is to define the maximal response capability of the system (E_m) and estimate

---

BOX 3.3

Fitting dose—response data to the Black—Leff model.

Under the correct circumstances, experimental dose-response data may be fit to the Black—Leff operational model to yield estimates of affinity (K_A) and efficacy (τ) for any agonist. Two essential parameters for this process are an independent estimate of E_m and an estimate of the affinity of the agonist; this latter parameter can be easily determined for a partial agonist as it will be approximated by the EC_{50}. The data is then fit to the simple adsorption isotherm to determine the slope of the curve (n):

$$\text{Response} = \frac{[A]^n \text{Max}}{[A]^n + EC_{50}^n} \tag{3.4}$$

These procedures will yield three of the four parameters necessary to start fitting to the equation for the Black—Leff model for all slopes of dose-response curve. This equation is:

$$\text{Response} = \frac{[A]^n \tau^n E_m}{[A]^n \tau^n + ([A] + K_A)^n} \tag{3.5}$$

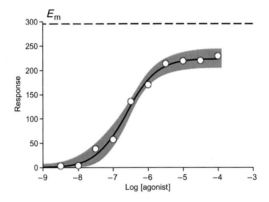

Least squares fitting by computer then yields a better estimate of K_A and a value for efficacy (τ), thereby completing the determination of all parameters needed to predict efficacy in other tissues.

---

n, the slope factor of the dose-response curve. If a series of agonists all yield the same observed maximal response in a given preparation, this generally supports the postulate that the common observed maximal response is a reasonable estimate of E_m (it would be likely that all of the agonists are full agonists yielding the maximal response of the system).

The slope of the dose-response curve can be obtained by independent fitting of the adsorption isotherm with no required added data (see Box 3.3). The second step is to obtain an estimate of K_A; if the ligands are partial agonists, then the EC_{50} (obtained from step 1) can be used as a first estimate of K_A to be subsequently used for the computer fitting of data to the Black–Leff equation (for variable n; see Box 3.3). For a full agonist, the K_A must be estimated to some value greater than EC_{50}. The third is to fit the data to the model equation (see Fig. 3.5).

For high-efficacy full agonists (high τ values), the maximal response will reflect the point at which the agonist saturates the stimulus-response capability of the cell and not the 100% receptor occupancy point. In fact, there are numerous cell systems where powerful, high-efficacy agonists produce a100% maximal tissue response by occupying only a small fraction of the available receptors. Once the maximal tissue

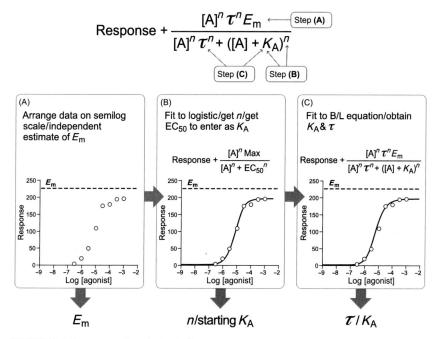

FIGURE 3.5 Fitting the Black–Leff operational model to data. Step (A) arranges the data on a semilogarithmic scale for response (vs dose of agonist); a maximal response of the system must be identified or assumed. Step (B) fits the data to a simple logistic function to yield the slope of the curve (n) and a measure of the location parameter along the concentration axis (EC_{50}). Step (C) then refits the data to the Black–Leff equation (shown at the top of the figure) using the predetermined values of E_m, n, and estimating the K_A as the EC_{50} (in cases where the agonist is a partial agonist). In cases where the agonist is a full agonist, a value higher than the EC_{50} is used. This procedure yields an estimate of the efficacy (τ).

response is attained, occupancy of the remaining receptors by the agonist only serves to make the agonist more potent (i.e., the concentration-response curve shifts to the left along the concentration axis). For high-efficacy agonists where the maximal cellular response can be obtained with a low level of receptor occupancy, the receptors occupied beyond the point where the maximum is attained are referred to as being "spare" (also referred to as "receptor reserve" or "spare receptor capacity"). The maximal response of most tissues to powerful natural agonists (neurotransmitters, hormones) is produced by partial activation of the total receptor population on the cell surface; the remaining receptors appear to be "spare" and in fact participate in making the tissue more or less sensitive to the agonist. For example, the ileum of guinea pigs produces a maximal force of isometric contraction to the natural agonist histamine by activation of only 3% of the available receptors [2]. Therefore, in practical terms, 97% of the receptor population can be removed or inactivated with no decrease in the maximal response to histamine (albeit there is a loss in the sensitivity to histamine). The term "receptor reserve" has been historically associated with the tissue (it involves the number of receptors in a given tissue and the efficiency with which they are coupled to the stimulus-response machinery of the cell). However, the intrinsic efficacy of the agonist is intimately involved in the magnitude of receptor reserve. Thus, the magnitude of the receptor reserve for two different agonists will be different; the agonist with the higher efficacy will have a greater receptor reserve, that is, one agonist's spare receptor is a weaker agonist's essential one.

It should be noted that there is an infinite combination of efficacies and affinities that can fit a given model to a dose-response curve for a full agonist, therefore, no unique estimate of τ and/or K_A can be obtained. However, the ratio τ/K_A is a unique parameter for a full agonist and for this reason, $\mathrm{Log}(\tau/K_A)$ values are valuable parameters to gage the strength of an agonist to produce a response—see Box 3.4.

The major application of the Black–Leff operational model is the prediction of agonism in tissues. Specifically, there are many circumstances where the *ratio* of efficacy of two agonists (as ratios of τ values) is a *tissue-independent* measure of relative efficacy, which can be measured in one test tissue and applied to all tissues. This is an important aspect of experimental pharmacology, as drugs are almost always tested and developed in one type of system for use in another (i.e., the therapeutic one). Reliance on tissue-dependent measures of drug activity (i.e., pEC_{50}, maximal response) is capricious and difficult to apply to the therapeutic environment without a tool, such as the operational model to negate the effects of tissue type.

In general, once the ratio of τ and K_A values is defined for two agonists in one system, and assuming that the mechanism of response

BOX 3.4

Log(τ/KA) as an index for agonism.

Agonist activity involves the maximal response that any given agonist can impart to a tissue and also its potency (location parameter along the concentration axis of the dose-response curve). These are complex functions of agonist affinity (K_A) and efficacy (τ) in terms of the operational model and maxima and potency can vary independently depending on the sensitivity of the system. A single parameter that captures the power of an agonist to produce response in any tissue is Log(τ/K_A). Ratios of this parameter are independent on the receptor expression level in any tissue and capture both the efficacy and affinity of the agonist. As shown in the curves for carbachol (filled circles) and oxotremorine (open circles) the ΔLog(τ/K_A) value of 0.42 remains constant in a sensitive tissue (solid lines) or in the same tissue where the receptors have been reduced by chemical alkylation (broken lines)-data redrawn from Ref. [3]. This value can be obtained by fitting the Black–Leff operational model to dose-response curves but it also, under some circumstances, can be obtained from a single ratio Log (max./EC$_{50}$).

$$\text{Maximum} = \frac{\tau^n E_{max}}{(\tau^n + 1)} \qquad (3.6)$$

$$\text{EC}_{50} = \frac{K_A}{((2+\tau^n)^{1/n} - 1)} \qquad (3.7)$$

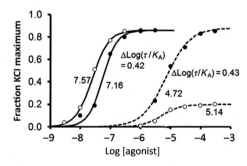

As described by Black et al. [4], the maxima and EC$_{50}$ of agonist dose-response curves are given by expressions of τ and K_A. It can be seen from the equations shown above that if the slope of the agonist dose-response curve is not significantly different from unity, then ΔLog(max./EC$_{50}$) = ΔLog(τ/K_A).

production for both agonists is the same; these ratios can define the relative responses to those agonists in any tissue. There are a few key pieces of data required for this process. This will be illustrated with two hypothetical agonists, Agonist A (a reference standard) and Agonist B (a new test agonist). The first requirement is that the test system must be suitable to yield dose-response curves to both agonists (see Fig. 3.6, Panel 1); the Black−Leff operational model is fit to the data to yield estimates

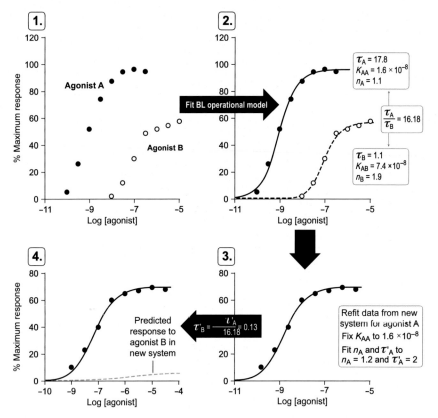

FIGURE 3.6 Measuring the relative efficacy of two agonists. Panel 1 shows dose-response curves for agonists A and B. The Black−Leff operational model is fitted to these data points (see Fig. 3.5) to yield estimates of τ and K_A for each agonist. The ratio of the τ values should be a molecular system-independent parameter unique to the agonists. Panel 3 shows data from another system for one of the agonists. This is fit to the Black−Leff model to yield a τ value for this system. It will be assumed that the τ for the second agonist will adhere to the ratio of τ values found in the first system. This predicts that the τ for the second agonist in this system will be 0.13. The predicted response to agonist B is obtained by back-calculating response according to the Black−Leff model with the designated K_A and τ values.

of K_A and τ for each agonist (Fig. 3.6, Panel 2). From this procedure, a ratio for τ_A/τ_B is obtained; this is a molecular property that is unique to both of these agonists and links agonism produced by each in any system. The next requirement is that a dose-response curve be obtained in the system for which the prediction will be made; the assumption is that the curve for the reference agonist (Agonist A) is observed in this system (Fig. 3.6, Panel 3). The Black—Leff model is fit to the data for the reference agonist in this system. It is assumed that the affinity of the agonist will be the same in the test system and this new system. With this procedure, a new τ'_A value is obtained. Then, using the affinity for the test agonist (Agonist B) obtained from the test system and a predicted efficacy τ'_B equal to $\tau_B \times$ the ratio of efficacies for the two agonists calculated in the test system (τ_A/τ_B), a predicted new efficacy for Agonist B is used in the Black—Leff equation to predict the responses to agonist B in the new system (Fig. 3.6, Panel 4). In the particular example shown, it is seen that little response to the test agonist would be predicted from the calculated ratio of efficacies (τ_A/τ_B) estimated in the test system.

This is a powerful tool to predict agonism that has value in predicting in vivo activity from in vitro data. Assuming that the pharmacokinetics of the agonists are adequate to yield exposure of the target to the agonists in vivo (see chapters: Pharmacokinetics I: Permeation and Metabolism, and Pharmacokinetics II: Distribution and Multiple Dosing), predictions using the Black—Leff operational model can detect test agonists that would not warrant testing in high-resource in vivo assays. For example, Fig. 3.7 shows data for a reference agonist (Agonist A) and a test Agonist B ($\tau_A/\tau_B = 5/0.3 = 16.7$). Testing of the reference Agonist A in the in vivo system showed that a 6.25-fold loss of sensitivity occurs from testing in the in vitro test system compared to the in vivo system. Assuming comparable pharmacokinetics (an important assumption), the Black—Leff operational model predicts that considerably less agonism will be observed in the in vivo system with Agonist B.

This result is intuitively obvious from the profiles of these agonists since it is clear that Agonist B is less efficacious and potent than Agonist A in the test system. Specifically, it is clear that a 6.25-fold loss of sensitivity in the systems would impact Agonist B more than Agonist A in terms of observed agonism. However, the power of this method extends beyond such obvious predictions. As seen in Fig. 3.2, the response to an agonist becomes depressed as the concentrations approach the K_A. Therefore, in cases where the affinity of the test agonist is higher than the affinity of the reference agonist, but the efficacy is lower, surprising profiles can result in systems with lowered sensitivity. Fig. 3.8 shows a system whereby the test agonist is actually

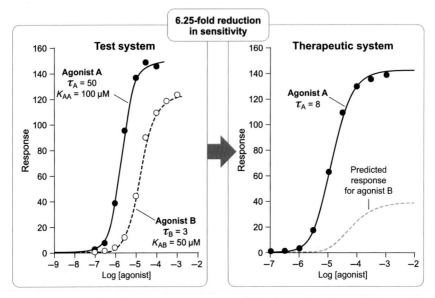

FIGURE 3.7 Prediction of relative responses to agonists in a therapeutic system 6.25-fold less sensitive than the test system. The relative τ values for agonists A and B were found to be $\tau_A/\tau_B = 16.7$ (left panel). The curve to agonist A furnishes the τ for the system in the right panel, indicating the 6.25 decrease in sensitivity. Thus the τ values for agonist B divided by this ratio predict the τ in that system to predict the curve of agonist B (broken line).

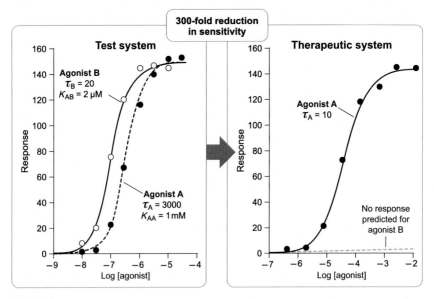

FIGURE 3.8 Prediction of agonism in a system after a 300-fold loss in sensitivity from the test system. Agonist B has a higher affinity but lower efficacy than agonist A. Nevertheless, the higher affinity causes agonist B to be more potent than agonist A in the test system. However, in the 300-fold less sensitive system, the low efficacy of agonist B prevents any agonism being observed, so there is a striking reversal of effects with agonist A being more active than agonist B. This type of reversal could not be predicted without quantifying the relative affinities and efficacies of the two agonists.

more potent than the reference agonist. However, this increased potency is due to a higher affinity, not a higher efficacy ($\tau_A/\tau_B = 150$). Therefore, in an in vivo system where the reference Agonist A is $1/300$ as active, the surprising prediction that the response to Agonist B will disappear is made from application of the Black–Leff operational model (see Fig. 3.8).

Receptor selectivity

Since receptors control so many cellular functions, the drugs that activate them must be selective for the processes for which they are designed, i.e., activate only the target receptors and no others. For instance, M1 subtype-selective muscarinic receptor agonists are proposed to be effective in improving cognition in Alzheimer's disease, but they must not show equal activity at the other four muscarinic subtype receptors (M2, M3, M4, and M5). Receptor selectivity is measured through EC_{50} potency ratios for full agonists but this method cannot be applied to the comparison of full to partial agonists. As shown in Fig. 3.2, as one of the agonists becomes a partial agonist in the system, the ratio of EC_{50} values for the two agonists changes and becomes system-dependent. When this occurs, the potency ratio is an unreliable measure of selectivity. However, a useful and system-independent measure of relative agonist activity is available in the form of $\Delta Log(\tau/K_A)$ values (see Box 3.4). When both agonists are full agonists, the $\Delta Log(\tau/K_A)$ is the ratio of EC_{50} values as with conventional methods. However, when one or both are partial agonists, the $\Delta Log(\tau/K_A)$ value remains a system-independent parameter and can be used to gage selectivity. Fig. 3.9 shows a hypothetical selective muscarinic M1 agonist that is more potent than acetylcholine for M1 receptors and less potent than acetylcholine on M2 through M5 receptors. Differences in sensitivity of the various tissues used to measure the various subtype activities are accounted for by direct comparison to acetylcholine in each tissue (see $\Delta Log(\tau/K_A)$ values in the table for Fig. 3.9). The activity of the agonist on the various receptor subtypes, compared to acetylcholine, is shown as the geometric shape within the pentagram defined by the standard acetylcholine activity in Fig. 3.9. The selectivity is then obtained by comparison of $\Delta Log(\tau/K_A)$ values for each receptor subtype in the form of $\Delta\Delta Log(\tau/K_A)$ values, and this is shown visually as the square defined by the activity of acetylcholine for each subtype in Fig. 3.9.

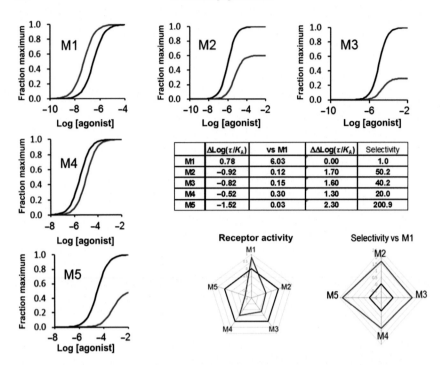

FIGURE 3.9 Calculation and expression of receptor selectivity. Dose-response curves to a hypothetical muscarinic M1 selective agonist for cognition in Alzheimer's disease in five functional receptor systems for the five muscarinic receptor subtypes are shown; red curves are the test agonist and black curves the curves to acetylcholine in the same system. The relative agonist activity of the test agonist, compared to acetylcholine, is calculated as a value of $\Delta Log(\tau/K_A)$ for each subtype (see table column 2). The antilog of these values are shown in the third column (i.e., the test agonist is $6.03\times$ more active than acetylcholine for M1 receptors but $0.12\times$ as active for M2 receptors). A visualization of this pattern of activity is shown by the pentagram labeled "Receptor Activity." The selectivity of the test agonist for the M1 receptor subtype is calculated through $\Delta\Delta Log(\tau/K_A)$ values (column four of table); the relative receptor activity for the M1 subtype is chosen as the reference. Thus, $\Delta\Delta Log(\tau/K_A)$ for M2 is given as $\Delta Log(\tau/K_A)_{M1} - \Delta Log(\tau/K_A)_{M2} = 0.78 - (-0.92) = 1.7 = \Delta\Delta Log(\tau/K_A)$. The antilog of $\Delta\Delta Log(\tau/K_A)$ values are the numerical selectivities of the agonist over the other receptor subtypes compared to the agonists' M1 activity (selectivity for M2 receptors $= 10^{1.7} = 50.2$).

Biased agonist signaling

As discussed in the previous chapter, if the receptor is linked to multiple signaling pathways then the nature of the receptor active state stabilized by the agonist determines, which of these signaling pathways are activated. The corollary to this idea is that, if two agonists stabilize different receptor states, then they may also emphasize different signaling pathways, that is, these will produce biased signaling with respect to each other—see Box 2.7. Such biased signaling may have significant therapeutic ramifications and provide agonists with improved qualities of efficacies. The identification of which signaling pathways may be beneficial and which may not is an active area of therapeutic pharmacology and often involves the application of gene knock-outs—see Box 2.8.

Once a favorable signaling bias is identified, a means to optimize such a profile is required; this involves quantifying the biased efficacy so that medicinal chemistry can be used to change the relative efficacy mediated by the agonist. Bias is quantified in exactly the same way as efficacy is quantified, namely through the Black–Leff operational model. However, the assays are customized so that the various signaling pathways can be measured separately. Under these circumstances, the efficacy and affinity of the agonist for each signaling pathway can be quantified through separate values of τ and K_A (see Fig. 3.10) and then these can be used to determine the relative activity of the agonist on each pathway. Fig. 3.11 shows an example of the quantification of the bias of the chemokine CCL3L1 toward the internalization of the CCR5 receptor over the activation of inositol phosphate production. This procedure requires an internal

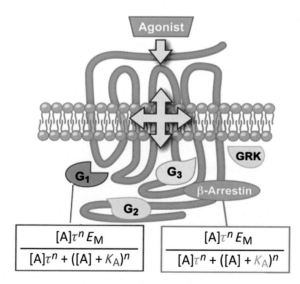

$$\frac{[A]\tau^n E_M}{[A]\tau^n + ([A] + K_A)^n} \qquad \frac{[A]\tau^n E_M}{[A]\tau^n + ([A] + K_A)^n}$$

FIGURE 3.10 The Black–Leff operational models can be used to quantify the effects of agonists on specific signaling pathways. Thus, with the appropriate assay, the τ and K_A values for G protein activation and, separately, for β-arrestin activation can be quantified through measurement of Log(τ/K_A values). *Source: Redrawn from T.P. Kenakin, Pharmacological onomastics: what's in a name? Br. J. Pharmacol. 153 (2008) 432–438 [5].*

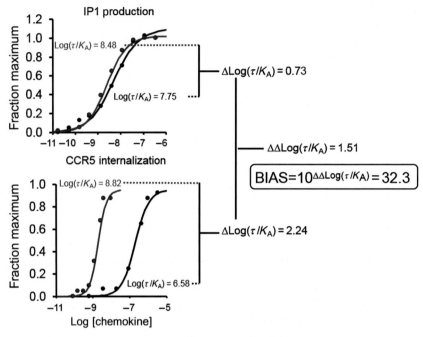

FIGURE 3.11 Dose-response curves for inositol phosphate production (IP1 production) and CCR5 receptor internalization for two chemokines acting on the CCR5 receptor; CCL3L1 in red and CCL3 in black. The power of these agonists to induce the response are calculated through $Log(\tau/K_A)$ values. The relative power of each agonist to produce each response is calculated for each assay as $\Delta log(\tau/K_A)$. Finally, the relative power of CCL3L1 to induce internalization (over IP1 production) as compared to CCL3 is given as $\Delta\Delta Log$ (τ/K_A). It can be seen from this example that CCL3L1 is 32.3 times more powerful in producing receptor internalization (over IP1 production). *Source: Data taken from T.P. Kenakin, C. Watson, V. Muniz-Medina, A. Christopoulos, S. Novick, A Simple Method for Quantifying Functional Selectivity and Agonist Bias ACS Chem. Neurosci. 3 (2012) 193–203.*

reference to be used to cancel the effects of assay sensitivity and other tissue effects, that is, the responses are scaled as $Log(\tau/K_A)$ values by comparison to an internal reference to yield $\Delta Log(\tau/K_A)$ values; in this example, the reference agonist is the chemokine CCL3. These are then further compared across signaling pathways to yield $\Delta\Delta Log(\tau/K_A)$ values and the bias of a ligand toward a given pathway is $10\Delta\Delta Log$ (τ/KA). As shown in Fig. 3.11, the chemokine CCL3L1 produces 32.threefold more CCR5 internalization (as compared to CCL3) than IP1 production. In this case biased signaling may be linked to a favorable profile in that chemokine-induced internalization of CCR5 receptors can have therapeutic ramifications for AIDs therapy—see Box 3.5.

BOX 3.5

Biased efficacy delays progression to AIDS

The chemokine receptor CCR5 is the anchoring protein for HIV-1 allowing it to infect cells. One mechanism to delay HIV-1 infection is through the internalization of CCR5 into the cell, thereby removing it from the cell surface [6]. As shown in Fig. 3.11, the chemokine CCL3L1 is over 30-fold biased toward internalization of CCR5 over other chemokines, such as CCL3, and it has been shown that CCL3L produces pronounced CCR5 internalization of the receptor. After HIV-1 infection, a robust CCL3L1 presence in the body has been shown to greatly increase survival and delay the onset of AIDs [7]. As shown below, after HIV-1 infection, patients with multiple copies of the gene coding for CCL3L1 have a much greater rate of survival over the patients who have a low gene copy number. CCR5 internalization through exogenous chemokines, such as PSC-RANTES has been proposed as a viable preventative against HIV-1 infection [8].

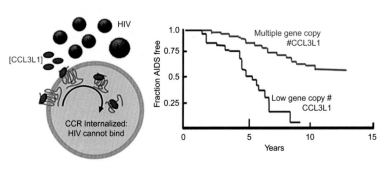

As discussed above, biased signaling can be a therapeutically advantageous strategy, but it can also confound traditional measures of agonist activity. For example, if two agonists differentially activate multiple signaling pathways in cells, then the emphasis the cell puts on those pathways to generate cellular metabolism responses can control agonist selectivity. Under these circumstances, the cell type can modify bias, which can lead to cell type heterogeneity in agonist potency ratios. For example, Box 3.6 shows the modification of the relative selectivity of biased agonists for the human calcitonin receptor when the receptor is recombinantly expressed in two different cell lines. It can be seen from

---

BOX 3.6

When cells take control

Agonist potency ratios can be constant, if the receptor stimulus is monotonic in nature, that is, a single pathway is involved. However, many receptors are pleiotropically linked to multiple signaling pathways, and this can lead to variation in potency ratios with cell types for biased agonists. For example, the human calcitonin receptor is pleiotropically linked to Gs, Gi, and Gq proteins, and the agonists are biased with respect to the G proteins they emphasize in signaling. This can lead to cell type dependence with respect to agonist potency ratios. As shown above, human calcitonin receptors transfected into two different host cells lines yield very different relative potencies for porcine (filled circles), human (open circles), calcitonin, and rat CGRP (open triangles).

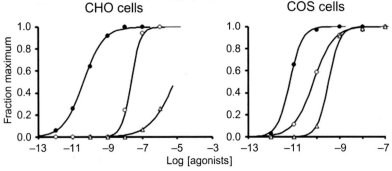

Data redrawn from L. Christmanson, P. Westermark, C. Betsholtz, Islet amyloid polypeptide stimulates cyclic AMP accumulation via the porcine calcitonin receptor. Biochem. Biophys. Res. Commun. 205 (1994) 1226–1235 [9].

---

this example that the relative potencies of the agonists are drastically different when the receptor is present in COS versus CHO cells.

In addition, if an agonist activates multiple signaling pathways and is biased with respect to that activation, then differences in the relative activity may be found depending on which signaling pathway is chosen for comparison. For example, Box 3.7 shows two estimates of β_2- versus β_1-adrenoceptors selectivity for the bronchodilator agonist clenbuterol. While comparisons of responses for cyclic AMP show a 500-fold selectivity for β_2- over β_1-adrenoceptors, this drastically reduces to 5.8, if β-arrestin is chosen as the response.

BOX 3.7

Choice of response affects selectivity

The selectivity of an agonist is given by a comparison of dose-response curves to the agonist in two systems; as shown in Fig. 3.9, $\Delta Log(\tau/K_A)$ values can be used for this purpose. However, if the agonist(s) are biased with respect to the signaling pathways they activate in the cell, then the choice of response can affect the final determination of selectivity. For example, clenbuterol is a bronchodilator useful in the treatment of asthma through a selective bronchiole smooth muscle relaxation via β_2-adrenoceptors over a debilitating cardiovascular response mediated by β_1-adrenoceptors. If cyclic AMP (A) (Gαs protein) is used as the index of response, clenbuterol is a robust 500-fold selective for β_2- over β_1-effects. However, if β-arrestin (B) is used as the response, then the selectivity diminishes to 5.eightfold [10]. This is because clenbuterol is biased toward G protein signaling for β_2-adrenceptors and biased toward β-arrestin for β_1-adrenoceptor signaling.

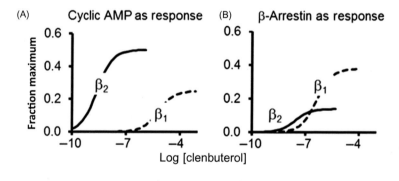

Descriptive pharmacology: III

Continuing the theme of a progressive characterization of the drug effect of molecules through pharmacologic procedures, Fig. 3.12 shows the next step in quantifying observed full or partial agonism. Specifically, the estimation of the affinity and relative affinity of a test agonist theoretically could lead to the ability to predict agonism to that test agonist in any system. At this time, it should be stressed that there are two overriding assumptions in this procedure. The first is that the concentrations used on the abscissa axis of the dose-response curves

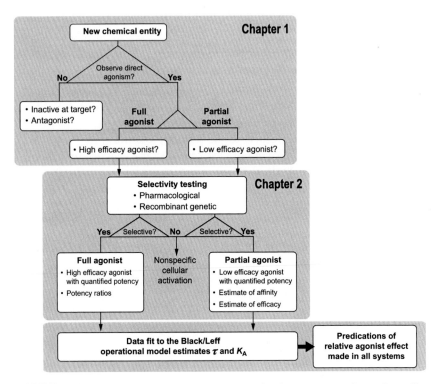

FIGURE 3.12 Continuation of logical progression for determination of new drug effect (from Fig. 2.11). Agonist dose-response curves are fit to the Black–Leff operational model to yield estimates of affinity (K_A) and efficacy (τ). These can be used to predict agonism in other systems.

(whether in vitro or in vivo) accurately reflect the concentration present at the target interface. The second is that the mechanism of action of the test and reference agonists in producing a response is identical. If either of these assumptions is not true, then dissimulations between predicted and observed agonism will occur.

Summary

The sensitivity of cells to directly activating molecules (agonists) depends upon the intrinsic properties of the molecule (affinity and intrinsic efficacy) and the cell system (receptor number and efficiency of receptor coupling). The operational model allows ascription of molecular properties (affinity in the form of K_A and efficacy in the form of τ);

this model allows prediction of agonist effect in different tissues from ratios of K_A and τ obtained for agonists. For agonists that activate receptors that are pleiotropically linked to multiple signaling pathways, there is a distinct possibility that different agonists will emphasize different pathways with respect to each other (i.e., show biased signaling). This can lead to better-defined efficacy for therapeutic applications but also ambiguity in estimates of selectivity.

Questions

3.1. Why did Black and Leff use the Michaelis–Menten equation as the basis for signal transduction in the operational model?

3.2. Describe how the operational model parameter τ characterizes both the intrinsic efficacy of the agonist and the sensitivity of the system.

3.3. A given agonist A was found to have a receptor reserve of 90% in a given tissue system. What does this mean? Another agonist B had a reserve in the same tissue of only 40%; what properties of agonists A and B could lead to this result?

3.4. Agonist potency ratios can be used for the comparison of only full agonists to assess relative receptor selectivity; what technique can be used to compare molecules when one is a full and the other a partial agonist?

3.5. A potency ratio between two agonists was once considered a general descriptor of the overall general relative activity of those two agonists in all systems; why is this now not the case?

References

[1] J.W. Black, P. Leff, Operational models of pharmacological agonist, Proc. R. Soc. Lond. [Biol]. 220 (1983) 141.

[2] M. Nickerson, Receptor occupancy and tissue response, Nature. 178 (1956) 697–698.

[3] T. Kenakin, C. Watson, V. Muniz-Medina, A. Christopoulos, S. Novick, A simple method for quantifying functional selectivity and agonist bias, ACS Chem. Neurosci. 3 (2012) 193–203.

[4] J.W. Black, P. Leff, N.P. Shankley, An operational model of pharmacological agonism: the effect of E/[A] curve shape on agonist dissociation constant estimation, Br. J. Pharmacol. 84 (1985) 561–571.

[5] T.P. Kenakin, Pharmacological onomastics: what's in a name? Br. J. Pharmacol. 153 (2008) 432–438.

[6] M. Mack, B. Luckow, P.J. Nelson, J. Cihak, G. Simmons, P.R. Clapham, Aminooxypentane-RANTES induces CCR5 internalization but inhibits recycling: a novel inhibitory mechanism of HIV infectivity, J. Exp. Med. 187 (1998) 1215–1224.

[7] E. Gonzalez, H. Kulkarni, H. Bolivar, A. Mangano, R. Sanchez, G. Catano, The influence of CCL3L1 gene-containing segmental duplications on HIV-1/AIDS susceptibility, Science 307 (2005) 1434–1440.

[8] O. Hartley, H. Gaertner, J. Wilken, D. Thompson, R. Fish, A. Ramos, Medicinal chemistry applied to a synthetic protein: development of highly potent HIV entry inhibitors, Proc. Natl. Acad. Sci. USA. 101 (2004) 16460–16465.

[9] L. Christmanson, P. Westermark, C. Betsholtz, Islet amyloid polypeptide stimulates
cyclic AMP accumulation via the porcine calcitonin receptor, Biochem. Biophys. Res.
Commun. 205 (1994) 1226–1235.

[10] I. Casella, C. Ambrosio, M.C. Gro, P. Molinari, T. Costa, Divergent agonist selectivity
in activating β1- and β2-adrenoceptors for G-protein and arrestin coupling, Biochem.
J. 438 (2011) 191–202.

Drug antagonism: orthosteric drug effects

By the end of this chapter, readers should be able to quantify the effects of antagonists to yield empirical measures of antagonist potency. They will also be able to relate patterns of antagonism produced by orthosteric antagonists (those producing steric hindrance of agonists) to mechanisms of

Pharmacology in Drug Discovery and Development
DOI: https://doi.org/10.1016/B978-0-443-14124-9.00021-5

antagonist action. Readers will then be able to use these mechanisms to apply the appropriate mathematical analysis to yield estimates of true system-independent antagonist potency that transcend cell type and measuring system.

Bimolecular systems

The previous chapters discussed the binding of a molecule to a protein target to cause a change in cellular function (agonism); in these cases, the system consists of a single molecule interacting with a target in the cell. There are a large number of pharmacologically relevant interactions that involve *two molecules*; one causing a change of cellular function and the other interfering with that action. For example, Fig. 4.1 shows a synaptic cleft where a neurotransmitter molecule A is released from the neuron to act on the postsynaptic membrane containing receptors for that neurotransmitter; molecule B can be added to the system to modify the interaction of A with the target. There are two pharmacologically relevant outcomes, namely that the response to A can be increased or diminished (see Fig. 4.1). If the

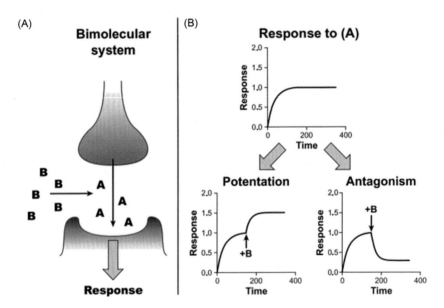

FIGURE 4.1   Schematic diagram of a physiological system consisting of a neuron releasing an agonist A and the addition of an external compound B. If B has an affinity for the target, the response to A can be increased (potentiated) or blocked. Potentiation would be an allosteric mechanism (discussed in the chapter: Allosteric Drug Effects); antagonism is the subject of this present chapter.

response is increased this could be due to an interference in the disposition of A in the synaptic cleft (inhibition of transport) or allosteric alteration of the target to increase responsiveness. This latter topic will be discussed in Chapter 5, Allosteric Drug Effects. This present chapter discusses the inhibition of the response to A. Implicit in this discussion is the understanding that the effects seen are specific for the drug target being considered, that is, the molecule does not produce nonspecific toxic or other effects on the cell system to modify the cell sensitivity to the agonist.

New terminology

The following new terms will be introduced in this chapter:

- *Allosteric*: Describing an interaction mediated by the binding of a molecule to a protein at a distinct site to affect the interaction of that protein with another molecule binding at a different site.
- *Antagonism*: The process of inhibition of an agonist-driven cellular response by another molecule.
- *Competitive antagonism*: A specific model of receptor antagonism whereby two molecules compete for a single binding site on the receptor, and the kinetics of binding of both the agonist and antagonist are rapid enough to allow mass action to control the relative proportions of receptor bound to agonist and antagonist.
- *Hemi-equilibrium*: A condition where there is an insufficient amount of time for complete re-equilibration of agonist and antagonist for a population of receptors according to mass action. This results in a selectively noncompetitive effect at high-agonist receptor occupancies, causing a partial depression of the maximal response to the agonist.
- *Insurmountable*: Describing a pattern of agonist dose-response curves whereby the maximal response to the agonist is depressed.
- *Noncompetitive*: Describing antagonism resulting from a system whereby the antagonist does not dissociate from the receptor rapidly enough to allow competition with the agonist.
- *Orthosteric*: A steric interaction whereby molecules compete for binding at the same site on a protein.
- *pA2*: Minus logarithm of the molar concentration of an antagonist that produces a twofold shift of the agonist dose-response curve.
- *pIC50*: Minus logarithm of the molar concentration of antagonist that produces a 50% inhibition of a defined agonist effect.
- *pKB*: Minus logarithm of the equilibrium dissociation constant of the antagonist-receptor complex.
- *Schild analysis*: The application of the Schild equation to a set of dextral displacements produced by a surmountable antagonist; if the

Schild plot is linear with a slope of unity the antagonism fulfills criteria for simple competitive antagonism.
- *Surmountable*: Describing antagonism whereby the agonist dose-response curve is shifted to the right with increasing addition of antagonist, but where the maximal response is not altered.

What is drug antagonism?

This chapter will deal with molecules that bind to the target to interfere with agonists producing response; this is the process of *antagonism*. There are many therapeutically relevant conditions where an antagonist would be useful, as in cases of inappropriate, excessive or persistent agonism (i.e., inflammation, gastric ulcer) or diseases where remodeling of systems leads to normal agonism becoming harmful (cardiovascular disease). Conceptually, antagonism could be envisioned as the binding of the antagonist to a target to hinder the binding or function (or both) of an agonist. The three factors that control the extent of antagonism are:

- the quantity of antagonist bound (*potency*);
- the location of the binding relative to the binding of the natural agonist (*mechanism*);
- the persistence of antagonist binding (*antagonist kinetics*).

It is worth considering each of these important factors when discussing therapeutically relevant antagonism.

Antagonist potency

Potency refers to the amount of antagonism in a system for a given concentration of antagonists. The relevant parameter for this is the affinity of the antagonist for the protein target (as defined by Langmuir adsorption binding isotherm; see Eq. 2.1). Unlike agonism, estimates of antagonist potency should not be cell-type dependent, and thus these are chemical terms that can be measured in a test system and the result applied to all systems, including the therapeutic one. The affinity of an antagonist quantified as the equilibrium dissociation constant of the antagonist-protein complex, can be measured in an appropriate in vitro system either directly (if a means to trace the protein-bound antagonist species can be quantified, such as in radiolabeled binding assays) or indirectly through interference of agonist activity in a functional assay. This latter approach is preferable as it is what the antagonist will do in vivo that is important. In addition, there are numerous cases where physical binding of molecules and their effect on physiological responses can differ. The desired parameter in this case is referred to as the pK_B, namely the negative logarithm of the equilibrium dissociation constant of the antagonist-protein complex. To measure antagonist potency in an in vitro functional assay, comparisons are made between the dose-response curve of the agonist produced in the absence of antagonist, and then again in the presence of antagonist (usually for a range of antagonist concentrations). The resulting pattern of curves is then utilized in an appropriate model defined by the proposed mechanism of action of the antagonist. It should be noted that the antagonism must be shown to be specific for the biological target in question (see Fig. 4.2); it will be assumed that the observed antagonist effects are specific for the target.

There are two effects an antagonist can have on the dose-response curve to an agonist: depression of maximal response and dextral displacement of the curve (or both; see Fig. 4.3). Both of these effects reflect a diminution of the sensitivity of the system to the agonist in the presence of the antagonist, thus higher concentrations of agonist are required to produce a response in the presence of the antagonist. Different mechanisms of antagonism can produce varying amounts of shift and depression of maxima of the dose-response curves. This can also vary with the type of agonist used to produce response and the sensitivity of the functional system used to measure the effect. For this reason, the pattern(s) of antagonism seen in vitro cannot reliably be used to identify the mechanism of action; in fact, the reverse is true. Once a mechanism of action is identified, the appropriate model is applied to the data to characterize antagonist potency (pK_B values).

Mechanism(s) of receptor antagonism

There are two molecular mechanisms operable for the antagonism of responses to endogenous hormones, neurotransmitters, or autacoids:

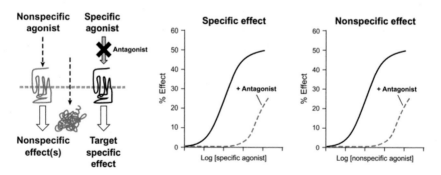

FIGURE 4.2   Determining specificity of antagonism. Nonspecific effects are suggested if the test antagonist blocks the effect of a nonspecific stimulant of the cell (i.e., acting through another receptor or otherwise elevating response biochemically).

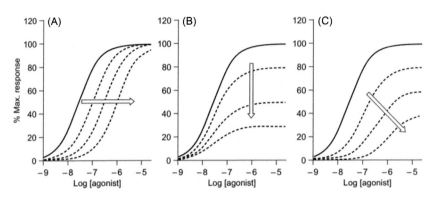

FIGURE 4.3 Orthosteric target antagonism can take the form of a shift to the right of the agonist dose-response curve (A), a depression of the maximal response to the agonist (B) or a mixture of the two effects.

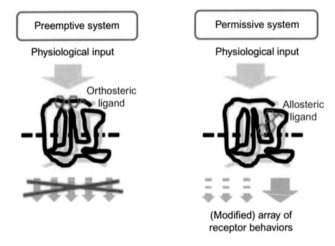

FIGURE 4.4 Two mechanisms of interaction of ligands with receptors. A preemptive system is created by the orthosteric binding of an antagonist to the agonist binding site. This precludes agonist binding and therefore blocks all receptor actions mediated by agonist binding. In contrast, allosteric interaction, where the antagonist binds to a site separate from the agonist binding site, is a permissive system in that it is still possible for the agonist to bind and produce action at the receptor. Allosteric mechanisms are discussed fully in Chapter 5, Allosteric Drug Effects.

orthosteric or allosteric binding. Orthosteric antagonism (see Fig. 4.4) is where the antagonist binds to the same site as the endogenous agonist and precludes agonist binding to the protein. This mechanism is preemptive, in that occupancy of the site by the antagonist prevents all actions of the agonist. The second mechanism (allosteric; see Fig. 4.4) is where the antagonist and agonist bind to separate binding sites on the protein, and the interaction between them occurs through a change in conformation of the protein. This type of mechanism is permissive in that some (or even all) actions of the agonist can still be produced when the antagonist is bound. However, some characteristics of the agonist response are modified, such as potency and/or efficacy. Orthosteric antagonism is the most simple and will be discussed in this present chapter; allosteric mechanisms will be discussed in Chapter 5, Allosteric Drug Effects.

Orthosteric (competitive and noncompetitive) antagonism

As discussed in Chapter 2, Drug Affinity and Efficacy, the binding of a molecule to a protein is a stochastic process, meaning that at any one instant there will be a population of protein binding sites where the antagonist is tightly bound to the protein and another where it has momentarily diffused away from the binding site, leaving it open for binding to other molecules. Thus the probability of another molecule (e.g., an agonist) binding to the same site in the presence of the antagonist will be determined by the amount of time the antagonist is momentarily not bound to the protein (determined in turn by the affinity and concentration of the antagonist) and the concentration and affinity of the agonist. Thus it can be seen that in such a system of competition, a very high concentration of agonists theoretically could bind to all of the sites and the maximal response to the agonist would be attained even in the presence of the antagonist. This idea is captured in a simple equation presented by John Gaddum (see Box 4.1), known as the Gaddum equation for competitive kinetics. Specifically, this equation relates the fractional receptor occupancy by a molecule A (ρ_A) to the concentration A (denoted C_A, referring to the concentration normalized as a fraction of the equilibrium dissociation constant of the A−receptor complex), and the normalized concentration of another drug B competing for the same site on the receptor (see Derivations and Proofs, Appendix A.5) [1]:

$$\rho_A = \frac{C_A}{1 + C_A + C_B} \tag{4.1}$$

Therefore in a completely competitive situation, where the binding of both the antagonist and agonist are rapid, the dose-response curve to the agonist will be shifted to the right in the presence of the competitive antagonist and very high concentrations of the agonist will produce the original maximal response (obtained in the absence of antagonist) even in the presence of the antagonist. The shift to the right of the agonist curve

BOX 4.1

The Gaddum equation

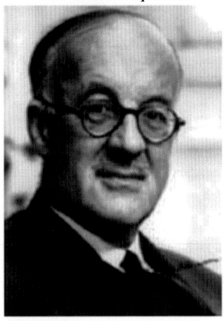

Sir John Gaddum (1900−65)

John Henry Gaddum (1900−65) was a British pharmacologist who did a great deal to propagate quantitative pharmacology. Educated at Cambridge, Gaddum became a medical student at University College London, where he applied for and won a post at the Wellcome Research Laboratories. There, he wrote his first paper on quantitative drug antagonism. After working for the influential pharmacologist Sir Henry Hallet Dale and later chairing the Department of Pharmacology at Cairo University, Gaddum returned to University College London to head the Department of Pharmacology. At this time, he presented a short communication to the Physiological Society in 1937 entitled "The quantitative effects of antagonistic drugs" [1], which contained the famous "Gaddum equation":

$$\rho_A = \frac{C_A}{1 + C_A + C_B}$$

where ρ_A is the fractional receptor occupancy by drug A in the presence of another drug B that competes for the binding of A at the receptor. The terms C_A and C_B refer to the normalized (divided by the equilibrium dissociation constants of the drug-receptor complexes) concentrations of a drugs A and B, respectively. It can be seen that if $C_A \gg C_B$, then the total occupancy of the receptor will revert to a situation identical to that where only molecule A is present, that is, it will compete with B to the extent that B no longer occupies the receptor.

reflects the lower probability of the agonist producing a response in the presence of the obstructing antagonist; this probability is increased with increased agonist concentration, therefore, the curve reappears at higher concentrations of agonist. The magnitude of the shift in the dose-response curve is proportional to the degree of antagonism and relates to the concentration of the antagonist present and its affinity. Schild and colleagues (see Box 4.2) used this fact to devise a method to measure the affinity of competitive antagonists, in a procedure since given the name "Schild analysis" for the construction of a "Schild plot" [2].

The procedure for doing this is shown in Fig. 4.5. The first step is to define the sensitivity of the system to the agonist (obtain a control dose-response curve). Then, the preparation is preequilibrated with a defined concentration of the antagonist; this ensures that the receptors and antagonist come to a binding equilibrium according to the Langmuir isotherm. Then, the sensitivity of the tissue is measured again in the presence of the preequilibrated antagonist, and the shift in the curve is used to estimate the antagonist potency.

For Schild analysis, this is done repeatedly with a range of antagonist concentrations, and then an array of shifts of the control curve produced by a matching array of antagonist concentrations is used to estimate the affinity of the antagonist. The shifts are quantified as ratios of the EC_{50} of the agonist in the presence and absence of the antagonist; these are referred to as dose ratios ($Dr = EC_{50[antagonist]}/EC_{50[control]}$). It can be shown that the $Log(Dr - 1)$ values for a range of concentrations of antagonist [B] have a linear relationship according to the "Schild equation" (see Box 4.2):

$$Log(DR - 1) = Log[B] - pK_B \qquad (4.2)$$

where pK_B is the negative logarithm of the equilibrium dissociation constant of the antagonist-receptor complex; this parameter is a system-independent measure of the potency of a competitive antagonist. An example of this type of analysis is given in Fig. 4.6. It should be noted that for there to be confidence in the veracity of pK_B as a true measure of antagonist potency, the Schild plot (line according to Eq. 4.2) should be linear and have a slope of unity.

At this point, it is worth discussing that another practical method of quantifying the potency of competitive, and indeed nearly any other kind of, antagonist. As discussed in Chapter 1, Pharmacology: The Chemical Control of Physiology, the Langmuir adsorption isotherm shows that the concentration of antagonism equal to K_B (K_{eq} in the binding isotherm) occupies 50% of the receptor population. It can be shown that occupancy of 50% of the receptor population by the antagonist will necessitate a doubling of the concentration of the agonist to produce the same level of response obtained in the absence of antagonist. This means that in the

BOX 4.2

H. O. Schild and the "Schild Equation"

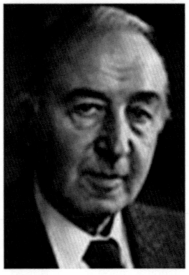

Heinz Schild (1906–84)

Heinz Schild took Gaddum's equation for competitive binding and ingeniously extended it to provide a tool for the measurement of the potency of a competitive antagonist-blocking agonist response. The key to this is the application of the null assumption, which state that equal responses to an agonist emanate from equal levels of receptor occupancy by that agonist. This allows the response to a concentration of an agonist A (C_A), measured in the absence of an antagonist B, to be represented by ρ_A. This is the receptor occupancy by A, as given by the Gaddum equation, to be represented (since equal responses are being compared) by the response of the same agonist obtained in the presence of the antagonist:

$$\rho_A = \frac{C_A}{1 + C_A} = \frac{C_A'}{1 + C_A' + C_B}$$

The concentration of agonist in this latter situation (denoted C_A') will be greater in the presence of the antagonist since it must overcome the competition by antagonist. Cross multiplication and dividing the entire expression by C_A results in the Schild equation where C_A'/C_A is denoted by the equiactive dose–ratio Dr:

Schild Equation

$$\frac{C_A'}{C_A} = C_B + 1 = \frac{[B]}{K_B} + 1 = DR$$

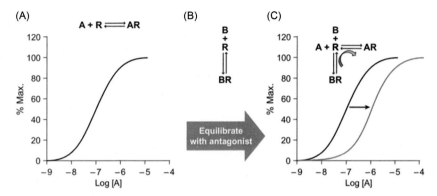

FIGURE 4.5 The process of assessing receptor antagonism. (A) The sensitivity of the system to the agonist is measured through observation of an agonist dose-response curve. (B) After the agonist is removed, the tissue is equilibrated with a given concentration of antagonist. (C) In the presence of the antagonist, the sensitivity to the agonist is again measured with an agonist dose-response curve.

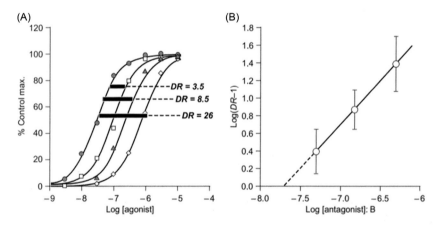

FIGURE 4.6 Schild analysis. (A) Dose-response curves to the agonist are obtained in the absence and presence of various concentrations of the antagonist. The resulting shifts to the right of the agonist dose-response curves are converted to dose ratios (Dr) and utilized in the Schild equation (Eq. (4.2)) to construct a Schild regression (shown in panel (B)). Thus a regression of $\text{Log}(Dr - 1)$ values for a given array of antagonist concentrations provides a linear regression (ideally with a slope of unity) the intercept of which is $-\text{p}K_B$.

presence of this concentration of antagonist, the dose ratio for the agonist will be 2. This can be seen from the Schild equation, where at $Dr = 2$, Log $[B] = -\text{p}K_B$. The concentration that produces a twofold shift to the right of the agonist dose-response curve is thus a characteristic measure of potency (being an estimate of the K_B or the concentration producing 50% receptor occupancy); it is referred to as the $\text{p}A_2$, specifically the negative logarithm of the molar concentration of antagonist that produces a twofold shift to the right of the agonist dose-response curve. The pA_2 can readily be calculated by measuring the shift to the right produced by a single concentration of antagonist (as long as it is ≥ 2), and calculating the pA_2 through the relationship (see Box 4.3):

$$pA_2 = \text{Log}(DR - 1) - \text{Log}[B] \tag{4.3}$$

BOX 4.3

Estimation of competitive antagonist potency through the pA_2

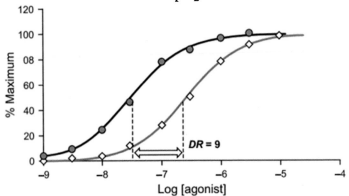

In practical terms, all that is required to estimate the potency of a simple competitive antagonist is the determination of the effect of a single concentration of the antagonist on an agonist dose-response curve. As shown in the figure to the right, a control dose-response curve to an agonist (filled circles) is shifted to the right in the presence of a $1\,\mu M$ concentration of antagonist [B]; see the curve denoted by open circles. The magnitude of the dose ratio (Dr) is given by the ratio of the EC_{50} concentrations of agonist in the presence of antagonist (in this case 270 nM) and absence of antagonist (in this case 30 nM); thus for this example, $Dr = 270/30 = 9$. According to the pA_2 calculation from Eq. (4.3) the pA_2 is:

$$pA_2 = \text{Log}(9 - 1) - \text{Log}(1\mu M) = 0.9 - (-6) = 6.9$$

This is a unique estimate of this antagonist's potency, meaning that a molar concentration of $10^{-6.9} = 126$ nM shifts the dose-response curve by a factor of 2 and binds to 50% of the receptors in any tissue.

In general, it is not prudent to simply obtain a pA_2 estimate and assume that it represents the true affinity as a pK_B; a complete Schild analysis allows observation of the criteria for true competitive inhibition, namely that the regression should be linear and have a slope of unity. If these conditions are not met, then the pA_2 is an empirical measure of antagonist potency, which can still be of value, but may not equal the true pK_B.

Schild analysis was presented as a linear transform at a time when fitting data to models was more difficult than it is in the present day. An alternative to using the linearly transformed Schild analysis approach is to fit the raw data directly to the model for simple competitive antagonism. This is represented by an equation yielding the response to the agonist [A] in the presence of a concentration of antagonist [B] in the following form:

$$\text{Response} = \frac{([A]/EC_{50})^n \text{Max}}{([A]/EC_{50})^n + ([B]/K_B)^n + 1} \tag{4.4}$$

where n is the slope parameter for the agonist dose-response curve, Max is the maximal asymptote of the agonist dose-response curve, EC_{50} is the concentration of agonist producing the half-maximal response, and K_B is the desired parameter, namely the equilibrium dissociation constant for the antagonist-receptor complex. An example of direct fitting of dose-response data to the competitive model is shown in Fig. 4.7.

Three methods of measuring the affinity of a competitive antagonist have been discussed: pA_2 as an empirical measure (Eq. 4.3); pK_B from Schild analysis (Eq. (4.2)); and pK_B through direct fitting to Eq. (4.4). In all of these cases, no useful data can be obtained until the antagonist is present in the receptor compartment at a concentration that occupies $\geq 50\%$ of the receptors (this produces $Dr = 2$). Lower concentrations than this will produce little change in the agonist dose-response curve and thus yield no data for calculation. When testing an antagonist of unknown potency, this poses a problem in terms of which concentration should be first equilibrated with the preparation to yield useful data. For this reason, when unknown antagonists are to be tested, another strategy, namely determining the pIC_{50}, is used. This strategy preactivates the system with an agonist and then adds a range of concentrations of antagonist; then the resulting effect on the elevated basal response is measured. Fig. 4.8 shows how preequilibration of the system with an EC_{50} of agonist yields an inverse sigmoidal curve, which then can be used to estimate the pIC_{50}, namely the negative logarithm of the molar concentration of antagonist that reduces the agonist response by

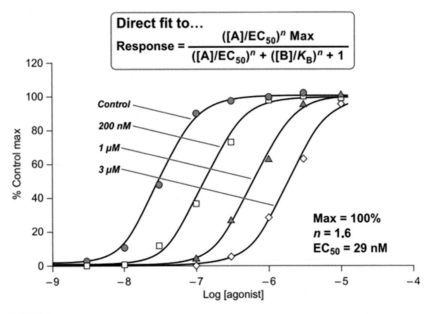

FIGURE 4.7 Direct fitting of data to the simple competitive model of antagonism (Eq. (4.4)) to yield, in this case, a pK_B for the antagonist of 7.25.

50%. It can be seen that considerably fewer data points are required for this estimate. The pIC_{50} for a competitive antagonist then can be used to calculate the pK_B for the antagonist through a correction equation given as (see Derivations and Proofs, Appendix A.6) [3]:

$$pK_B = -\text{Log}\left[\frac{IC_{50}}{((2+([A]/EC_{50})^n)^{1/n}-1}\right] \qquad (4.5)$$

It should be noted that Eq. (4.5) is valid only for those antagonists that produce surmountable antagonism; if the antagonism is insurmountable, then a different relationship will be operative between the pIC_{50} and the pK_B (*vide infra*).

Slow dissociation kinetics and noncompetitive antagonism

For true competitive kinetics to be operative, the antagonist that has been preequilibrated with the receptors must dissociate quickly enough for the agonist present in the receptor compartment to bind according to mass action (Fig. 4.9A). If this does not occur, the antagonist will occupy an inordinately high percentage of the receptors and antagonism will dominate. This percentage of receptors could be high enough to prevent

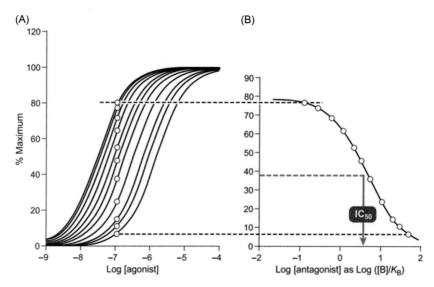

FIGURE 4.8 Effects of a simple competitive antagonist on an agonist dose-response curve (left panel); open circles show the effects of the antagonist on a selected dose of agonist that produces 80% maximal response in the absence of the antagonist. Right panel shows the responses to that same selected dose of agonist as a function of the concentrations of competitive antagonist producing the blockade. It can be seen that an inverse sigmoidal curve results (pIC$_{50}$ curve). The value of the abscissa corresponding to the half-maximal ordinate value of this curve is the IC$_{50}$, namely the molar concentration of antagonist that produces half-maximal inhibition of the defined agonist response.

the agonist from producing a maximal response, thus an insurmountable effect on the agonist dose-response curve will result (Fig. 4.9B). This is sometimes also referred to as "pseudo-irreversible" antagonism because the antagonist is essentially irreversibly bound to the receptor within the time frame relevant for the production of response by the agonist. This often results in a depressed maximal response in the agonist dose-response curve. The degree of maximal response depression depends on the number of receptors needed to induce response in the cell preparation, that is, the magnitude of the receptor reserve (see chapter: Predicting Agonist Effect). If the cell is extremely sensitive to the agonist, such that only a small fraction of the receptor population needs to be activated to produce tissue maximal response, then even an irreversible antagonist may shift the curve to the right with little depression of maximum, that is, if only 7% of the receptors are needed for maximal response, then irreversibly blocking 80% of the receptors will still enable the agonist to produce a maximal response.

On the other hand, if the cell is not very sensitive to the agonist and 100% of the receptors are needed for the production of a maximal

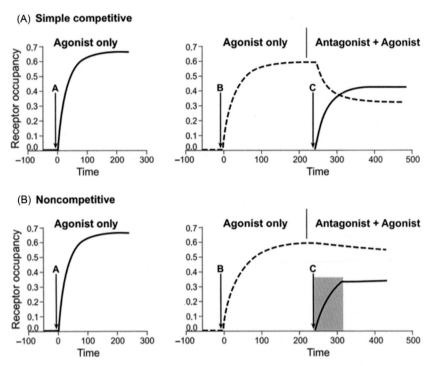

FIGURE 4.9 The kinetics of reequilibration of agonists, antagonists and receptors. (A) For simple competitive antagonist systems, where there is sufficient time for re-equilibration between receptors. The reduction in antagonist receptor occupancy (dotted line) rapidly adjusts as the agonist binds to receptors (solid line). (B) For a slowly dissociating antagonist (broken line), the agonist binding is biphasic, characterized by an initial rapid phase (where the agonist binds to open receptors), and a slow phase whereby the agonist must deal with a slowly dissociating antagonist. The gray rectangle represents the window of opportunity to measure agonist response in the presence of the antagonist; if this is less than the time required for complete re-equilibration of agonist, antagonist, and receptors then the agonist receptor occupancy will be less than would be defined by true competitive interactions.

response, an irreversible antagonist will immediately produce a depression of the maximal response to the agonist. These different scenarios are shown in Fig. 4.10. In cases of true noncompetitive orthosteric blockade where the maximal response to the agonist is depressed by all concentrations of antagonist, the pIC_{50} can be obtained as for competitive antagonists (Fig. 4.8) and the resulting pIC_{50} is essentially equal to the pK_B (see Fig. 4.11). This obviates the use of a correction factor, such as that provided by Eq. (4.5).

So far, two kinetic extremes of orthosteric antagonist action have been discussed; a rapidly dissociating antagonist that allows true competitiveness between agonist and antagonist to result and a slowly dissociating antagonist (essentially irreversible) that causes the antagonist

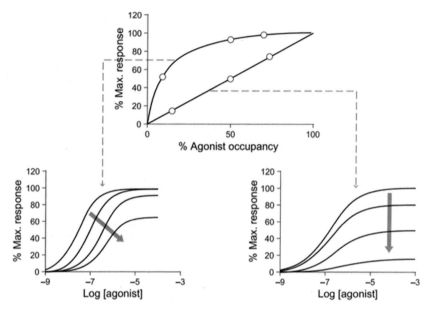

FIGURE 4.10   The effects of a noncompetitive antagonist in two different tissue systems. The top left panel is a system possessing a receptor reserve for the agonist (100% response can be obtained by occupancy of 70% of the receptors). Therefore noncompetitive (pseudo-irreversible) blockade of receptors will result in dextral displacement of the agonist dose-response curve with no depression of maximal response until concentrations of antagonist that block >70% are present. The response system to the right has no reserve for the agonist (note the linear relationship between percentage agonist occupancy and response). Under these circumstances, the noncompetitive antagonist will produce a depression of the maximal response to the agonist at all concentrations.

to eliminate a certain fraction of the receptor from consideration of agonism. There are a large number of systems, referred to as "hemi-equilibria," that fall in between these extremes. Here, the antagonist partially dissociates from the receptors in the presence of the agonist causing only the high concentrations of the agonist (those requiring high-receptor occupancies) to be subjected to irreversible blockade. Under these circumstances, the dose-response curves to the agonist are shifted to the right by the antagonist but may have a truncated (essentially "chopped") maximal response (see Fig. 4.12). In these cases, the potency of the antagonist can be estimated with a pA_2 and/or Schild analysis on the parallel shifted portions of the curves.

The main reason for noting the patterns of antagonism produced by orthosteric antagonists with various rates of offset kinetics is to determine the correct method of estimating antagonist potency. As discussed previously, all antagonisms can be estimated with a pIC_{50}, but there are circumstances where this empirical quantity differs from the correct pK_B

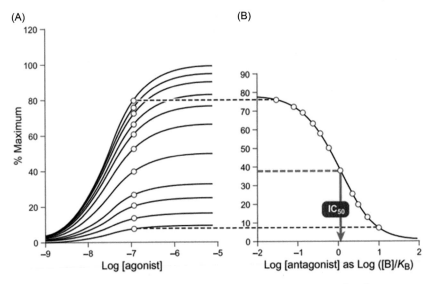

FIGURE 4.11 Effects of a noncompetitive antagonist on an agonist dose-response curve (left panel); open circles show the effects of the antagonist on a selected dose of agonist that produces an 80% maximal response in the absence of the antagonist. The right panel shows the responses to that same selected dose of agonist as a function of the concentrations of competitive antagonist producing the blockade. It can be seen that an inverse sigmoidal curve results (pIC_{50} curve). The value of the abscissa corresponding to the half-maximal ordinate value of this curve is the IC_{50}, namely the molar concentration of antagonist that produces half-maximal inhibition of the defined agonist response. The same pIC_{50} curve would be obtained for any level of response.

(notably with simple competitive antagonists). The pA_2 can also be a useful estimate, but a full analysis of a range of concentrations of antagonists in a Schild analysis is needed to ensure the identity of the pA_2 with the pK_B. Finally, a direct fit of curves for a simple competitive antagonist can yield an estimate of pK_B (Fig. 4.7). For true noncompetitive (insurmountable) antagonism, where the maximal response to the agonist is depressed, directly fitting experimental data requires a more explicit model than that available for simple competitive antagonism (i.e., Eq. 4.4). Specifically, a noncompetitive model based on the Black–Leff operational model (see chapter: Predicting Agonist Effect) can be used according to the equation shown below (Derivations and Proofs, Appendix A.7):

$$\text{Response} = \frac{[A]^n \tau^n E_m}{[A]^n \tau^n + (([A]+K_A)([B]/K_B+1))^n} \tag{4.6}$$

where K_A and τ are the affinity and efficacy of the agonist [A], E_m is the maximal response of the system, n is a slope fitting parameter, and K_B

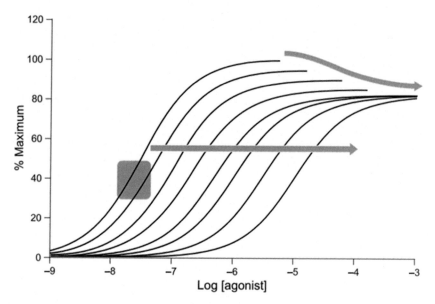

FIGURE 4.12 Antagonist hemi-equilibrium. Shown are the effects of increasing concentrations of a competitive antagonist in a system, where there is insufficient time for complete re-equilibration between agonist, antagonist, and receptors within the time frame available to measure response to the agonist in the presence of the antagonist. This type of system is characterized by a depression of maximal response to a new steady-state level below that of the control curve but greater than zero. The antagonist potency can be estimated with Schild analysis or through estimation of the pA_2 (shaded rectangle).

is the equilibrium dissociation constant for the antagonist [B]. An example of the application of Eq. (4.6) to fitting data is shown in Fig. 4.13.

While the pattern of curves for antagonism observed in vitro is relevant to the quantification of antagonist potency, it is not as important in therapeutic use. Specifically, the production of competitive (surmountable) versus noncompetitive antagonism can simply be a function of the way the antagonist is studied. The key factor here is the time allowed for the collection of agonist response in the presence of antagonist. If this time is short and insufficient for reequilibration of agonist, antagonist, and receptors to occur, then noncompetitive antagonism will result. For example, a truncated time for response collection is operative in measuring transient calcium release, a rapid process. Thus many antagonists produce noncompetitive antagonism in this type of assay. The very same antagonist may produce surmountable simple competitive antagonism (parallel shift to the right of curves with no depression of maximum) in another assay that allows a longer time for agonist, antagonist, and receptor to re-equilibrate. Reporter assays, which incubate the ligands for 24 hours while gene expression takes place, are one such assay; thus a given antagonist may be noncompetitive in

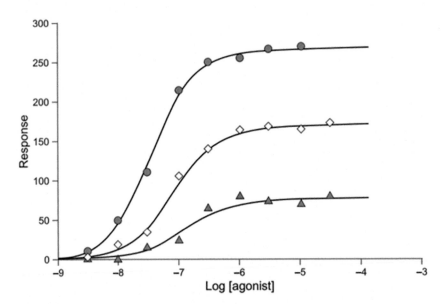

FIGURE 4.13 Dose-response curves obtained in the presence of increasing concentrations of a noncompetitive antagonist fit to the model for noncompetitive antagonism (Eq. 4.6).

a calcium transient assay and surmountably competitive in a reporter assay (see Fig. 4.14).

The ultimate aim of these experiments is to utilize antagonists in vivo for therapeutic advantage. Under these circumstances, the antagonist will enter a system already activated by the agonist (much as in a pIC_{50} experiment) and produce a reduction in the basal response. Once the antagonist diffuses out of the receptor compartment (through whole body clearance; see chapter: Pharmacokinetics II: Distribution and Multiple Dosing), the basal response will be regained provided the steady-state function of the system has not otherwise changed. Since it would be postulated that most physiological systems will operate in a region sensitive to changes in the endogenous agonist concentration (lower region of the dose-response curve), the effects of antagonists on the high-concentration end of the agonist dose-response curve probably are not relevant to whole body physiology. Fig. 4.15 shows the in vivo effect of an antagonist on a basal agonist response.

Fig. 4.16 shows the in vivo responses of a simple competitive (surmountable) and a noncompetitive (insurmountable) antagonist; it can be seen that the in vivo effects are nearly identical. Therefore the determination of competitive versus noncompetitive mechanisms in vitro is important only from the point of view of using the correct model to measure the pK_B.

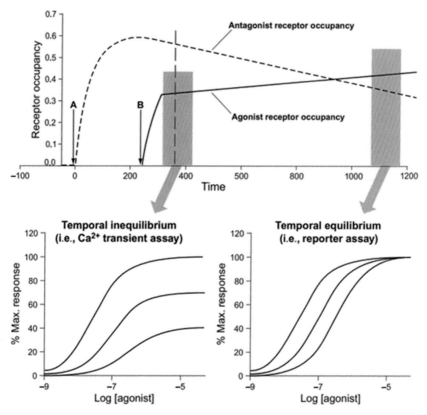

FIGURE 4.14 Effect of different time periods to measure agonist response (in the presence of a slowly dissociating orthosteric antagonist) shown in top panel. Panel on the left shows observed antagonism when the period for measurement of response is too short for complete re-equilibration (noncompetitive antagonism is observed). Panel on the right shows the same system when sufficient time for the slowly dissociating antagonist is allowed for proper reequilibration between agonist, antagonist and receptors. Under these circumstances, simple competitive antagonism is observed.

Irreversible antagonists

If the antagonist has no appreciable rate of offset from the receptor (but simply irreversibly binds to the receptor never to dissociate), then a K_B cannot be measured because a steady-state of a constant fraction of occupied receptor cannot be attained. This is because, as long as the antagonist is not depleted from the medium, it will continue to inactivate the receptors until there are no more receptors left in the tissue to inactivate. In essence, the onset of an irreversible antagonist is a chemical reaction that runs to completion when either the antagonist or receptors are depleted. Since, K_B = rate of offset/rate of onset, then $K_B \rightarrow 0$ as equilibration with

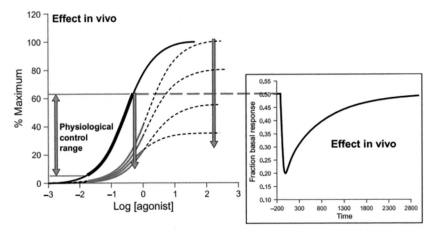

FIGURE 4.15   Effects of an antagonist in vivo where a level of basal activity is present. The dose-response curve to the endogenous agonist will be shifted to the right and/or depressed by the antagonist; the panel on the right shows the observed response in vivo. As the antagonist enters the receptor compartment and binds, the elevated basal response is depressed; as the antagonist washes out of the receptor compartment, the response returns.

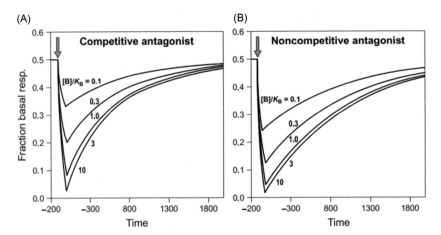

FIGURE 4.16   In vivo effects (see Fig. 4.15) of a competitive versus a noncompetitive antagonist on endogenous elevated basal response.

antagonist progresses (the rate of offset is essentially $= 0$). Fig. 4.17 shows two antagonists producing apparent noncompetitive antagonism as they are equilibrated with the tissue for increasing periods of time. Unlike the reversible antagonist, which takes the tissue to a submaximally blocked state (depressed maximum dose-response curve, which does not change with further equilibration time), the truly irreversible antagonist blocks the response until a dose-response relationship for the agonist cannot be

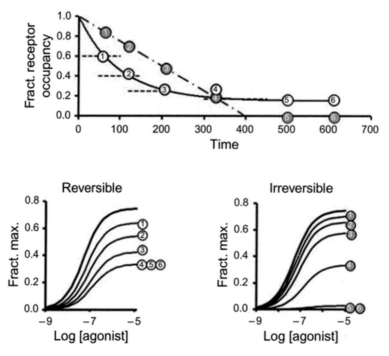

FIGURE 4.17   Irreversible receptor blockade. Top panel shows diminution of agonist receptor occupancy with a reversible noncompetitive antagonist (solid line) and an irreversible antagonist (broken line). Six time points (noted with the numbered circles) are chosen and the dose-response curve to the agonist is shown in the presence of the reversible (left panel) and irreversible (right panel) antagonists. The circled numbers next to the dose-response curves refer to the timepoints for antagonist onset. While, the reversible antagonist comes to a steady state by timepoints 4–6, the irreversible antagonist continues to depress response until no response to the agonist can be obtained. The lack of nonzero steady-state denotes the irreversibility of the antagonism.

attained. When noncompetitive receptor antagonism is observed it should be confirmed that submaximal states of inhibition can be attained and that a K_B can be measured to differentiate pseudo-irreversible antagonism from truly irreversible antagonism.

Target disposition as a method of antagonism

The pharmacologic outcome of irreversible antagonism is the complete elimination of agonist response; this is reflected in severe dextral displacement of agonist dose-response curves and/or concomitant depression of the maximal response to the agonist. In essence, this is formally identical to the physical removal of the drug target. There are conditions where this could be a viable mechanism of action to achieve drug antagonism, especially in the case of so-called "undruggable" targets. There are nearly 650,000 "undruggable" protein-protein interactions (PPIs) in the human interactome that can potentially be considered novel therapeutic targets and only 2% of these have been targeted with drugs. PPIs are considered to be undruggable because they don't have well-defined binding pockets but rather have contact surfaces that are usually flat, featureless, and relatively large, interacting through electrostatic and hydrophobic interactions, hydrogen bonds, and van der Waals forces over less well-defined, larger areas.

In fact, undruggable proteins have contact surfaces that are usually flat, featureless, and relatively large, interacting through electrostatic and hydrophobic interactions, hydrogen bonds, and van der Waals forces over less well-defined, larger areas. In this energetic context, a small molecule usually fails to compete with natural partners, mainlybecause of its size and the limited number of interactions. Many of these proteins are involved in pathophysiology and their removal would be beneficial opening the question "can we inhibit nonenzymatic proteins by triggering their degradation?"

One method to do this is through Proteolysis Targeting Chimeras (PROTACs). These are unique three domain hybrids (ligand binding domain ("warhead") for a target protein, ligand binding domain for E3 ubiquitin ligase and a linker joining the two domains). PROTACs produce a knockdown of the targeted protein by directing the protein to Nature's natural waste disposal system, namely the ubiquitin-proteosome system—see Fig. 4.18.

Therefore the challenge is to design therapeutics that target noncatalytic proteins to trigger their degradation. Traditional inhibitors must bind tightly to targets, not the case with degraders and their effects rely on event-driven rather than occupancy-driven pharmacology. Protacs produce a knockdown of the targeted protein by directing the protein to the ubiquitin-proteosome system. This has proven to be a useful strategy for the degradation of various types of target proteins related to a number of diseases including cancers, viral infections, immune disorders, and neurodegeneration. For example, JQ1 binds the cancer protein BRD4 to the ubiquitin system through an E3 ubiquitin ligase ligand; levels of BRDR4 are more efficiently reduced by the PROTAC in JQ1 resistant-derived tumors than just the JQ1 molecule. The improved reduction of BRDR4 shown results in the MDA-MB-231R-derived tumors—see Box 4.4. PROTAC not only eliminates the catalytic functions of enzymes, such as kinases in cancer but also promotes the destruction of the kinase; this eliminates the noncatalytic scaffolding functions of these enzymes (i.e., focal adhesion kinases, FAK; conventional kinase inhibitors do not inhibit all FAK functions). This technique also offers the advantage of improved duration of effects; however, possible limitations involve the large molecular size of PROTACs molecules and added expense of synthesis.

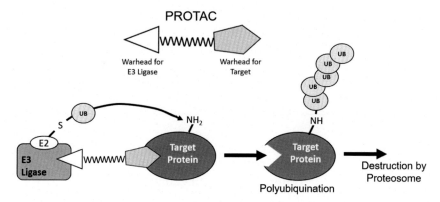

FIGURE 4.18 Protacs molecules are comprised of a hybrid structure with a binding site for the targeted protein and an attached ubiquitin E3 ligase; these bind to a target protein and then promote the ubiquitinylization of the protein through the ligase to produce a species that is targeted for destruction by the proteosome. PROTACs produce a knockdown of the targeted protein by directing the protein to this natural waste disposal mechanism, namely the ubiquitin-proteosome system.

BOX 4.4

Undruggable drug targets—PROTACs: harnessing nature's waste disposal systems

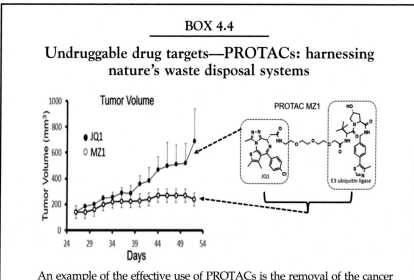

An example of the effective use of PROTACs is the removal of the cancer target BRD4. The war head JQ1 binds BRD4 to the ubiquitin system through an E3 ubiquitin ligase ligand to lower levels of BRDR4 in JQ1 resistant-derived tumors by MZ1 more efficiently than just the JQ1 molecule. From Del Mar Noblejas-López M, Nieto-Jimenez C, Burgos M, Gómez-Juárez M, Montero JC, Esparís-Ogando A, Pandiella A, Galán-Moya EM, Ocaña A (2019) Activity of BET-proteolysis targeting chimeric (PROTAC) compounds in triple negative breast cancer. J Clin Cancer Res. 38: 383.

Another strategy is to affect the disposition of pathological molecules. For instance, CGRP is released and causes contraction of intracranial blood vessels to cause migraine headaches. Antibodies that bind CGRP are used to scavenge CGRP and prevent it from causing activation of cranial vessel CGRP receptors in the treatment of migraine—see Box 4.5.

BOX 4.5

CGRP-antibodies create a natural vacuum cleaner to relieve migraine headache

One hypothesis for the cause of migraine headaches is that trigeminal nerves release Calcitonin Gene-Related Peptide (CGRP) that goes on to dilate intracranial nerves to cause migraine pain. A novel approach to alleviating this effect is to administer antibodies that strongly bind CGRP into an inactive complex that cannot produce vasodilatation.

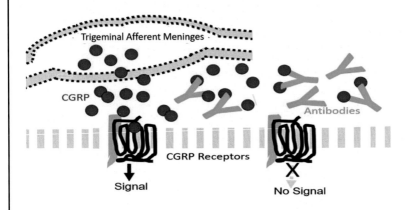

Partial and inverse agonists

As discussed in Chapter 1, Pharmacology: The Chemical Control of Physiology, affinity and efficacy are generated by the same thermodynamic properties of the molecule; thus if a molecule has affinity for a given protein, it is likely to have some kind of efficacy as well. Efficacy is the ability of the molecule to bind to and stabilize selective protein states, and to shift the equilibrium between protein states. Depending on the types of receptor states produced, this could result in a receptor with properties different from those of the unbound receptor. In terms of cell signaling, this difference could take the form of increased cellular activity (positive agonism) or a decrease in elevated basal activity (inverse agonism). This latter condition occurs when the cell contains a critical mass of receptors already in an activated state; this could be because of a mutation or high-receptor expression. It is useful to think of the receptor population in any cell as a mixture of conformations (termed an "ensemble") with some preferred low-energy conformations and others mediating cellular activity. Most systems are preset to the "inactive" conformations of receptors, thus the baseline cellular activity is low. A given antagonist could have preferred affinity for this "inactive" state or have a low affinity for an active state; these preferred affinities will shift the equilibrium of the ensemble toward those preferred states and thus lead to an observed cellular response.

First, we will consider partial agonism. If the predominant species of receptor in the cell are in the inactive state, then an antagonist with positive efficacy has the potential to activate these receptors, and produce a measurable response. Fig. 4.19 shows the effect of a range of concentrations of partial agonist on the responses to a full agonist. The elevated baseline shows the intrinsic activation of the system by the partial agonist.

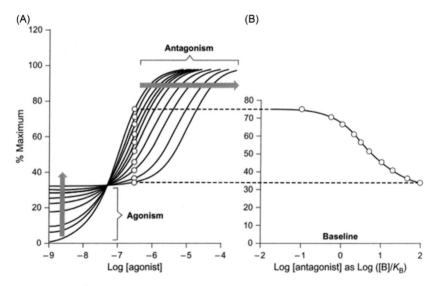

FIGURE 4.19 The effect of a partial agonist on the dose-response curve to an agonist. The partial agonist produces a direct response due to a low level of positive efficacy and it also shifts the dose-response curve to the agonist to the right. This competitive antagonist effect is the result of competition between the high efficacy agonist and lower efficacy partial agonist. The activity of the partial agonist as an antagonist can be determined with a pIC_{50} curve (panel on the right); note how the direct effect of the partial agonist produces an elevated baseline for the pIC_{50} curve. The shift to the right of the agonist dose-response curve can be used in Schild analysis to determine the pK_B.

The shift to the right of the full agonist dose-response curve shows how the partial agonist with lower efficacy occupies the receptor and blocks the effect of the more efficacious full agonist; thus a dual nature of partial agonists is revealed. They can function as agonists in sensitive systems, but they can also function as antagonists of highly efficacious agonists. It is this dual nature of partial agonists (specifically with the β-adrenoceptor partial agonist dichloroisoproterenol) that intrigued James Black and his team at ICI and led them to discover and develop beta-blockers (see Box 4.6). The dextral displacement of the full agonist dose-response curves furnishes dose ratio values that can be used in Schild analysis to determine the pK_B of the partial agonist. Whether a given partial agonist will produce a measurable direct response in a given system or not depends upon the intrinsic efficacy of the antagonist molecule and the sensitivity of the system. Box 4.7 shows how two systems of differing sensitivity show the dual nature of the β-adrenoceptor partial agonist prenalterol.

Another type of shift in protein conformational equilibrium leads to an opposite effect, namely inverse agonism. As noted, receptor proteins exist in collections of conformations and some of these spontaneously formed active states may produce a cellular response (referred to as "constitutive activity"). One method of quantifying this effect is through an "allosteric constant" designated L, which is the spontaneous ratio of active receptor state (denoted $[R_a]$) and inactive receptor state ($[R_i]$) with the relation $L = [R_a]/[R_i]$. Thus a value of $L = 10^{-4}$ indicates that for every 10,000 receptors, one may be spontaneously in the active state at any one time. There are conditions, such as receptor mutation or receptor overexpression (e.g., cancer), where this ratio can lead to an elevated basal response. In the case of receptor overexpression, if a tumor cell expresses 1000 times more receptors on the cell surface, it can be seen that a receptor with $L = 10^{-4}$ may now produce an ambient level of 1000 active-state receptors, possibly enough to produce an elevated basal cellular response. An antagonist with a preferred affinity for the active state will now reverse this elevated basal effect and produce a depression of the cellular basal level of response. Fig. 4.20 shows the effect of an inverse agonist on dose-response curves of a full agonist in a system demonstrating elevated-constitutive activity. It should be noted that this same molecule will produce simple competitive blockade (i.e., effects, such as those shown in Fig. 4.6) in cells with no constitutive activity. In this sense, the term inverse "agonist" is a misnomer, since these really are antagonists. However, since the reversal of elevated basal response can be seen as an overt change in cellular state, the term agonist has been used to describe these molecules.

It can be seen from Fig. 4.20 that the constitutively elevated basal effect is depressed by the inverse agonist, but the dose-response curves to the

---

BOX 4.6

Partial agonists: drugs with two faces

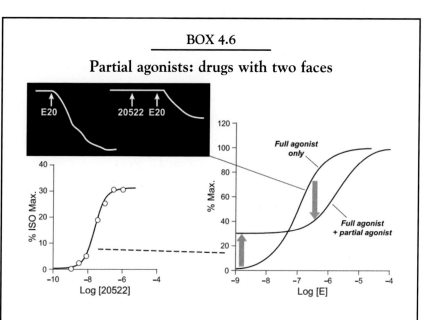

Partial agonists can cause activation of a quiescent system and antagonism of response in a system activated by a more efficacious agonist. This dichotomous behavior intrigued James Black (see Box 2.6) who noticed that dichloroisoproterenol (then known as Lilly 20522) blocked the effects of isoproterenol (see black tracing) in guinea pig trachea (redrawn from Powell and Slater [4]) but otherwise was known to stimulate receptors like isoproterenol, but to a lesser extent. An example of this latter activity is shown in the dose-response curve for GTP-γS activation, where 20522 produces a 30% maximal response to isoproterenol (redrawn from Ambrosio et al. [5]). This apparently conflicting activity can be seen from the complete dose-response curves for an agonist in the absence and presence of a partial agonist. At lower values of basal activity, the stimulatory effect of the partial agonist is seen, whereas at higher response values, the antagonism by the partial agonist dominates. Understanding this effect led Black and his team to develop the first beta-blockers.

---

full agonist are shifted to the right. Under these circumstances, this dextral displacement of the curves can be used for Schild analysis to calculate a pK_B for antagonism. When discovered for 7TM receptors by Costa and Herz (see Box 4.8) [4], inverse agonism appeared to be an anomaly. However, as more constitutively active systems became available for experimentation, it became clear that, as theoretically predicted, inverse

BOX 4.7

Partial agonist efficacy as an electric battery

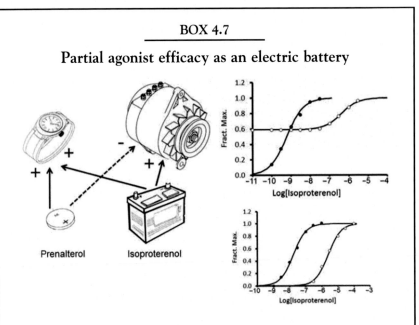

Data redrawn from T.P. Kenakin, D. Beek, Is prenalterol (H133/80) really a selective beta-1 adrenoceptor agonist? Tissue selectivity resulting from differences in stimulus-response relations. J. Pharmacol. Exp. Ther. 213 (1980) 406—413 [6] and T.P. Kenakin, D. Beek, Relative efficacy of prenalterol and pirbuterol for beta-1 adrenoceptors: measurement of agonist affinity by alteration of receptor number. J. Pharmacol. Exp. Ther. 229 (1984) 340—345 [7].

As discussed in Chapter 2, Drug Affinity and Efficacy and Chapter 3, Predicting Agonist Effect, efficacy is both a tissue- and drug-related property. Therefore whether a given agonist will produce a response or not depends on (1) the sensitivity of the tissue and (2) the intrinsic efficacy of the agonist. This latter property can be likened to a battery driving electrically driven devices. Thus a low level of intrinsic efficacy would be a small battery capable of driving a small device such as a watch (sensitive tissue) but not capable of driving a larger device, such as the starter engine to a car (insensitive tissue). Such is the case for prenalterol, a low-efficacy β-adrenoceptor agonist. In an insensitive tissue such as desensitized rat left atrium (panel B), prenalterol functions as a competitive antagonist and does not produce direct agonist itself. In contrast, it does produce a direct agonism in a more sensitive tissue (nondesensitized rat atria—panel A) to show the typical profile of antagonism by a partial agonist.

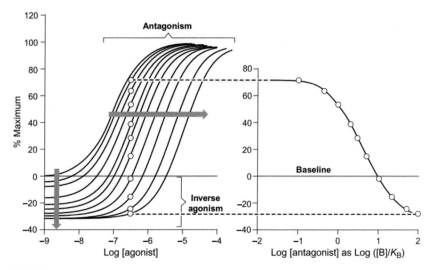

FIGURE 4.20 The effect of an inverse agonist on the dose-response curve to an agonist. If the receptor system is constitutively active then the baseline response will be spontaneously elevated. The inverse agonist produces a direct reversal of this elevated basal response due to a low level of negative efficacy; the inverse agonist also shifts the dose-response curve to the agonist to the right. The activity of the inverse agonist as an antagonist can be determined with a pIC_{50} curve (panel on the right); note how the direct effect of the inverse agonist produces a baseline for the pIC_{50} curve that is lower than the constitutively elevated baseline. The shift to the right of the agonist dose-response curve can be used in Schild analysis to determine the pK_B.

agonism is the most prevalent form of antagonism and the depression of basal responses becomes evident for these molecules only when the assay allows constitutively elevated activity to be observed. However, there are a subclass of antagonists that presumably have similar affinities for $[R_a]$ and $[R_i]$ to the point that no change in basal effect is produced, even in constitutively active systems; this subclass of antagonist is referred to as "neutral." It is not clear to what extent inverse agonism is a therapeutically relevant drug property, since most cell systems do not appear to be constitutively active. However, in cases where they are (i.e., tumor growth), inverse agonists and neutral antagonists will have different properties. In addition, inverse agonism has been linked in some systems to antagonist tolerance upon chronic administration (see Box 4.9).

If an antagonist molecule produces a receptor conformation with a lower intrinsic ability to produce a response than the spontaneously formed receptor active state ($[R_a]$), then an intriguing reversal of observed activity can occur. Specifically, such a molecule will produce positive activation of the receptor under normal circumstances but inverse agonism in cases where there is a high level of constitutive

BOX 4.8

The discovery of inverse agonism

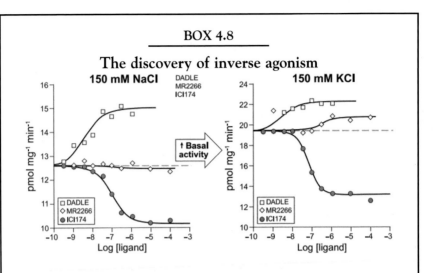

Although negative agonism was noted for benzodiazepine receptors some years earlier, a paper by Costa and Herz [8] was the first to demonstrate inverse agonism for seven transmembrane receptors. Working with opioid receptors in NG-108 cells, they showed that elevation of the basal response through changes in ionic media revealed a clear negative response to the peptide ICI174. Notably, the weakly positive response to Mr2266 was not obvious until the basal response and assay sensitivity were elevated to a higher level with 150 mM KCl. These data clearly showed how the observation of ligand efficacy depends on the setpoint of the assay. Increased sensitivity of the assay is optimal for demonstrating positive agonism (note Mr226 in 150 NaCl) and increased basal response is optimal for showing inverse agonism (ICI174 in 150 KCl). Although considered an oddity when first published, inverse agonism is now seen to be a very common phenomenon by other researchers as they test antagonists in constitutively active (elevated basal response) assays.

activity; such molecules are referred to as "protean agonists," named after the Greek mythological god Proteus, who could change his shape at will (see Box 4.10).

Antagonist effects in vivo

The interplay of the potency of a molecule as it induces antagonism and its intrinsic efficacy (either positive for partial agonists or negative

BOX 4.9

Inverse agonism can lead to tolerance

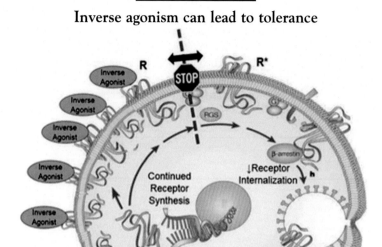

Inverse agonists are ligands that selectively bind to the inactive state of the receptor. If any receptor happens to be in an active state spontaneously, then an inverse agonist will reverse the resultant constitutive activity. However, the main pharmacological effect of inverse agonists is receptor antagonism, that is, inverse agonists will block the effect of agonists and the effect on constitutive activity is only relevant, if the system is spontaneously active. There is a property of inverse agonists that may be therapeutically relevant in nonconstitutively active systems. In normal physiological systems, there is a steady-state membrane surface level of receptors present to mediate signaling that results from a constant synthesis from within the cell and an internalization after receptor activation and phosphorylation. If receptor activation is interrupted, the continuing receptor synthesis can lead to an increase in the steady-state level of receptors on the cell surface and a concomitant elevation in the sensitivity of the cell to agonists.

For example, it was known that patients on antiulcer therapy with histamine H2 blockers became tolerant upon chronic treatment [9]; this tolerance was linked to elevated histamine receptor levels on the parietal cell [10]. Subsequent work showed that patients on the inverse agonist cimetidine, used for treatment of gastric ulcers through blockade of histamine H2 receptors, became tolerant after chronic treatment [11].

continued

BOX 4.9   (cont'd)

This suggests that in some cases, inverse agonists, by virtue of the fact that they stabilize the inactive state of the receptor, can upon chronic use cause elevation of receptor levels on the cell surface and this, in turn, can cause escape from chronic receptor antagonism. While this may not occur with all inverse agonists, it is a drug property that has been linked to tolerance and thus should be determined for a new antagonist.

BOX 4.10

Protean agonists

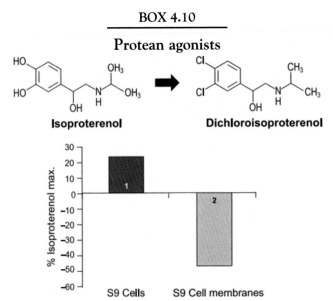

Considering efficacy as the stabilization of a distinct ensemble of receptor conformations with the ability to induce a response, it should be noted that spontaneously formed receptor active states responsible for constitutive activity (elevated basal responses) also have an intrinsic efficacy (ability to induce response). In early formulations of receptor theory, it was assumed that agonists simply enrich levels of the naturally occurring active state(s), but subsequent research showed that many ligands can induce unique receptor conformations with varying levels of ability to produce cellular effect. If agonist stabilization produces an ensemble of lower efficacy to induce response than the naturally occurring receptor active state, then a phenomenon referred to as "protean" agonism can occur [15]. Named after the Greek mythological sea god Proteus, who could change his shape at will, protean agonists, such as dichloroisoproterenol are positive agonists in normal systems and inverse agonists in constitutively active systems. As shown by Chidiac and coworkers [16] in the graph below, DCI produces positive agonism in S9 cells. When membranes are produced from these cells that are spontaneously active and have an elevated basal response, DCI produces negative effects instead.

for inverse agonists), and the ambient basal response of the system in vivo (either through the presence of an endogenous agonist or through constitutive activity) can combine to produce a complex array of observed effects in vivo. Fig. 4.21 shows the possible outcomes of such molecules to in vivo systems of varying endogenous activation. In general, a rich array of potential therapeutic effects can be achieved through judicious choice of efficacy in candidate antagonist molecules.

Antagonists with multiple activities

This chapter mainly describes the steric hindrance of endogenous agonists, that is, orthosteric antagonism. However, such a mechanism does not preclude the molecule from inducing other effects on receptors that produce responses concomitant with antagonism. Positive and/or inverse agonism are two of these occurring through the stabilization of different receptor conformations, which then go on to interact with signaling elements in the cell. However, beyond these effects, there is no reason a priori that an antagonist will not have other biological activities and these may interfere with the expression of receptor blockade. One such effect is shown by the muscarinic receptor antagonist ambenonium, which has self-canceling effects of potentiation of acetylcholine response through blockade of acetylcholinesterase and reduction of acetylcholine response through muscarinic receptor blockade (see Box 4.11). These effects can combine to yield a concentration range for this drug that erroneously suggests that it has no effect; one way to separate such multiple effects is through the observation of pharmacological responses. This principle relies on the notion that two separate processes, (such as acetylcholinesterase blockade and receptor blockade) may well have different time courses and thus before a self-cancellation of steady-state effect can occur, the approach to a steady-state will unveil the separate processes; as shown in Box 4.11, this is the case with ambenonium.

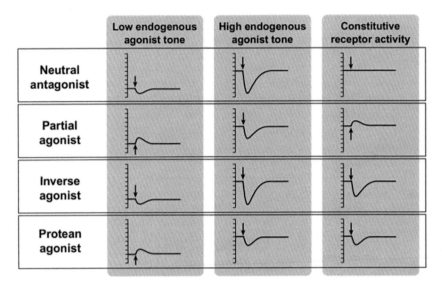

FIGURE 4.21   The in vivo effects of various antagonists. A neutral antagonist will block endogenous agonism but will have no effect on constitutively active agonism. A partial agonist may elevate the response under conditions of low endogenous activation but block the effects of high-endogenous agonism. A partial agonist will elevate the response in a constitutively activated system, if the level of constitutive activity is low. An inverse agonist will depress all responses whether it is due to endogenous agonism or constitutive receptor activity. A protean agonist will elevate the response in conditions of low activation but will block the effects of both high-endogenous agonism or constitutively elevated response.

Descriptive pharmacology: IV

Chapter 1, Pharmacology: The Chemical Control of Physiology, Chapter 2, Drug Affinity and Efficacy, and Chapter 3, Predicting Agonist Effect, discussed the effects of molecules that directly alter the cellular function (agonists). Fig. 4.22 shows two possible effects of molecules that, when added to a bimolecular system (reference agonist plus test molecule), can alter the effect of a reference agonist. Increases in response are discussed further in Chapter 5, Allosteric Drug Effects. If response is diminished, then some form of antagonism is operative. As with agonism (see chapter: Drug Affinity and Efficacy, Agonist Selectivity), the selectivity of the antagonism must be determined to differentiate effects from nonspecific toxic or depressant activity. This can be done readily by demonstrating that no antagonism is produced to agonists of other receptors in the same preparation.

Fig. 4.23 shows the possible array of responses to a purported antagonist and the resulting classifications of activity deduced from the observed

Real time unravels multiple drug activities

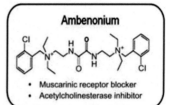

Ambenonium

- Muscarinic receptor blocker
- Acetylcholinesterase inhibitor

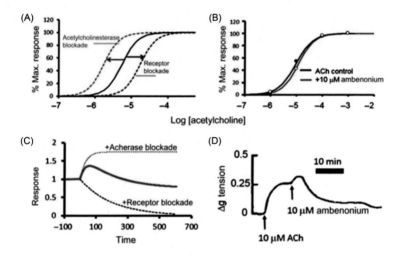

Data redrawn from T.P. Kenakin, D. Beek, Self-cancellation of drug properties as a mode of organ selectivity: the antimuscarinic effects of ambenonium. J. Pharmacol. Exp. Ther. 232 (1985) 732–740 [12].

Drugs frequently have more than one activity; in the case of the antimuscarinic antagonist ambenonium, these produce conflicting pharmacologic effects. Specifically, this molecule potentiates acetylcholine response through blockade of acetylcholinesterase [13], an enzyme that degrades acetylcholine and reduces response through blockade of muscarinic receptors [14] (see Fig. A). As shown in Panel B, 10 μM ambenonium appears to have little effect on the dose-response curve to acetylcholine.

However, multiple processes can be further separated through real time kinetics, that is, the processes may produce balancing equilibrium effects but the rates at which that condition is achieved may differ. This may serve to separate the two drug activities. For instance, Panel C shows the effect of a drug that potentiates acetylcholine response with a rate faster than it blocks the receptor response; the real time emergence of the effect shows the two phase action in red. This appears to be the case for ambenonium, which shows the two phase response in real time in Panel D.

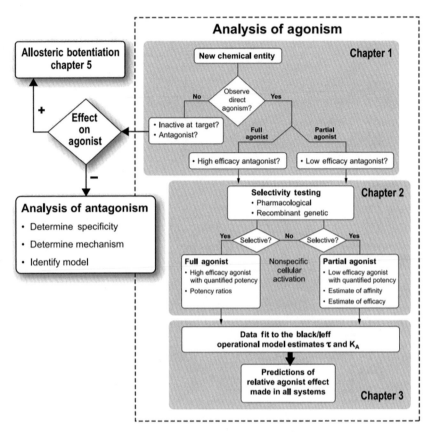

FIGURE 4.22   Descriptive pharmacology; schematic diagram of logic used to characterize drug effect. The characterization of agonism is shown in the area bounded by the dotted line (as described in chapters: Pharmacology: The Chemical Control of Physiology, Drug Affinity and Efficacy, and Predicting Agonist Effect). If no direct agonism is observed then the new chemical entity should be tested in a bimolecular system consisting of the test compound and an endogenous agonist. If the level of endogenous agonism is elevated, then the test compound most likely is an allosteric positive modulator; these are discussed in Chapter 5, Allosteric Drug Effects. If the endogenous agonism is depressed, then analysis continues to determine the mode of antagonism.

response; these effects can be classified by the respective effects of the molecule on the basal assay response and the maximal response of the assay to a full agonist. If the molecule blocks the effects of powerful full agonists, but also increases the basal response of an assay in its own right, then it is a partial agonist (assuming it produces surmountable antagonism of the full agonist effect). Under these circumstances, the dextral displacements of the full agonist dose-response curve can be used in Schild analysis to determine the pK_B. If the molecule decreases basal response, and especially if it can be

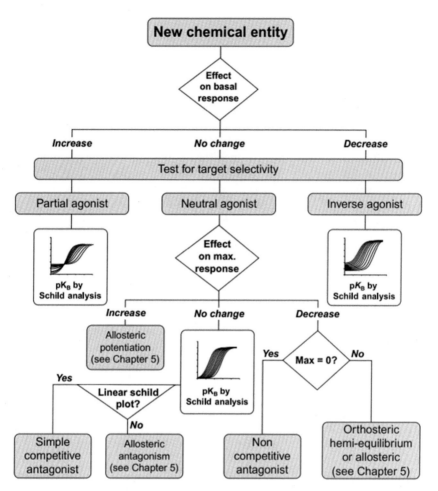

FIGURE 4.23 A schematic diagram depicts the logic used to determine the mode of action and potency of an antagonist. It is assumed that relevant procedures are used to determine that the antagonism is specific for the target (see Fig. 4.2). The antagonist may elevate basal response, in which case it would be analyzed as a partial agonist. Similarly, if the molecule depressed basal activity it would be analyzed as an inverse agonist. If no effects on basal response are observed then the antagonism is classified in terms of the effects on the maximal responses to the agonist. If no effect on maximal response is observed, then a Schild analysis is done to test for linearity of the Schild plot and adherence to the model of simple competitive antagonism. If the Schild plot is curvilinear, then further tests are done to determine possible allosteric antagonism (see chapter: Allosteric Drug Effects). This is also the case if the antagonist produces an increased maximal response to the agonist. If the maximal responses to the agonist are depressed, then the nature of this depression is explored further. Specifically, the degree to which the maximal response is depressed is examined; if the maximal response can be completely depressed to baseline, then an orthosteric noncompetitive antagonism is suggested (although it is still possible that a high level of negative cooperativity in a negative allosteric modulator could also cause this; see chapter: Allosteric Drug Effects). If the antagonism reaches a new steady state beyond which no further antagonism occurs, then a negative allosterism is suggested (see chapter: Allosteric Drug Effects). If the maximal response is depressed to a new steady state but further dextral displacement of the curve occurs, then an orthosteric hemi-equilibrium is suggested.

determined that the basal response is constitutively elevated through spontaneous receptor activity, then it is likely that the molecule is an inverse agonist. Under these circumstances, the pK_B can be estimated through Schild
analysis, as discussed in the section Orthosteric (Competitive and
Noncompetitive) Antagonism in this chapter.

Finally, a molecule may produce no effect on basal response, but may
otherwise antagonize the responses to a full agonist. If the maximal response
to the full agonist is not affected, then this would be consistent with simple
competitive antagonism. The potency of the antagonist (as a pK_B) could
then be estimated with Schild analysis. If an increase in the maximal
response is produced by the molecule, then it is an allosteric modulator (see
chapter: Allosteric Drug Effects). If the molecule produces a depression of
the maximal response, then a number of possibilities arise. The depression of the maximum could be concentration-dependent and complete
(i.e., a sufficiently high concentration of the antagonist will reduce the
maximal response to zero). Under these circumstances, the effect could
be a pseudo-irreversible orthosteric noncompetitive blockade or an allosteric antagonism. Data can be fit to the noncompetitive model to yield a
pK_B under these conditions. If the depression of maximal response
reaches a limiting value and no further antagonism is produced by higher concentrations of antagonist, this suggests allosteric antagonism (see
chapter: Allosteric Drug Effects). If the maximal response is depressed to
a limiting value greater than zero, but increasing concentrations of antagonist further shift the curve with a newly depressed maximum, this suggests a hemi-equilibrium state whereby a mixed pseudo-irreversible and
competitive blockade is produced. Under these circumstances, Schild
analysis can be used to estimate the pK_B.

Summary

- There are two possible modes of action of antagonism; orthosteric
  blockade (occlusion of the agonist binding site) and allosteric
  modulation.
- Antagonism is characterized by the quantity of antagonist bound
  (*potency*), the location of the binding relative to the binding of the
  natural agonist (*mechanism*), and the persistence of antagonist binding
  (*antagonist kinetics*).
- The relative rates of dissociation of the antagonist from the receptor,
  the rate of association of the agonist with the receptor, and the length
  of time available to achieve equilibrium determine whether
  surmountable or insurmountable blockade will be observed.

- Simple competitive blockade occurs when there is sufficient time to achieve equilibrium; it is characterized by parallel shifts to the right of the agonist curves with no depression of maximum.
- Competitive antagonism is quantified with a pK_B value determined through Schild analysis.
- If the rate of dissociation of the antagonist is slow it can effectively irreversibly block a portion of the receptor population and a depression of the maximal response to the agonist can result.
- A mixture of the above effects can occur whereby a portion of the receptors are essentially irreversibly blocked; this is referred to as hemi-equilibrium and results in partially depressed maxima with shifts to the right of the curve(s).
- Estimates of antagonist potency can be obtained for all modes of antagonism through a pA_2 value and/or a pIC_{50} of the antagonism of a fixed agonist effect.
- Antagonists can produce low levels of positive response (partial agonists) or depression of basal responses elevated by constitutive receptor activity (inverse agonists).
- Surmountable versus insurmountable antagonism has little relevance to antagonism in vivo since a reduction in basal response is the main effect observed in these systems.

References

[1] J.H. Gaddum, The quantitative effects of antagonistic drugs, J. Physiol. Lond. 89 (1937) 7P–9P.

[2] O. Arunlakshana, H.O. Schild, Some quantitative uses of drug antagonists, Br. J. Pharmacol. 14 (1959) 48–58.

[3] P. Leff, I.G. Dougall, Further concerns over Cheng–Prusoff analysis, Trends Pharmacol. Sci. 14 (1993) 110–112.

[4] C.E. Powell, I.H. Slater, Blocking of inhibtory adrenergic receptors by a dichloro analog of isoproterenol, J. Pharmacol. Exp. Ther. 122 (1958) 480–488.

[5] C. Ambrosio, P. Molinari, F. Fanelli, Y. Chuman, M. Sbraccia, O. Ugur, Different structural requirements for the constitutive and agonist-induced activities for the β2-adrenergic receptor, J. Biol. Chem. 280 (2005) 23464–23474.

[6] T.P. Kenakin, D. Beek, Is prenalterol (H133/80) really a selective beta 1 adrenoceptor agonist? Tissue selectivity resulting from differences in stimulus-response relations, J. Pharmacol. Exp. Ther. 213 (1980) 406–413.

[7] T.P. Kenakin, D. Beek, Relative efficacy of prenalterol and pirbuterol for beta-1 adrenoceptors: measurement of agonist affinity by alteration of receptor number, J. Pharmacol. Exp. Ther. 229 (1984) 340–345.

[8] T. Costa, A. Herz, Antagonists with negative intrinsic activity at δ-opioid receptors coupled to GTP-binding proteins, Proc. Natl. Acad. Sci. USA. 86 (1989) 7321–7325.

[9] C.U. Nwokolo, J.T.L. Smith, C. Gavey, A. Sawyerr, R.E. Pounder, Tolerance during 29 days of conventional dosing with cimetidine, nizatidine, famotidine or ranitidine. Aliment, Pharmacol. Ther. 4 (suppl) (1990) 29–45.

[10] C.U. Nwokolo, J.T. Smith, A.M. Sawyerr, R.E. Pounder, Rebound intragastric hyper-acidity after abrupt withdrawal of histamine H2 receptor blockade, Gut 32 (1991) 1455—1460.

[11] M.J. Smit, R. Leurs, A.E. Alewijnse, J. Blauw, G.P. Van Nieuw Amerongen, Y. Van De Vrede, Inverse agonism of histamine H2 antagonist accounts for upregulation of spontaneously active histamine H2 receptors, Proc. Natl. Acad. Sci. USA. 93 (1996) 6802—6807.

[12] T.P. Kenakin, D. Beek, Self-cancellation of drug properties as a mode of organ selec-tivity: the antimuscarinic effects of ambenonium, J. Pharmacol. Exp. Ther. 232 (1985) 732—740.

[13] A. Arnold, A.E. Soria, F.K. Kirchner, A new anticholinesterase oxamide, Proc. Soc. Exp. Biol. Med. 87 (1954) 393—394.

[14] J.H. Brown, G.T. Wetzel, J. Dunlap, Activation and blockage of cardiac muscarinic receptors by endogenous acetylcholine and cholinesterase inhibitors, J. Pharamcol. Exp. Ther. 223 (1982) 20—24.

[15] T.P. Kenakin, Protean agonists: keys to receptor active state? Ann. N. Y. Acad. Sci. 812 (1997) 116—125.

[16] P. Chidiac, T.E. Hebert, M. Valiquette, M. Dennis, M. Bouvier, Inverse agonist activ-ity of β-adrenergic antagonists, Mol. Pharmacol. 45 (1994) 490—499.

CHAPTER

5

Allosteric drug effects

OUTLINE

By the end of this chapter, the reader will know the characteristic properties of allosteric molecules and how they interact with proteins. In addition, the reader will know strategies for identifying allosterism and the reasons why this is relevant to drug discovery. Specifically, these involve the unique therapeutic properties of allosteric modulators.

Pharmacology in Drug Discovery and Development
DOI: https://doi.org/10.1016/B978-0-443-14124-9.00013-6

Finally, the reader will learn how to use pharmacologic tools to quantify the allosteric behavior of molecules for use in studies aimed at optimizing allosteric activity.

Introduction

Conventional concepts about drug discovery center on the assumption that a drug must have an affinity for a naturally physiologically relevant site on a biological target. For instance, antimuscarinic antagonists, such as scopolamine are targeted toward the acetylcholine-binding site on the acetylcholine receptor. Similarly, many kinase inhibitors are targeted toward the natural ATP-binding site of kinases. These systems, as discussed in Chapter 4, Drug Antagonism Orthosteric Drug Effects, can be thought of as "orthosteric" in nature since steric hindrance may play an important role in the mechanism of action. Allosteric molecules can bind to virtually any site on the target protein and affect its activity; this greatly expands the possible therapeutic opportunities for a given target. This may be an extremely important approach, as it is known that if a molecule is bound to the protein at any site the conformational movement of that protein may be affected (*vide infra*). These effects are allosteric and have become a very important part of new drug discovery.

New terminology

The following new terms will be introduced in this chapter:

- α: Denoted within the standard model for functional allosterism quantifying the effect of an allosteric modulator on the affinity of a protein for another molecule.
- β: Denoted within the standard model for functional allosterism quantifying the effect of an allosteric modulator on the efficacy of an agonist binding to a receptor protein.
- *Cooperativity*: The effective interaction between the two cobinding allosteric molecules on the protein, that is, the effect of one of the ligands on the affinity and efficacy of the other.
- *Ensemble*: A collection of protein conformations visualized as a snapshot in time in a dynamic system whereby the protein spontaneously samples an enormously large library of conformations.
- *Modulator (allosteric)*: A molecule that cobinds with another on a protein to affect the behavior of the protein toward the cell and the cobinding ligand.
- *Negative allosteric modulator (NAM)*: An allosteric modulator that antagonizes agonist activation of a receptor, that is, reduces the

affinity and/or efficacy of an agonist for a receptor (an allosteric antagonist).

- *Positive allosteric modulator (PAM)*: An allosteric modulator that promotes agonist activation of a receptor, that is, increases the affinity and/or the efficacy of an agonist for a receptor.
- *Probe dependence*: Variation of activity of an allosteric modulator as it modifies the protein interaction with various probes (radioligands, agonists).

Protein allosterism

Allosteric interactions on proteins, such as receptors and ion channels occur through the binding of a molecule to the protein to affect its free energy of conformation. This subsequently affects the behavior of the protein toward the cell, other proteins, and ligands. The change in behavior occurs through a change in the conformation of the protein. The energy of the protein changes upon ligand binding no matter how relatively small the molecule is in relation to the protein. There are a number of proposed mechanisms for protein allostery, ranging from the existence of low-energy pathways between binding sites (allosteric "hot wires") to the stabilization of global protein conformations. A major milestone in the consideration of protein behavior was given by Koshland [1] who described how structured enzymes (modeled by the historical "lock-and-key" model of rigid proteins) accommodated substrates through the movement of amino acid residues ("induced fit"; see Box 5.1).

For receptors, this induced-fit model is less applicable than the conformational selection model discussed in Chapter 2, Drug Affinity and Efficacy (see Fig. 2.6 and Box 2.5), which describes the stabilization of global protein conformations through ligand binding. Receptors and other protein drug targets are complex macromolecules that exist in a multitude of tertiary inter

convertable conformations (shapes). At any one instant, a collection of protein molecules will have a selection of different conformations of similar free energy; these collections are called ensembles. As discussed in Chapter 2, Drug Affinity and Efficacy, the binding of a ligand initiates a process of conformational selection within the ensemble where the ligand preferentially binds to the conformations for which it has the highest affinity at the expense of others. The process of conformational selection by allosteric ligands is discussed in Box 5.2. If the enriched protein species mediates cellular response, then the ligand is an agonist. In this chapter, ligands that produce a conformational change to affect the behavior of the protein toward other molecules will be considered; these molecules are referred to as *allosteric modulators*.

BOX 5.1

Koshland and induced fit into proteins

In 1894 Emil Fischer accounted for the extraordinary specificity of enzyme-substrate interactions with a description of a strict geometric complementarity; this idea became famous as a "lock-and-key" hypothesis for recognition between molecules and proteins. While this explained enzyme recognition of substrates, it did not account for the stabilization of a new state of the enzyme referred to as the "transition state" needed to induce enzyme catalysis. Daniel Koshland, working at the University of California, Berkely, recognized that proteins are flexible structures and hypothesized that they accommodate the substrate by molding their shape around it; the substrate may also change its shape to optimize a conformation ideal for catalysis. This idea, referred to as "induced fit," overturned a 100-year-old view of how enzymes function and paved the way for allosteric theories of enzyme and receptor mechanisms.

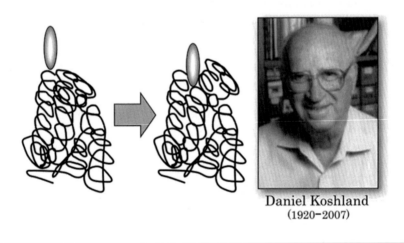

Daniel Koshland
(1920−2007)

Protein allostery describes the process of *cooperativity* between binding sites, that is, the binding of a molecule at one site on the protein alters the subsequent interaction of the protein with other molecules binding at other sites. One of the earliest models of allosterism in proteins, termed the Monod−Wyman−Changeux model [5], describes the binding of molecules to proteins made up of multiple subunits, whereby the binding of a molecule to one subunit alters the subsequent binding of molecules to other subunits. Fig. 5.1 shows the binding of a

BOX 5.2

Do proteins make conformations they don't normally know how to make?

When a ligand binds to a receptor protein and the conformation of that receptor changes, it may not be clear if the ligand has actually actively changed the shape of the protein (conformational induction) or if the ligand has stabilized that conformation from an array of conformations that the protein already makes (conformational selection). In terms of energetics, it is predicted that the energy required for a protein to make a conformation it does not already know how to make is inordinately high. In addition, there is a kinetic rationale for conformational selection over induction in biological systems. Specifically, the timecourse for the various transitions shown in the figure are given by the integration of the differential equations $d[AR]/dt = k_1[A][R] - k_1[AR]$ and $d[AR^*]/dt = k_2[AR] - k_2[AR^*]$ [3]. A reasonable assumption considers that the interaction between the ligand and the inactive receptor will be weak, leading to a guideline parameter for k_1 of $10^4\,M^{-1}s^{-1}$. Conformational changes within proteins being on the order of $10^2\,s^{-1}$ lead to a half time for the formation of $[AR^*]$ of 2.5 hours (it would take a day to reach equilibrium). In contrast, conformational selection yields a half time of 80 seconds. Conceptually, it is difficult to differentiate induction from the selection of an extremely rare preexisting conformation and there is evidence to suggest that some allosteric conformations may be rare and not often spontaneously formed by the protein. Specifically, the inordinately long times required to achieve steady states for allosteric enzyme inhibitors [4] have been explained in terms of the rarity of the allosteric conformation chosen by the allosteric ligand, that is, the ligand has nowhere to bind until the rare conformation is formed by the spontaneous dynamics of the protein ensemble.

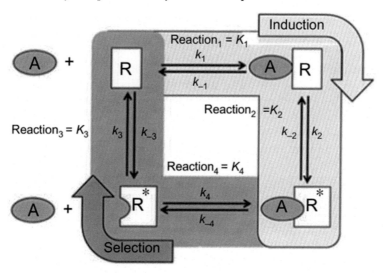

Source: *Figure redrawn from: T. Kenakin, New concepts in pharmacological efficacy at 7TM receptors: IUPHAR review 2. Br. J. Pharmacol. 168 (2013) 554–575* [2].

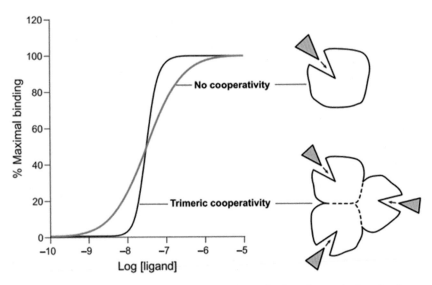

FIGURE 5.1 Dose-response curve for the binding of a ligand to a single subunit protein according to the Langmuir isotherm (Eq. 2.1, curve in gray marked "no cooperativity") and to a protein made up of three identical cooperatively linked subunits (black curve labeled "trimeric cooperativity"). For the trimer the binding of the ligand to one subunit promotes the binding to the second and the third, causing the binding curve to be steeper than that for a monomer.

molecule to a single subunit and to a trimeric protein consisting of three subunits, where the binding of each promotes the binding of the next (positive cooperativity). This produces a steep curve with a slope greater than unity for the Hill coefficient. Such binding behavior can be advantageous in physiology; for example, the tetrameric cooperativity of oxygen binding to hemoglobin optimizes the delivery of oxygen to tissues (see Box 5.3).

Allosteric ligands bind to their own site on the protein. This opens the possibility of also binding the endogenous ligand as a cobinding ligand. This geographical distinction between binding sites was one of the first features of allosterism to be discovered. Specifically, the modification of biosynthetic enzyme activity, through the binding of a structurally unrelated downstream product of biosynthetic pathways (as in the case of the biosynthesis of isoleucine [6]), was one of the first indications that proteins, such as enzymes can bind molecules at multiple sites to modify their activity (Fig. 5.2). The binding of molecules to separate sites leads to a permissive system (whereby the action of one of the ligands may not necessarily preclude the action of another); this can facilitate an interaction between the endogenous ligand and the modulator. It also means that the behavior of the modulator-bound protein can

---

BOX 5.3

Allostery at work: cooperative binding of oxygen to hemoglobin

Hemoglobin is a tetrameric protein that binds and transports four oxygen molecules per unit and then releases them to myoglobin. The binding of oxygen to hemoglobin is allosterically cooperative, in that the binding of each oxygen molecule facilitates the binding of the next. As shown on the curve to the right, this produces a steep binding curve ideal for oxygen binding, transport, and release. It can be seen from these curves that oxygen readily binds to hemoglobin at the high pO_2 values in the lung (100 torr). However, in tissues with lower oxygen levels (pO_2 20–40 torr) the cooperative binding of oxygen to hemoglobin causes the oxygen binding to drop off sharply. This allows hemoglobin to release oxygen to myoglobin. It can be seen that the noncooperative binding of oxygen to myoglobin causes it to be more tightly bound in this region of oxygen tension (20–40 torr).

The cooperative binding of oxygen is caused by the interaction of the four subunits of hemoglobin, whereby the binding of an oxygen molecule to one subunit increases the affinity of the remaining subunits for oxygen.

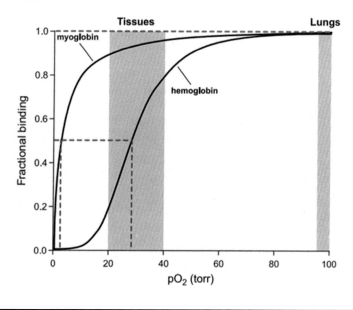

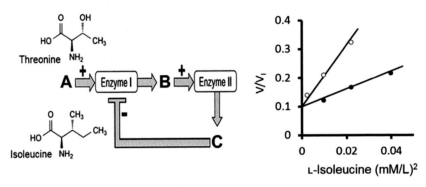

FIGURE 5.2 Negative feedback inhibition by the product of an enzyme cascade. The product of enzyme II (compound C; isoleucine) is structurally different from substrate A (threonine), yet inhibits enzyme I through an allosteric site. Panel on right shows the inhibition of the utilization of threonine in threonineless mutants of *Escherichia coli* by isoleucine in the presence of 10 mM (open circles) and 20 mM l-threonine (redrawn from [4]). This system is optimal for control of output since the overall product then controls the initial rate of the reaction cascade.

vary for different cobinding ligands. This is one of the most important features of allostery, namely, *probe dependence*. If the endogenous ligand is thought of as a probe of receptor function, then a given allosteric modulator can have *different* effects on different probes. The second important feature of allostery is *saturation of effect*. Unlike competitive mechanisms where effects can continue as long as different quantities of the interactants are added to the system, allosteric effects cease when the allosteric site on the protein is saturated. These properties of probe dependence and saturation of effect will surface repeatedly throughout this chapter as the specific properties of allosteric modulators are discussed.

Allosteric phenotypes

In general, there is no way to predict the effects of an allosteric ligand. It is possible that, upon binding an allosteric ligand, a receptor may have altered affinity (through a cooperativity term α), efficacy (through a cooperativity term β), or be directly stimulated by the modulator to produce a response (through an allosteric efficacy term τ_B)—see Fig. 5.3. Moreover, there are no constraints as to the combinations of properties that can be given to the receptor, that is, α may be $>$ or $<$, β may be $>$ or $<$ and efficacy τ_B will be subject to the normal constraints of agonism (tissue sensitivity—see Box 4.5).

Fig. 5.4A shows the effect of an allosteric modulator on the affinity of full and partial agonists; an increased affinity causes a shift to the left of

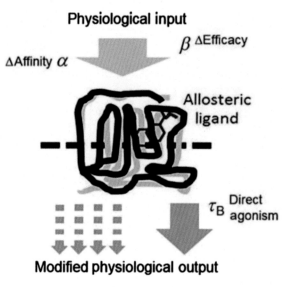

Physiological input

β ΔEfficacy

ΔAffinity α

Allosteric ligand

τ_B **Direct agonism**

Modified physiological output

FIGURE 5.3   Three characteristic parameters of allosteric ligands. Considering a receptor receiving physiological input (i.e., binding of neurotransmitter or hormone to mediate physiological response), the allosteric ligand can alter the affinity of the endogenous agonist through a cooperativity term α, modify the efficacy of the endogenous agonist through a cooperativity term β, or itself produce direct agonism through a positive allosteric efficacy denoted τ_B. There are no constraints on the direction or magnitude of any of these effects for any given allosteric ligand-endogenous agonist pair.

the dose-response curve, and a decreased affinity causes a shift to the right. Fig. 5.4B shows the effect of allosteric changes in the efficacy of full and partial agonists. In this case, increased efficacy will shift the curve to a full agonist to the left, whereas for a partial agonist, it will produce an increase in the maximal response. Similarly, a decreased efficacy can shift the dose-response curve to a full agonist with a high receptor reserve to the right or, in cases of smaller receptor reserves, depress the maximal response. For a partial agonist, which by definition has no receptor reserve, a decrease in efficacy will depress the maximal response (see Fig. 5.4B). At this point, it is worth considering how these properties of allosteric modulators can lead to unique drug behaviors therapeutically.

Considering all possibilities leads to 17 combinations of parameters but for all practical considerations, three phenotypes of receptor activity (with two agonist variants) emerge.

Thus if $\alpha\beta < 1$, negative allosteric modulation results and the ligands are referred to as negative allosteric modulators (NAMs)—see Fig. 5.5A. If $\alpha\beta > 1$, then potentiation of response occurs and these ligands are referred to as positive allosteric modulators (PAMs)—Fig. 5.5B.

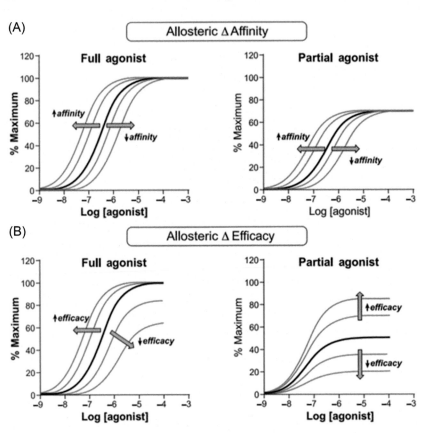

FIGURE 5.4 The various possible effects of an allosteric modulator on the response to an agonist. Panel A: Changes in the affinity of the receptor for both full and partial agonists result in shifts along the concentration axis of the dose-response curves (to the left for increased affinity and to the right for decreased affinity). Panel B: Effects of modulator-induced increases or decreases in agonist efficacy differ for full and partial agonists. Since, the system cannot show further increased maximal responses to a full agonist, modulator-induced increased efficacy results in shifts to the left of the dose-response curve to a full agonist. For a partial agonist, the maximal response will increase. With a decrease in efficacy, the maximal response to a partial agonist will decrease. This may also occur for a full agonist, although this will depend on the magnitude of the receptor reserve for the full agonist (i.e., see Fig. 4.10). Therefore if there is a high receptor reserve for the full agonist, a modulator-induced decrease in efficacy may result in a shift to the right of the dose-response curve with little depression of maximum. If the receptor reserve is small, then a modulator-induced decrease in efficacy will result in a depression of the maximal response.

A unique phenotype emerges, if $\alpha > 1$ and $\beta < 1$ to yield PAM-antagonists (Fig. 5.5C). These phenotypes can also be seen with concomitant positive agonism to give NAM-agonists (Fig. 5.5D) and PAM-agonists (Fig. 5.5E). These phenotypes confer unique modifications of physiological signaling, which can be exploited for therapeutic purpose.

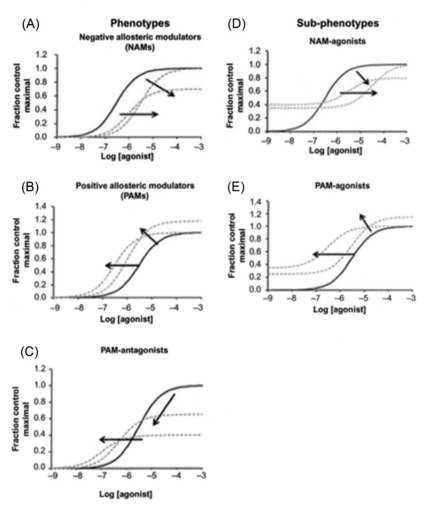

FIGURE 5.5 Phenotypic profiles for allosteric receptor ligands. Arrows represent direction of response in the presence of allosteric modulation. (A) NAMs decrease agonist response through a dextral displacement of dose-response curves and/or a depression of maximal response. (B) PAMs potentiate responses through sinistral displacement of curves and/or increased maximal responses. (C) PAM-antagonists produce sinistral displacement of curves and depression of maxima. (D) NAM-agonists produce NAM effects with concomitant direct agonism. (E) PAM-agonists produce PAM effects with concomitant agonism. *NAM*, negative allosteric modulator; *PAM*, positive allosteric modulator.

There are no a priori rules for how a given allosteric modulator will affect the action of receptor probes. If the responsiveness of the receptor is reduced to a given probe, then the molecule is an *allosteric antagonist* (see Fig. 5.3). It should be noted that the principle of probe dependence

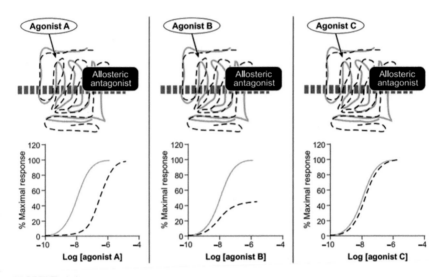

FIGURE 5.6   Probe dependence of an allosteric antagonist for three agonists A, B, and C. The modulator produces surmountable antagonism of responses to agonist A, a non-competitive antagonism of responses to B, and no effect at all on responses to agonist C. Such behavior is characteristic of allosteric modulators.

dictates that different probes may be affected in different ways. Thus an allosteric antagonist may block some agonists but not others (Fig. 5.6).

An example of where this type of behavior may have therapeutic relevance is in the use of allosteric antagonists of HIV-1 entry for AIDs—see Box 5.4. The pattern of antagonism can vary from being surmountable to being insurmountable. A discerning feature of allosteric antagonists is that they can produce a maximal asymptotic effect (when the allosteric site is fully occupied); the maximal effect they have on a receptor system is determined by cooperativity factors (*vide infra*). This fact can be used to differentiate allosteric antagonism from orthosteric antagonism.

For example, a given surmountable allosteric effect may produce shifts to the right of the agonist dose-response curve that come to a maximal value (see Fig. 5.7A). Under these circumstances, Schild analysis in such a system produces a distinct curvature of the Schild plot (Fig. 5.7B).

The use of this concept to identify allosterism is discussed later in this chapter. Some allosteric modulators can also increase the responsiveness of protein targets; these are referred to as PAMs (see Fig. 5.8). The effects of PAMS are also subject to probe dependence—see Fig. 5.8.

As noted earlier, allosteric systems are permissive in that the endogenous agonist may still interact with the receptor; in fact, the relevant species for therapy is the receptor with both the endogenous agonist and the allosteric modulator bound to the receptor. This is in contrast to orthosteric systems where there is never a receptor species with both the

BOX 5.4

Allosteric probe dependence provides a therapeutic advantage in AIDs therapy

As discussed in Chapter 3, Predicting Agonist Effect (see Box 3.5), chemokines internalize the CCR5 receptor, which is used for HIV-1 to infect cells. Therefore an intrinsic advantage would be gained with an antagonist of HIV-1 binding to the receptor that otherwise allowed chemokines, such as CCL3L1 to internalize the receptor. Allosteric antagonists have the capability of being probe-dependent and thus show differential blockade of different probes of the CCR5 receptor. In this case, an allosteric HIV-1 entry inhibitor that preferentially blocked HIV-1 binding over CCL3L1-induced receptor internalization would be predicted to be advantageous. Such probe dependence is seen with the two allosteric HIV-1 inhibitors TAK779 and TAK652. While TAK779 shows preferential potency for the blockade of CCL3L1-induced receptor internalization over HIV-1 entry, TAK652 shows a more favorable profile of greater potency for HIV-1 entry over CCL3L1-induced internalization. This degree of added selectivity may allow ambient chemokines to internalize CCR5 receptors (and thus reduce HIV-1 infection) as well as directly blocking HIV-1 binding to the receptor.

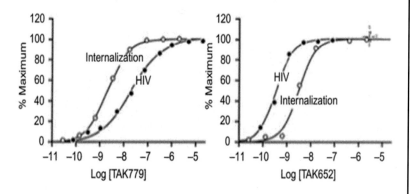

Source: *Data redrawn from: V.M. Muniz-Medina, S. Jones, J.M. Maglich, C. Galardi, R.E. Hollingsworth, W.M. Kazmierski, et al., The relative activity of "function sparing" HIV-1 entry inhibitors on viral entry and CCR5 internalization: is allosteric functional selectivity a valuable therapeutic property? Mol. Pharmacol. 75 (2009) 490–501 [7].*

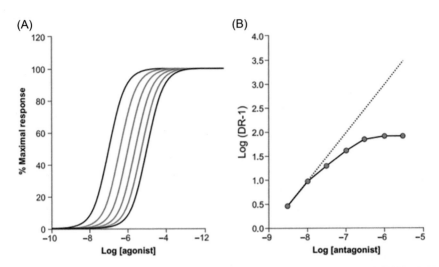

FIGURE 5.7   Surmountable allosteric antagonism. Panel A shows the limited antagonism produced by an allosteric antagonist; the limit of antagonism is reached when the
concentration of modulator fully saturates the allosteric binding site. This limit of dextral
displacement of the dose-response curves is reflected in a downward curvature in the
Schild regression (Panel B); such curvilinear Schild regressions are characteristic of surmountable allosteric antagonists.

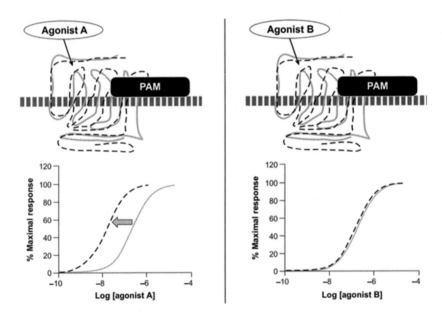

FIGURE 5.8   Probe dependence of a positive allosteric modulator (PAM) for two agonists
A and B. While the modulator potentiates responses to agonist A, no effect is seen on agonist B. As with allosteric antagonism, such behavior is characteristic of allosteric modulators.

antagonist and the agonist bound simultaneously. The permissive nature of allosteric systems opens the possibility that the allosteric ligand will induce biased signaling, that is, the natural quality of the endogenous agonist efficacy will change with allosteric modulation. Box 5.5 shows this effect on the signaling of prostaglandin D2 by the NAM indole$_1$.

BOX 5.5

Negative allosteric modulators (NAMs) induce biased signaling in natural systems

Negative and positive allosteric modulators may allow the natural endogenous agonist to interact and produce receptor effects even when the NAM or PAM is bound to the receptor. This opens the possibility that the natural signaling will be modified, that is, the quality of efficacy of the natural agonist will be allosterically altered. In the example below, the NAM Indole1 binds to the CRTH2 receptor to confer signaling bias on the natural agonist prostaglandin D2 (PDG2). Specifically, it is known that under normal circumstances, PDG2 binds to the receptor to activate Gi protein and also β-arrestin. Upon binding of indole1, only the β-arrestin response to PDG2 is blocked; the ability of PDG2 to activate Gi protein is not altered. Thus in the presence of indole$_1$, the quality of PDG2 efficacy is changed.

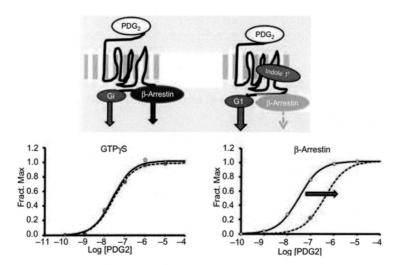

Source: *Data redrawn from: J.M. Mathiesen, T. Ulven, L. Martini, L.O. Gerlach, A. Heinemann, E. Kostenis, Identification of indole derivatives exclusively interfering with a G protein independent signaling pathway of the prostaglandin D2 receptor CRTH2. Mol. Pharmacol. 68 (2005) 393–402 [8].*

At this point, it is worth considering how these properties of allosteric modulators can lead to unique drug behaviors therapeutically.

Unique effects of allosteric modulators

To discuss the unique effects of allosteric modulators, it is first useful to consider orthosteric antagonists. These are molecules that preclude access of other molecules, such as agonists, to the receptor; these types of preemptive systems lead to the same maximal result, namely, an inactivated (or in the case of partial agonists, a partially activated) receptor to all agonism. In contrast, allosteric molecules are permissive in that they potentially allow interaction of the protein with other molecules; the result of an allosterically modulated system can be different for different agonists. This property of saturation of effect cause allosteric modulators to have a unique range of activities. These are:

The potential to alter the interaction of very large proteins

A hallmark of large protein-protein effects is that they probably involve multiple areas of interaction. Under these conditions, an orthosteric ligand (one that alters only a single region of the protein) would be predicted to be minimally effective. However, an allosteric ligand that stabilizes a new global conformation of the protein (see Fig. 5.9) has the potential to alter the position of numerous areas of the protein, and thereby affect large protein-protein interactions. An example of this type of effect is the blockade of the interaction of the chemokine CCR5 receptor and the HIV-1 virus coat protein gp120 (both large proteins) by the allosteric ligand aplaviroc (1/200 the size of the proteins) to prevent HIV-1 infection [9].

The potential to modulate but not completely activate and/or inhibit receptor function

The saturation of the allosteric effect upon complete occupancy of the allosteric site allows allosteric modulators to produce limited effects on target proteins. For example, an allosteric antagonist may produce only a maximal 10-folds decrease in the affinity of the receptor for a given agonist (Fig. 5.10A). As can be seen from Fig. 5.10A, a pIC_{50} plot (see chapter: Drug Antagonism Orthosteric Drug Effects) under these conditions yields a curve that does not reach the baseline. This is a hallmark of the allosteric antagonist modulators that have limited maximal effects on receptors. The same net effect can be seen with allosteric antagonists that reduce the efficacy of receptor agonists (see Fig. 5.10B). Thus it can

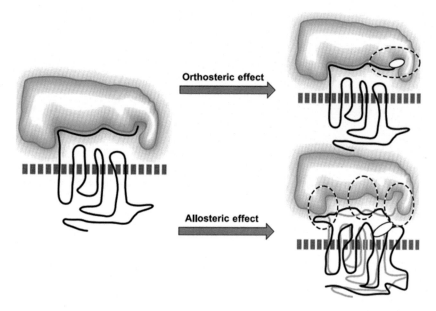

FIGURE 5.9 Disruption of the interaction of two proteins with multiple points of inter-action. Top panel shows how an orthosteric molecule may interfere with protein-protein interaction at the site of binding. Bottom panel shows how stabilization of different global protein conformation can alter numerous regions of the protein to correspondingly affect numerous regions of interaction between the proteins.

be seen that, unlike an orthosteric antagonist, an allosteric antagonist modulator can reduce the responsiveness of a target without completely blocking its function. Another feature of saturability is that it can disas-sociate the length of time of target blockade from the degree of block-ade, that is, high doses of a limited allosteric antagonist can allow a strategy whereby the production of a pool of drug gives a long-lasting effect without overdose (see Box 5.6).

Preservation of physiological patterns

While direct agonism produces blanket activation of systems, PAMs potentiate the existing responses in proportion to the natural physiological tone. This may be important in regions, such as the brain, where failing complex patterns of neurological signaling may need to be augmented (as in diseases, such as Alzheimer's).

Reduction in side effects

A PAM produces no direct effect, but rather has an action only when the system is active through the presence of the natural agonist.

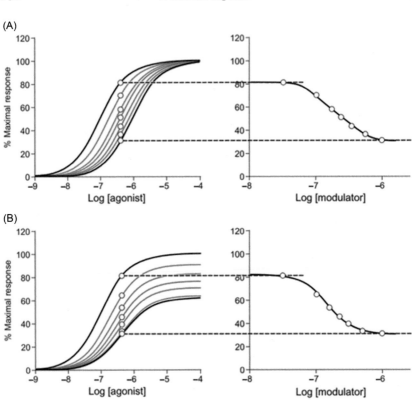

FIGURE 5.10 pIC$_{50}$ curves for allosteric antagonists that produce limited maximal blockade of functional effects. (A) The pIC$_{50}$ curve for a surmountable allosteric antagonist that produces a limited maximal shift to the right of the agonist dose-response curve may have a maximal value of inhibition that is above the baseline value of no agonism. (B) The same effect can occur with a noncompetitive allosteric modulator that produces a limited maximal blockade.

Under these conditions, it would be expected that a lower side-effect profile for the PAM would be observed.

Can produce texture in antagonism

While orthosteric antagonists all produce a common end product upon saturation of binding (namely, an inoperative biological target), allosteric antagonists produce antagonism through alterations of protein conformation, and these need not be identical. Under these circumstances, different allosteric modulators could produce pharmacological blockade through the production of different protein conformations. This may be of importance in diseases, such as AIDs where it is expected that HIV-1 viral mutation will eventually lead to tolerance to

---

BOX 5.6

High target coverage without overdose

The fact that allosteric effects are saturable (the effect stops when the allosteric site is fully occupied) can lead to a maximal asymptote for antagonism. This can, in turn, lead to a dissociation between the intensity of the effect and duration of action. Specifically, to achieve a long-lasting effect, high doses of an antagonist must be used. With an orthosteric antagonist, this will, in turn, produce a large maximal effect, which may lead to toxic interactions. In contrast, an allosteric antagonist achieves a self-limiting maximal effect. Increasing the dosage of such a molecule will not produce an overdose, but will rather prolong the effect in vivo.

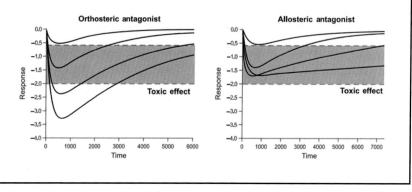

---

an HIV-1 entry inhibitor as the virus mutates to a form that can utilize the allosterically modified receptor. Therapy with a different allosteric modulator (one that produces a different conformation) could overcome this viral resistance.

Can have separate effects on agonist affinity and efficacy

There is no a priori rule to dictate that allosteric changes need to be in the same vectorial direction (antagonism or potentiation). Thus it is possible to have an allosteric modulator that changes agonist affinity in one direction and efficacy in another (see Fig. 5.11). One particular combination of these activities can be useful, namely, an allosteric antagonist modulator that increases agonist affinity but decreases agonist efficacy. The outcome of this combination is an antagonist that becomes more potent with higher agonist concentrations, that is, the antagonist develops use dependence (see Box 5.7).

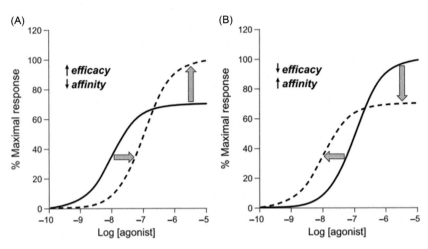

FIGURE 5.11 Effects of allosteric modulators that have opposite effects on agonist affinity and efficacy. (A) The allosteric ligand reduces agonist affinity and increases efficacy of a partial agonist; this will shift the dose-response curve to the right but increase maximal response. (B) A modulator that increases the affinity of the agonist but decreases the efficacy may shift the dose-response curve to the left (although the two effects may cancel to make this shift minimal) and will decrease the maximal response.

Allosteric modulators exercise "probe dependence"

Allosterism involves a change in the shape of the protein, and it is quite possible that a given change in shape could be catastrophic to the activity of one probe (i.e., agonist) but have no effect at all on another, especially if those probes bind to different regions of the protein. This has ramifications for the therapeutic application and also for the mode of discovery of allosteric modulators. In terms of the impact of probe dependence on the therapeutic application of allosteric modulators, the possibility exists that a given modulator could block or potentiate the endogenous agonist and have no effect on other receptor probes. For example, the CCR5 chemokine receptor mediates HIV-1 entry, leading to infection. However, activation of the CCR5 receptor by natural chemokines also offers protection against progression to AIDS after infection. Therefore an ideal HIV-1 entry inhibitor would block the utilization of CCR5 by HIV-1 but otherwise allow normal chemokine function for this receptor; this is possible with allosteric modulators. In support of this idea, varying relative activities of allosteric modulators for HIV-1 entry versus chemokine function have been noted experimentally [7]—see Box 5.4. In terms of how allosteric modulators are discovered and developed, this same probe dependence dictates that the endogenous ligand (i.e., the one that is targeted therapeutically) should be used in the screening and discovery process. For example, a PAM

BOX 5.7

Use dependence for allosteric antagonists

An allosteric antagonist stabilizes a unique receptor protein conformation, and this can lead to differences in the agonist affinity and/or efficacy. A modulator that increases the affinity of the agonist and decreases its efficacy can become more potent as the physiological system it is designed to block is driven to higher levels of activity; a "use dependence." This is due to the reciprocal nature of allosteric energy transfer. Thus just as the modulator increases the affinity of the agonist, so too will the agonist increase the affinity of the allosteric antagonist. Therefore the affinity of the antagonist will increase as the agonist concentration increases. Since, the presence of the antagonist on the receptor precludes activation by the agonist (the modulator decreases agonist efficacy), the antagonism will increase as the concentration of agonist increases. Thus the IC_{50} for blockade of a given level of response will decrease for the blockade of a higher level of response (i.e., see graph where the IC_{50} at 90% is $<IC_{50}$ at 50%). This type of activity is seen of the NMDA blocker ifenprodil [10] and the cannabinoid CB1 receptor blocker Org27569 [11].

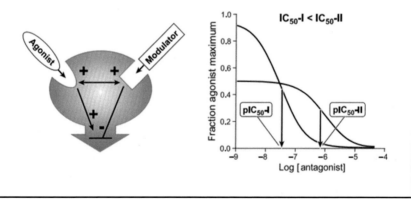

would be of use in augmenting a failing cholinergic neuronal transmission in Alzheimer's disease. However, the natural agonist (acetylcholine) is chemically unsuitable for use in a drug discovery screen and subsequent experiments. Under these circumstances, stable analogs, namely, carbachol and/or pilocarpine, are often used in the screening process. However, probe dependence predicts that the activity of allosteric ligands could be very different for natural versus synthetic ligands. For example, it has been observed that PAMs, such as LY2033298 cause agonist-dependent differential potentiation of different agonists, such as acetylcholine and oxotremorine [12]. This is also relevant to PAMs for targets with multiple natural agonists. For example, the antidiabetic PAM NOVO2 produces a fivefold potentiation of one of the natural agonists for the GLP-1 receptor GLP-1(7−36)NH_2, but a 25-fold potentiation of oxyntomodulin, another natural agonist for this receptor [13]. These data suggest that all agonists for a given receptor need to be tested when studying the effects of allosteric modulators.

Detecting allosterism

If a ligand potentiates endogenous signaling through binding to a target protein, it clearly is an allosteric ligand, that is, potentiation would occur only through the cobinding of endogenous agonist and modulator. However, for antagonists, it may not be immediately clear whether the effect is orthosteric or allosteric, since both mechanisms can produce surmountable or insurmountable blockade. There are two strategies that can be used to detect allosteric antagonism. The first is through elevation of the range of concentrations tested; this approach can be used to uncover saturation of effect (i.e., detect curvature in Schild regressions to observe a maximal plateau in antagonist effect). Fig. 5.12A shows the effect of a surmountable allosteric antagonist and how the shifts to the right of the dose-response curves differ from those of an equipotent orthosteric simple competitive antagonist. As shown in Fig. 5.4B, the saturation in the maximal shift to the right of the curve results in a curvilinear Schild regression. Fig. 5.12B shows a comparable saturation of effect for a noncompetitive (insurmountable) allosteric antagonist. In this case, an orthosteric antagonist will reduce the agonist response to baseline (zero response to the agonist) when given in a suitably high concentration, whereas an allosteric antagonist may not. The other approach to detecting allosterism is through probe dependence; testing as many agonists as possible may uncover agonist-related differences in effect.

To definitively confirm the allosteric effect, changes in the kinetics of interaction of the protein target with agonists and/or other probes (i.e., radioligands) must be determined, since such changes can only be produced by allosteric ligands. The basis for this mechanism is the chemical nature of the association (k_1) and dissociation (k_2) kinetics of ligands for protein receptors; both of these mechanisms depend on the tertiary conformation of the protein. Specifically, both k_1 and k_2 are unique for every protein conformation/ligand pairing; therefore, if a ligand produces a change in either k_1 or k_2 for another ligand, this can only occur through a change in the conformation of the protein.

If an allosteric ligand produces potentiation of effect, then the K_{eq} either for binding or effect will decrease, that is, the potency of the

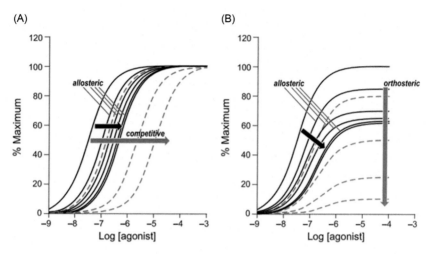

FIGURE 5.12 Saturation of allosteric effect. An allosteric antagonist modulator will have a limited maximal antagonism (although this may be quite large for some modulators), which may become evident when a wide range of concentrations of modulator are tested. (A) Whereas a simple competitive orthosteric antagonist will produce theoretically limitless shifts to the right of the agonist dose-response curve (broken gray lines), an allosteric modulator effect will cease when the allosteric site is saturated (black line curves). (B) Similarly, high concentrations of an orthosteric noncompetitive antagonist will depress the maximal response to an agonist to baseline values (broken gray lines), whereas an allosteric noncompetitive antagonist may block to a maximal effect above baseline (black line curves).

agonist will increase. Since, K_{eq} is k_2/k_1 (see chapter: Drug Affinity and Efficacy), potentiation (decrease in K_{eq}) can occur either through a decrease in k_2 (decrease in rate of dissociation) or an increase in k_1 (increase in rate of association), or some combination of these. The rate of dissociation of an agonist can be measured by viewing the decay of the response of the agonist after washing and the addition of a high concentration of antagonist. The antagonist is used to prevent rebinding of the agonist during the washout stage; under these circumstances, the decay of response reflects the k_2. Most PAM effects reflect decreases in k_2, as k_1 is often diffusion rate-limited (see Fig. 5.13).

Similarly, allosteric antagonism can result from either a decrease in k_1 or an increase in k_2; Fig. 5.14 shows the effect of increasing k_2 by a factor of five to produce a fivefold shift to the right of the agonist dose-response curve. The important concept in kinetic studies is the fact that a molecule must allow the agonist (probe of the receptor function) to bind in order to measure a change in rate of association or dissociation. Therefore by definition, only an allosteric molecule can alter the kinetics of agonist binding; an orthosteric molecule binds to the same site as the agonist and therefore does not allow agonist binding.

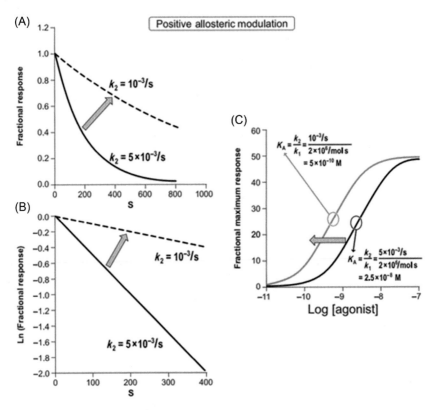

FIGURE 5.13 Alteration of kinetics of receptor dissociation by a positive allosteric modulator (PAM). Panel A shows the offset of receptor response to an agonist in the presence of a high concentration of a competitive antagonist; this reversal of response reflects the rate of dissociation of the agonist from the receptor (k_2). The solid line represents the system in the absence of the allosteric modulator; the dotted line shows the decrease in the offset rate (and subsequent decrease in the rate of dissociation) in the presence of the PAM. It can be seen that the k_2 value decreases by a factor of 5. Panel B shows the same plot on a log ordinate scale (fractional response expressed as the natural logarithm value). Panel C shows the effect of the PAM on the dose-response curve to the agonist. It can be seen that potentiation occurs (the agonist dose-response curve shifts to the left) as reflected by the decrease in k_2. In this experiment, the rate of association (k_1) does not change.

Quantifying allosteric effect

As with antagonism (see chapter: Drug Antagonism Orthosteric Drug Effects), allosteric effects can be quantified by comparing dose-response curves obtained in the presence of varying concentrations of allosteric modulators to behaviors predicted by quantitative models. The model

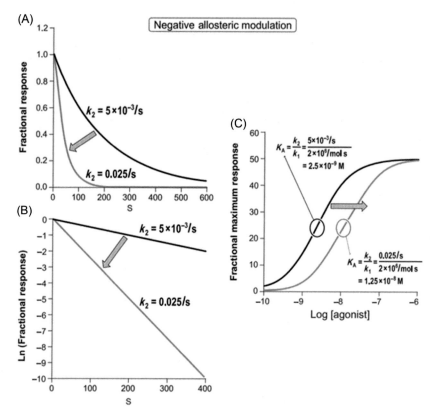

FIGURE 5.14 Alteration of kinetics of receptor dissociation by negative allosteric modulator (NAM). Panel A shows the offset of receptor response to an agonist in the presence of a high concentration of a competitive antagonist; this reversal of response reflects the rate of dissociation of the agonist from the receptor (k_2). The black line represents the system in the absence of the allosteric modulator; the gray line shows the increase in the offset rate (and subsequent increase in the rate of dissociation) in the presence of the NAM. It can be seen that the k_2 value increases by a factor of 5. Panel B shows the same plot on a log ordinate scale (fractional response expressed as the natural logarithm value). Panel C shows the effect of the allosteric modulator on the dose-response curve to the agonist. It can be seen that antagonism occurs (the agonist dose-response curve shifts to the right) as reflected by the increase in k_2. In this experiment, the rate of association (k_1) does not change.

that will be used is given below showing receptors (R), a receptor probe agonist (A), and an allosteric modulator (B):

Allosteric modification of the effect is quantified by the two cooperativity factors, α and β. As discussed previously, the term α quantifies the effect of the modulator B on the affinity of the receptor to A (and similarly, the reciprocal effect A has on the affinity of B). The term β quantifies the effect the modulator has on the efficacy of A. It can be seen from this model that an allosteric modulator cannot be characterized only by affinity (K_B^{-1}), but rather will also have a type of "efficacy" for the receptor and its interaction with A in the form of α and β. Accordingly, the following equation defines the response to an agonist (A) in the presence of an allosteric modulator (B) (see Derivations and Proofs, Appendix A.8) [14,15]:

$$\text{Response} = \frac{(\tau_A[A](K_B + \alpha\beta[B]))^n E_m}{(\tau_A[A](K_B + \alpha\beta[B]))^n + ([A]K_B + K_A K_B + K_A[B] + \alpha[A][B])^n}$$

(5.1)

where E_m is the maximal response capability of the system, τ_A is the efficacy of the agonist, K_A and K_B are the equilibrium dissociation constants of the agonist and modulator-receptor complexes, respectively, and n is a fitting factor for the curve. Just as for orthosteric antagonism, dose-response data is fit to Eq. (5.1) to yield values of K_B, α and $\beta$the characteristic descriptors of an allosteric modulator. For example, Fig. 5.15A shows the effects of an allosteric antagonist, which decreases both affinity ($\alpha = 0.3$) and efficacy ($\beta = 0.2$) of the agonist. Fig. 5.15B shows the effects of a PAM that increases the affinity ($\alpha = 20$) and efficacy ($\beta = 2$) of the agonist.

Allosteric modulators stabilize the conformational states of proteins and these may also have direct effects in their own right. Therefore the allosteric modulation can also be associated with direct agonism. Since a pure allosteric agonist binds to its own site on the protein and stabilizes an active state, this process can be independent of the process

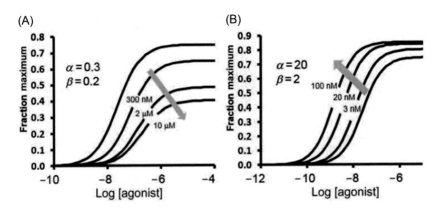

FIGURE 5.15   Fitting data to the model of allosteric function; Agonist $K_A = 300\,\text{nM}$, $\tau = 3$, $E_m = 100$ (Eq. 5.1). Panel A: Antagonism fit to the model for a negative allosteric modulator of $K_B = 100\,\text{nM}$, $\alpha = 0.3$, $\beta = 0.2$. Curves shown in the absence and presence of $300\,\text{nM}$ $2\,\mu\text{M}$ and $10\,\mu\text{M}$ negative modulator. Panel B: Data for a PAM of $K_B = 100\,\text{nM}$, $\alpha = 20$, $\beta = 2$. Curves shown in the absence and presence of $3\,\text{nM}$ $20\,\text{nM}$ and $100\,\text{nM}$ positive modulator.

of natural agonism produced by the endogenous agonist. The allosteric agonist may not interfere with the binding of the endogenous agonist, therefore, the resulting allosteric agonism will be additive to endogenous agonism; an example of this effect is shown in Fig. 5.16. However, since allosterism may produce a global change in the protein conformation, there is no priori reason why an allosteric agonist could not produce direct agonism along with a modified endogenous agonist response. Therefore just as with allosteric antagonists or PAMs, these changes could involve affinity (α) and/or efficacy (β). The model for description of agonist response in the presence of an allosteric modulator that may also produce direct agonism is (see Derivations and Proofs, Appendix A.9) [14,15]:

$$\text{Response} = \frac{(\tau_A[A](K_B+\alpha\beta[B])+\tau_B[B]K_A)^n E_m}{(\tau_A[A](K_B+\alpha\beta[B])+\tau_B[B]K_A)^n + ([A]K_B+K_AK_B+K_A[B]+\alpha[A][B])^n}$$

(5.2)

where the designations of the parameters are the same as for Eq. (5.1) with the addition that τ_B refers to the efficacy for direct agonism of the allosteric modulator.

Fig. 5.17A shows the effect of an allosteric agonist that also enhances the affinity ($\alpha = 20$) and efficacy ($\beta = 2$) of the endogenous agonist. It can be seen that in addition to a direct agonism, the responses to the endogenous agonist are enhanced. Fig. 5.17B shows the effect of an allosteric agonist modulator that reduces the affinity of the endogenous agonist ($\alpha = 0.2$; with no effect on efficacy $\beta = 1$). Interestingly, this type

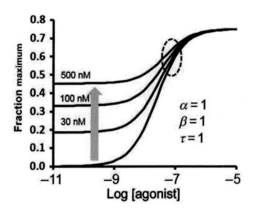

FIGURE 5.16 Fitting data to the model of allosteric function for modulator with direct agonist action for probe agonist $K_A = 100$ nM, $\tau = 3$, $E_m = 100$ (Eq. 5.2). Curves shown for the agonist alone and in the presence of an allosteric agonist of $K_B = 100$ nM, $\alpha = 1$, $\beta = 1$ and $\tau_B = 1$. Curves shown in the absence and presence of 30 nM 100 nM and 500 nM allosteric agonist.

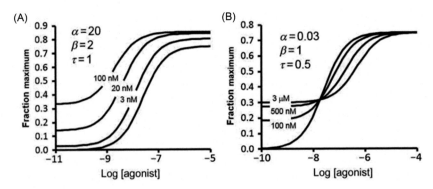

FIGURE 5.17 Fitting data to the model of allosteric function for modulator with the direct agonist action. For control probe agonist $K_A = 100$ nM, $\tau = 3$, $E_m = 100$ (Eq. 5.2). Panel A: Data for a PAM-agonist of $K_B = 100$ nM, $\alpha = 20$, $\beta = 2$ and $\tau_B = 1$. Curves shown in the absence and presence of 3 nM 20 nM and 100 nM PAM-agonist. Panel B: Antagonism fit to the model for a negative allosteric modulator with direct agonist activity of $K_B = 100$ nM, $\alpha = 0.3$, $\beta = 0.2$, $\tau_B = 0.5$. Curves shown in the absence and presence of 100 nM 500 nM and 3 μM negative modulator agonist.

of profile is very similar to that of a standard orthosteric partial agonist (see Fig. 4.18). To differentiate these profiles, the principles of saturation of effect and/or probe dependence would need to be applied.

The potency of an allosteric modulator is described by an affinity constant (pK_B) much like other antagonists. However, since the allosteric systems describe the energy of interaction between the two molecules acting on the protein, the effective affinity of the modulator is modified by the α factor provided by the cobinding ligand. Under these circumstances, it can be seen that different α factors for different ligands can lead to varying affinity, that is, the affinity of the modulator is contingent upon the nature of the cobinding ligand. Similarly, the functional effect of an allosteric modulator also depends upon the value of β, since this defines the effect of the modulator on the efficacy of the cobinding agonist. Therefore to fully characterize the allosteric effect of a modulator, values for the pK_B, α, and β and the identity of the cobinding must be designated. In practice, therapeutically targeted allosteric modulators usually deal with endogenous agonists; therefore a single set of pK_B, α, and β values for the endogenous ligand may be sufficient for characterization. However, in the case of multiple endogenous ligands (such as peptide receptors), complications may arise as the activity of the allosteric modulator may vary for different endogenous ligands. If probe dependence is *not* observed, it may be that the antagonist is still allosteric but that the wrong probes were utilized to detect the effect.

Descriptive pharmacology: V

A schematic diagram of the logic employed in the exploration of possible allosteric ligand effects is given in Fig. 5.18; it is governed by some key observations. The first observation describes the effect of the modulator on agonist response; if response is increased, then an allosteric effect is assumed since an orthosteric mechanism cannot accommodate this mechanism. Specifically, a molecule must cobind with the agonist to cause its potentiation. Under these circumstances, the dose-response curves can be fit to the allosteric model, specifically Eq. (5.1) if no direct modulator-agonist activity is seen and Eq. (5.2) if it is. The analysis is less straightforward if antagonism is observed. Under these circumstances the decision points identifying allosterism are based on conditional yes/no values. Specifically, if a distinct effect is obtained then allosterism is identified; if it is not, then it will be ambiguous in that allosterism may or may not be operative. For antagonism, if probe dependence is observed (i.e., the modulator blocks the effects of one agonist more than another), then allosterism is identified and Eqs. (5.1) and (5.2) can be applied. If no probe dependence is seen, it may be that

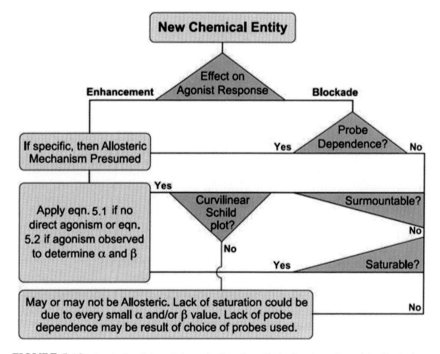

FIGURE 5.18   Logic for determining whether the effect of a given ligand is allosteric—see text.

the allosteric effect (if the antagonist is allosteric) is identical for the probes chosen for study. The next decision point comes from the observation of surmountability, that is, does the antagonist depress the maximal response? If not, then the antagonist is either an orthosteric simple competitive blocker or it is producing surmountable allosteric antagonism. Under these circumstances, the concentrations for blockade should be maximized to identify possible curvilinearity in the Schild plot (i.e., see Fig. 5.7B). If this is observed, allosterism is identified, and Eqs. (5.1) and (5.2) can be applied.

If depression of the maximal response is produced, then the concentrations of modulators can be increased to maximal values to try to identify saturation of effect (i.e., see Fig. 5.10B). If the antagonist brings the agonist's maximal response to baseline, then either the molecule is a noncompetitive orthosteric blocker or the values for β are small enough to completely negate agonism. If the depression of the maximum reaches an asymptotic limit (Fig. 5.10B), then allosterism is identified and Eqs. (5.1) or (5.2) can be applied.

Summary

The following concepts are discussed in this chapter:

- Allosteric systems are permissive in that two ligands bind to a protein (each to their own separate binding site) and affect the reactivity of the protein to each.
- This cobinding mechanism imparts unique features to allosteric modulators due to three distinct properties.
- The first unique property of allosterism is *saturability of effect*, that is, the allosteric modulation ends when the allosteric site is fully occupied.
- The second property is *probe dependence*, that is, the allosteric effect of a given modulator can be different for different cobinding ligands.
- The third property is that allosteric modulation can induce *separate effects* on cobinding ligand *affinity* and *efficacy*.
- While allosteric antagonism can appear to be simple orthosteric blockade, experiments can be done to identify possible saturation of effect and/or probe dependence to identify allosteric mechanisms.
- Only allosteric modulators can affect the kinetics of association or dissociation of cobinding ligands.
- Once allosterism has been identified as a mechanism, then comparison of data to an allosteric model can be used to identify characteristic parameters of the effect.

- These characteristics are: α (the effect of the modulator on the affinity of the cobinding ligand) and β (the effect of the modulator on the efficacy of the cobinding ligand).
- The magnitude of the effective pK_B (equilibrium dissociation constant of the modulator receptor complex) will depend on the nature of the cobinding ligand.

References

[1] D.E. Koshland, The active site of enzyme action, Adv. Enzymol. 22 (1960) 45–97.

[2] T. Kenakin, New concepts in pharmacological efficacy at 7TM receptors: IUPHAR review 2, Br. J. Pharmacol. 168 (2013) 554–575.

[3] H.R. Bosshard, Molecular recognition by induced fit: how fit is the concept? News Physiol. Sci. 16 (2001) 171–173.

[4] C. Tong, L. Churchill, P.F. Cirillo, T. Gilmore, A.G. Graham, P.M. Grob, Inhibition of p38 MAP kinase by utilizing a novel allosteric binding site, Nat. Struct. Mol. Biol. 9 (2002) 268–272.

[5] F. Monod, J. Wyman, J.P. Changeuz, On the nature of allosteric transitions, J. Biol. Chem. 12 (1965) 88–118.

[6] H.E. Umbarger, Evidence for a negative feedback mechanism in the biosynthesis of isoleucine, Science. 123 (1956) 848.

[7] V.M. Muniz-Medina, S. Jones, J.M. Maglich, C. Galardi, R.E. Hollingsworth, W.M. Kazmierski, The relative activity of "function sparing" HIV-1 entry inhibitors on viral entry and CCR5 internalization: is allosteric functional selectivity a valuable therapeutic property? Mol. Pharmacol. 75 (2009) 490–501.

[8] J.M. Mathiesen, T. Ulven, L. Martini, L.O. Gerlach, A. Heinemann, E. Kostenis, Identification of indole derivatives exclusively interfering with a G protein independent signaling pathway of the prostaglandin D2 receptor CRTH2, Mol. Pharmacol. 68 (2005) 393–402.

[9] C. Watson, S. Jenkinson, W. Kazmierski, T.P. Kenakin, The CCR5 receptor-based mechanism of action of 873140, a potent allosteric non-competitive HIV entry inhibitor, Mol. Pharmacol. 67 (2005) 1268–1282.

[10] J.N.C. Kew, G. Trube, J.A. Kemp, A novel mechanism of activity-dependent NMDA receptor antagonism describes the effect of ifenprodil in rat cultured cortical neurons, J. Physiol. 497 (3) (1996) 761–772.

[11] M.R. Price, G.L. Baillie, A. Thomas, L.A. Stevenson, M. Easson, R. Goodwin, Allosteric modulation of the cannabinoid CB1 receptor, Mol. Pharmacol. 68 (2005) 1484–1495.

[12] S. Suratman, K. Leach, P.M. Sexton, C.C. Felder, R.E. Loiacono, A. Christopoulos, Impact of species variability and "probe-dependence" on the detection and in vivo validation of allosteric modulation at the M4 muscarinic acetylcholine receptor, Br. J. Pharmacol. 162 (2011) 1659–1670.

[13] C. Koole, D. Wooten, J. Simms, C. Valant, R. Sridhar, O.L. Woodman, Allosteric ligands of the glucagon- like peptide 1 receptor (GLP-1R) differentially modulate endogenous and exogenous peptide responses in a pathway-selective manner: implications for drug screening, Mol. Pharmacol. 78 (2010) 456–465.

[14] T. Kenakin, New concepts in drug discovery: collateral efficacy and permissive antagonism, Nat. Rev. Drug Discov. 4 (2005) 919–927.

[15] F.J. Ehlert, Analysis of allosterism in functional assays, J. Pharmacol. Exp. Ther. 315 (2005) 740–754.

CHAPTER

6

Enzymes as drug targets

OUTLINE

Pharmacology in Drug Discovery and Development
DOI: https://doi.org/10.1016/B978-0-443-14124-9.00011-2

By the end of this chapter, students will understand how enzymes can be therapeutic drug targets. In addition to the four basic mechanisms of reversible enzyme inhibition, the topic of irreversible enzyme inhibition and enzyme activation will be discussed. Finally, the special cases of drug action on intracellular enzymes will be considered.

Introduction

Enzymes are nature's ubiquitous catalysts mediating thousands of biochemical reactions in the cell to control energy metabolism, oversee macromolecular synthesis, anabolic processes, regulate cell signaling, and control cell cycles. Enzymes also control the level of critical molecules in the cell. They do this by accelerating the rate of chemical reactions by lowering the reaction activation energy. Without such catalysts, these reactions would progress too slowly to sustain life. For example, without the presence of adenosine deaminase, the removal of the amine from adenosine would take 120 years (as opposed to the rate constant of activation of the enzyme of 370 seconds—an enhancement of 2.1×10^{12}-fold). Hundreds of enzymes control complex biochemical networks (many with strict fidelity to substrate type), although there are notable exceptions to this rule. Owing to their obvious key physiological role, enzymes are prime targets for therapeutic drug intervention.

New terminology

- *Catalysis*: The process of an enzyme producing a product from a bound substrate.
- *Competitive inhibition*: The inhibitor and substrate compete for the substrate binding site.
- *Covalent bond*: Chemical bond formed between the inhibitor and the enzyme through alkylation.
- *Irreversible inhibition*: The inhibitor has a negligible rate of dissociation from the enzyme once it binds.
- K_m: Michaelis—Menten constant referring to the sensitivity of an enzyme to a given substrate; it encompasses substrate binding and catalysis.

- *Mechanism-based inhibition*: The enzyme creates an active species through catalysis, which then goes on to alkylate the enzyme and inactivate it.
- *Mixed inhibition*: The inhibitor has different affinities for the enzyme and the enzyme-substrate complex.
- *Noncompetitive inhibition*: The inhibitor has equal affinity for the enzyme and the enzyme-substrate complex.
- *Substrate inhibition*: High concentrations of the substrate bind to different parts of the active site and enzyme activity is blocked.
- *Suicide inhibitor*: The inhibitor binds to the enzyme-active site and irreversibly inactivates the enzyme when it does so.
- *Tight-binding inhibitor*: The inhibitor has a negligible rate of dissociation from the enzyme once it binds, although the bond between the inhibitor and enzyme may not be covalent.
- *Uncompetitive inhibition*: The inhibitor binds only to the enzyme-substrate complex.
- V_{max}: The maximal rate of enzyme hydrolysis (characteristic for an enzyme-substrate pair).

Enzyme kinetics

The model used to describe enzyme kinetics is shown in Fig. 6.1A. Thus, a substrate binds to an enzyme (with a standard rate of association k_1 and dissociation k_2) and then a process of catalysis occurs (with a new rate constant k_{cat}), which results in a product (formed from the substrate) and regeneration of the enzyme. The enzyme, thus, acts as a catalyst to reduce the energy barrier that separates the substrate from the product (Fig. 6.1B). Enzymes can modify a single molecule or catalyze a reaction between two molecules; this can form a single product or there can be an exchange of atoms to produce two or more different products. The formal kinetic model used to describe enzyme reactions is the Michaelis—Menten model according to the equation (see Derivations and Proofs, Appendix A.10):

$$\text{Velocity} = \frac{[S]V_{max}}{[S] + K_m} \tag{6.1}$$

where [S] is the substrate concentration. V_{max} is the maximal rate of enzyme reaction and this, along with the magnitude of the amount of enzyme in the cell (and where it is located) describes the capacity of the enzyme system for catalysis. The K_m is a constant describing the

(A)

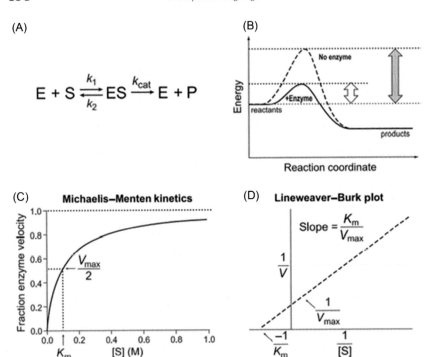

(B)

(C) Michaelis–Menten kinetics

(D) Lineweaver–Burk plot

FIGURE 6.1   Enzyme catalysis. (A) Scheme showing substrate [S] binding to enzyme [E] to form a complex [ES] which then, through k_{cat}, converts substrate to product [P] and initiates regeneration of enzyme E. (B) This can be seen as the enzyme functioning as a catalyst to lower the energy barrier for production of the product. (C) Graphical representation of the Michaelis–Menten equation for enzyme function Eq. (6.1). (D) Linear transformation of the Michaelis–Menten equation as published by Lineweaver and Burk (Eq. 6.3).

sensitivity of the enzyme reaction to substrate. In molecular terms, the K_m is further defined (see Fig. 6.1A) as:

$$K_m = \frac{k_2 + k_{cat}}{k_1} \tag{6.2}$$

The affinity of the substrate for the enzyme is described (as for binding in the Langmuir adsorption isotherm; see Eq. (6.1)) as $K_d = k_2/k_1$, but since this is not a static binding process (the reaction continues to the formation of product), k_{cat} must be included to describe the influence of catalysis on the binding process; k_{cat} is the collective rate constant for the forward progress of the chemical steps in catalysis. Therefore, K_d does not equal K_m unless $k_{cat} << k_2$.

Fig. 6.1C shows a graphical representation of Eq. (6.1); there are notable features in this relationship. For low substrate concentrations, enzyme velocity $\rightarrow (k_{cat}/K_m)[E][S]$ where $[E]$ is the enzyme concentration. Thus, the velocity of the reaction depends upon both the substrate concentration and the amount of enzyme present. Under these circumstances, the reaction resembles a bimolecular reaction with a pseudo second-order rate constant of k_{cat}/K_m. Efficient enzymes have values of k_{cat}/K_m approaching 10^8 to 10^{10}/M s (this becomes diffusion-limited). With high substrate concentrations ($[S] >> K_m$), the enzyme velocity is $V_{max} = k_{cat}[E]$. Under these circumstances, the rate of reaction depends only on the amount of enzyme present (unimolecular reaction with pseudo first-order rate constant k_{cat}).

The graphical relationship between substrate concentration and enzyme velocity according to the Michaelis–Menten equation Eq. (6.1) is shown in Fig. 6.1C. Here, it can be seen that the maximal velocity is V_{max} and the half-maximal velocity is the K_m (as a substrate concentration). Historically, a linear double reciprocal metameter of Eq. (6.1) has been used to analyze enzyme reactions according to the equation:

$$\frac{1}{V} = \frac{K_m}{[S]V_{max}} + \frac{1}{V_{max}} \qquad (6.3)$$

Termed as the Lineweaver–Burk equation, this yields a straight line with abscissal intercept of $-1/K_m$, an ordinate intercept of $1/V_{max}$, and a slope of K_m/V_{max} (see Fig. 6.1D). Before the widespread availability of computers able to fit data directly to nonlinear functions, linear transformations, such as the Lineweaver–Burk plot were used to estimate parameters; these could be calculated through linear regression analysis. However, the availability of techniques to fit data directly to the Michaelis–Menten equation has supplanted the use of linear transformations as the latter, being double reciprocal plots, can lead to seriously skewed estimates of parameters and are highly unreliable for the estimation of enzyme constants. It will be seen in future sections, however, that the Lineweaver–Burk plot can still be useful as an identifier of type of enzyme inhibition.

Enzymes as drug targets

Enzyme inhibitors have been used as therapeutic drugs throughout pharmacological history (see Box 6.1). There are numerous scenarios where drug intervention into an enzyme reaction can yield therapeutically favorable outcomes. These are:

BOX 6.1

From bitter bark to a universal remedy.

From the time of Hippocrates, (c.460–377 BC) extracts from the bitter bark and leaves of the willow tree were known to alleviate pain and fever. In 1828, a Professor of Pharmacy at the University of Munich isolated a tiny amount of yellow needle-like crystalline bitter-tasting crystals from willow bark, which he called salicin. In 1897, chemists at Bayer AG led by Arthur Eichengrün and Felix Hoffmann produced acetylsalicylic acid from salicin. Hoffmann gave the new compound to his father who was suffering from arthritis and noticed an improvement. The compound was patented in 1900, named "Aspirin" (the "A" from acetyl and spir from *Spiraea ulmaria*, the plant from which it was derived).

Long thought to act through the central nervous system, John Vane and Priscilla Piper tested aspirin at the Royal College of Surgeons in London and noted that it blocked the production of what later were found to be prostaglandins. Subsequent research showed that aspirin is an irreversible inhibitor of the enzyme cyclo-oxygenase through acetylation of a serine residue at the active site. This gives the molecule its analgesic, antiinflammatory, and antipyretic activity.

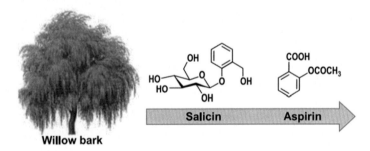

Willow bark   Salicin   Aspirin

Enzyme inhibition to alter levels of normal physiological cellular molecules

For example, the enzyme phosphodiesterase (PDE) degrades the physiologically active second messenger cyclic AMP in cardiac cells; this controls cardiac contractility and sinus rhythm. In failing hearts (congestive heart failure, CHF), a useful augmentation of contractility can be obtained by blocking the enzymatic degradation of cyclic AMP; PDE inhibitors such as milrinone are useful in CHF. Augmentation of cardiac contractility can also be gained from blockade of ATPase enzymes in heart muscle (e.g., using digitalis) and erectile dysfunction can be treated by blockade of cyclic GMP degradation by PDE V inhibition (sildenafil).

Blockade of enzyme activity that becomes pathophysiological

The renin-angiotensin system is intimately involved in blood pressure and fluid balance, and in conditions of hypertension, blockade of the angiotensin-converting enzyme by drugs, such as lisinopril lowers blood pressure. Similarly, aspirin blocks the enzyme cyclooxygenase to prevent the formation of inflammatory prostaglandins and thromboxane (see Box 6.1). Inhibitors of xanthine oxidase prevent this enzyme from producing excess amounts of uric acid in gout.

Blockade of an enzyme that exclusively takes part in a pathophysiological process

After HIV infection and in the progression process to AIDS, HIV-1 utilizes the enzyme HIV reverse transcriptase to catalyze the production of viral DNA from the viral RNA template to facilitate further infection; drugs such as AZT (azidothymidine) effectively block this process. Penicillin is a suicide substrate that selectively blocks the enzyme that controls bacterial wall integrity to selectively destroy bacteria with no harm to the host (see Box 6.2). Similarly, sulfa drugs, such as sulfanilamide block dihydropteroate synthetase to prevent bacteria from synthesizing the required folic acid; this is lethal to bacteria but not humans, providing a useful selective bacteriostatic action.

BOX 6.2

Penicillin: life saving suicide substrate.

Penicillins are molecules produced by molds in the Penicillium family. Their antibiotic activity was discovered in 1928 by Alexander Fleming, but penicillins were not widely used therapeutically until the 1940s. Penicillin act as suicide substrates of glycopeptide transpeptidase in bacteria. Thus, penicillin enters the active site as a substrate, but in the normal process of catalysis, it forms a covalent bond to permanently inactivate the enzyme. This enzyme is essential for bacterial wall cross-linking; thus, inactivation by penicillin disrupts bacterial integrity and causes death. There is no corresponding process in humans, therefore the biochemical reaction is unique to bacteria; this makes penicillin a valuable antibiotic. Some bacteria have developed penicillin resistance through the expression of an enzyme β-lactamase. This enzyme opens the four-membered ring of penicillins.

Blockade of hyperactivity from enzymes

Enzyme inhibitors can be selectively lethal to cells with varying levels of metabolic activity. For example, blockade of nucleotide synthesis by drugs such as methotrexate can be selectively lethal to rapidly growing cells carrying out DNA replication in tumors. In human breast cell tumors, the overexpression of HER2 can be countered by blockers of the tyrosine kinase ErbB2, such as herceptin.

There are many drugs that have inhibition of enzymes as their mechanism of action (see Table 6.1).

TABLE 6.1 Some drugs targeted for enzymes.

Compound	Target enzyme	Disease (indication)
Acetazolamine	Carbonic anhydrase	Glaucoma
Acyclovir	Viral DNA polymerase	Herpes
Agenerase	Viral protease	AIDS
Amprenavir	HIV protease	AIDS
Allopurinol	Xanthine oxidase	Gout
Argatroban	Thrombin	Cardiovascular disease
Aspirin	Cyclooxygenase	Inflammation/pain/fever
Amoxicillin	Penicillin binding proteins	Bacterial infection
Carbidopa	Dopa decarboxylase	Parkinson's disease
Celebrex	Cyclooxygenase-2	Inflammation/pain/fever
Clavulanate	β-Lactamase	Bacterial resistance
Combivir	Viral reverse transcriptase	AIDS
Digoxin	Na^+/K^+ ATPase	Congestive heart failure
Dutasteride	5-α-Reductase	Benign prostate hyperplasia
Efavirenz	HIV reverse transcriptase	AIDS
Epristeride	Steroid 5-α-reductase	Benign prostate hyperplasia
Etoposide	Topoisomerase II	Cancer
Fluorouracil	Thymidylate synthase	Cancer
Leflunomide	Dihydroorotate dehydrogenase	Inflammation
Levitra	Phosphodiesterase V	Erectile dysfunction
Lisinopril	Angiotensin-converting enzyme	Hypertension
Lovastatin	HMG-CoA reductase	Cardiovascular disease
Methotrexate	Dihydrofolate reductase	Cancer, immunosuppression
Nitecapone	Catechol-o-methyl transferase	Parkinson's disease
Norfloxacin	DNA gyrase	Urinary tract infection
Omeprazole	H^+/K^+ ATPase	Peptic ulcer
PALA	Aspartate transcarbamoylase	Cancer
Raltegravir	Viral integrase	AIDS
Relenza	Viral neuraminidase	Influenza
Sorbitol	Aldose reductase	Diabetic retinopathy
Tacrine	Acetylcholinesterase	Alzheimer's disease
Trazodone	Adenosine deaminase	Depression
Trimethoprim	Bacterial dihydrofolate reductase	Bacterial infection
Tykerb	ErbB-2/EGFR	Breast cancer

Unintentional but unavoidable drug-enzyme interactions

Every small-molecule drug that is tested in an animal or human system will be subject to enzyme interaction since liver enzymes are the main mechanism for detoxification of foreign chemicals. Therefore, whether a drug target is an enzyme or not, the molecular interaction with enzymes will need to be assessed in the drug development process. The main family of enzymes involved are the Cytochrome P450 group coded by 63 genes with many variants, but many other enzymes are also involved in hepatic metabolism of foreign substances- see Fig. 6.2.

The main safety issue with a new drug-hepatic enzyme interaction is the possibility of drug-drug interactions. For patients who are using a drug for therapy, a new drug has the potential to interfere with the metabolism of the existing therapeutic agent. In the context of a drug-drug interaction, the patient may be taking one drug (termed the "victim") and then have that balance altered by adding a new drug (termed the "perpetrator"). Thus, a dosage of the victim balanced with cytochrome P450 metabolism can have that steady-state metabolism altered, if the perpetrator interferes with metabolism, i.e., higher levels of the victim could ensue. There are two possible mechanisms for this effect:

1. Cosubstrate utilization of the enzyme: A reduction of enzyme activity will result by the added burden of the second substrate.
2. Pharmacologic inhibition of the enzyme; drug-drug interactions can occur if the new drug blocks metabolism of the previously administered drug.

Having cosubstrates is an almost inevitable consequence of multidrug therapy since there are a limited number of metabolizing enzymes and many more possible drug combinations; Table 6.2 shows the cross-over of substrates for some common Cytochrome P450 enzymes. A further consequence of cosubstrate mechanisms is the introduction of new pharmacologic

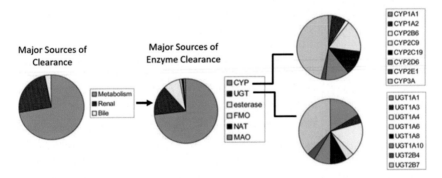

FIGURE 6.2 Mechanisms of drug removal: metabolism (enzymatic degradation, renal clearance, secretion into bile). The major enzymatic degradation mechanism is through cytochrome P450 enzymes and the UGT family of enzymes.

TABLE 6.2   Drugs utilizing common cytochrome P450 enzymes.

Enzyme	Substrate(s)
Cyp3A4	Amiodarone, Atorvastatin, Cimetidine, Clarithromycin, Clemastine, Clomipramine, Clotrimazole, Cyclosporine, Danazol, Diltiazem, Erythromycin, Felodipine, Fluconazole, Fluoxetine, Fluvoxamine, Glibenclamide, Ifosfamide, Indinavir, Itraconazole, Ketoconazole, Lovastatin, Metronidazole, Mibefradil, Miconazole, Midazolam, Nifedipine, Nelfinavir, Nevirapine, Nitrendipine, Norfloxacin, Omeprazole, Pravastatin, Propoxyphene, Quinidine, Ranitidine, Ritonavir, Rivastatin, Saquinavir, Sertindole, Sertraline, Simvastatin, Sulfinpyrazone, Tacrolimus, Tamoxifen, Tocainide, Troglitazone, Troleandomycin, Venlafaxine, Verapamil, Zafirlukast
Cyp2D6	Acebutolol, Amiodarone, Amitriptyline, Betaxolol, Bufuralol, Chlorpheniramine, Chlorpromazine, Cimetidine, Citalopram, Clomipramine, Desipramine, Flecainide, Fluoxetine, Fluphenazine, Flurbiprofen, Fluvoxamine, Haloperidol, Ketoconazole, Lomustine, Lovastatin, Mibefradil, Nefazodone, Norfloxacin, Paroxetine, Perhexiline, Pindolol, Pravastatin, Propafenone, Propranolol, Quinidine, Ranitidine, Ritonavir, Sertindole, Sertraline, Simvastatin, Thioridazine, Venlafaxine, Vinblastine, Vinorelbine
Cyp1A2	Caffeine, Ciprofloxacin, Clarithromycin, Diltiazem, Enoxacin, Erythromycin, Fluvoxamine, Isoniazid, Ketoconazole, Lansoprazole, Levofloxacin, Lidocaine, Lomefloxacin, Mexiletine, Norfloxacin, Ofloxacin, Phenacetin, Propofol
Cyp2C9	Amiodarone, Cimetidine, Diazepam, Diclofenac, Disulfiram, Fluconazole, Fluvoxamine, Itraconazole, Ketoprofen, Metronidazole, Omeprazole, Phenylbutazone, Pravastatin, Ritonavir, Simvastatin, Sulfinpyrazone, Tolbutamide, Troglitazone, Zafirlukast

activity into systems through active metabolites. Thus, in addition to a drug-drug interaction, the perpetrator could generate a pharmacologically active molecule to further complicate therapy; Table 6.3 shows some common drugs and the pharmacologically active metabolites they produce. Thus, the perpetrator could generate a secondary species that can itself induce a drug-drug interaction. Fig. 6.3 shows the number of drug-drug interactions produced by parent drugs and their pharmacological active metabolites.

The other possibility is that the perpetrator drug produces actual metabolizing enzyme inhibition; this would cause a drug-drug interaction in the form of an increase in the levels of the victim drug. Table 6.4 shows some substrate-perpetrator drugs where the perpetrator produces inhibition of the metabolizing enzyme for the victim to cause a drug-drug interaction. There are a number of ways a perpetrator drug could cause enzyme inhibition (vide infra) and in the conventional scenario whereby the two drugs compete for the enzyme active site, the levels of each drug are mutually antagonistic, i.e., a high level of victim will minimize the effect of the perpetrator and vice versa. However, there is a scenario where this can be reversed, namely uncompetitive enzyme inhibition whereby the perpetrator can only inhibit the enzyme

TABLE 6.3 Drugs generating pharmacologically active metabolites through Cytochrome P450 metabolism.

Drug	Metabolite	Drug	Metabolite
Acetylsalicylic acid	Salicylic acid	Isosorbide dinitrate	Isosorbide 5-monobitrate
Amitriptyline	Nortriptyline	Meperidine	Normeperidine
Carbamazepine	Carbamazepine 10, 11-epoxide	Morphine	Morphine 6-glucuronide
Chlordiazepoxide	Desmethyl chlordiazepoxide	Prazepam	Desmethyl Prazepam
Codeine	Morphine	Prednisone	Prednisolone
Diazepam	Desmethyl diazepam	Primidone	Phenobarbital
Enalapril	Enalaprilat	Procainamide	N-acetyl procainamide
Encainide	O-Desmethyl encainide	Sulindac	Sulindac Sulfide
Fluoxetine	Norfluoxetine	Verapamil	Norverapamil
Imipramine	Desipramine	Zidovudine	Zidovudine triphosphate

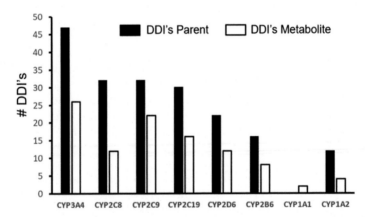

FIGURE 6.3 Number of drug-drug interactions (DDI) by parent drugs (filled bars) and their metabolites (open bars). Source: *Redrawn from J. Yu, Z. Zhou, J. Tay-Sontheimer, R.H. Levy, I. Ragueneau-Majlessi. Risk of clinically relevant pharmacokinetic-based drug-drug interactions with drugs approved by the U.S. Food and Drug Administration between 2013 and 2016. Drug Metab. Disp. 46 (2018) 835−845.*

TABLE 6.4 Cytochrome P450-induced drug-drug interactions.

Victim	Perpetrator (enzyme)
Paritaprevir	Ritonavir (Cyp3A)
Eliglustat	Ketoconazole (CYP3A4, CYP2D6); Paroxetine (CYP2D6); Fluconazole (CYP3A)
Ibrutinib	Ketoconazole (CYP3A); Erythromycin (CYP3A)
Grazoprevir	Lopinavir (CYP3A); Atanavir (CYP3); Darunavir, Ritonavir (CYP3A)
Naloxegol	Ketoconazole (CYP3A)
Dasabuvir	Gemfibrozil (CUP2C8)
Ivabradine	Josamycin (CYP3); Ketoconazole (CYP3A)
Simeprevir	Erythromycin (CYP3A)
Tasimelteon	Fluvoxamine (CYP1A2)
Pirfenidone	Fluvoxamine (CYP1A2)
Cobimetinib	Itraconazole (CYP3A)
Simeprevir	Ritonavir (CYP3A)
Flibanserin	Fluconazole (CYP3A, CYP2C19)
Venetoclax	Ketoconazole (CYP3A)

when the victim is engaged with the enzyme. In this situation, the perpetrator becomes more active in the presence of the victim, and thus, the potential for a drug-drug interaction actually reverses to a condition where high concentrations of the victim promote a higher drug-drug interaction by the perpetrator. The relationship between the victim and perpetrator to produce drug-drug interaction are shown in Fig. 6.4 for competitive, noncompetitive, mixed competitive, and uncompetitive enzyme inhibition.

Cytochrome P450 inhibition by drugs is further complicated by the fact that these are allosteric enzymes, a requirement since they must adjust to a wide range of substrates. A feature of allosteric enzymes is the phenomenon of probe dependence whereby given two substrates; the enzyme may have differing activity with each. This poses a problem for the prediction of drug-drug interactions in experimental studies. For example, Fig. 6.5 shows CYP3A4 inhibition by astemizole when three different substrates are used. It can be seen that when the substrates are, dibenzyl fluorescein (DBF) and (7-benzyloxy-4-trifluoromethylcoumarin) (BFC) are used, astemizole produces antagonism with an IC_{50} of $2-5$ μM. However, when the substrate is benzyloxy resorufin (BzRes), astemizole is much less potent ($IC_{50} \approx 1\mu$M), thus, illustrating allosteric probe

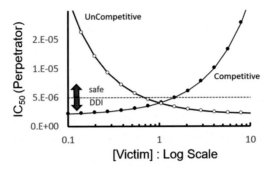

FIGURE 6.4   Potency of enzyme inhibitors (as an IC_{50} value, the concentration of inhibitor producing 50% inhibition of enzyme activity) as a function of competing cosubstrate concentration. The example shown indicates a competitive antagonist with an IC_{50} of 2 μM at low concentrations of substrate; as the concentration of substrate increases, the inhibition by the enzyme inhibitor decreases. For example, at a substrate concentration of 3 μM, the IC_{50} increases to 10 μM. In contrast, the reverse is true for an uncompetitive inhibitor, which becomes more potent with increasing concentrations of substrate. At low concentrations of substrate (i.e., 0.15 μM), the IC_{50} of the uncompetitive inhibitor is 22 μM; at 3 μM substrate, the IC_{50} is 3 μM.

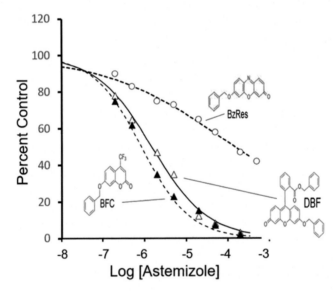

FIGURE 6.5   Blockade of CYP3A4 by astemizole when the enzyme acts on three difference substrates: BzRes (benzyloxy resorufin)—open circles, DBF (dibenzyl fluorescein)—open triangles and BFC (7-benzyloxy-4-trifluoromethylcoumarin)—filled triangles. *Source: Data drawn from D.M. Stresser, A.P. Blanchard, S.D.Turner, J.C.L. Erve, A.A. Dandeneau, V.P. Miller, C.L. Crespi. Substrate-dependent modulation of CYP3A4 catalytic activity: analysis of 27 test compounds with four fluorometric substrates. Drug Metab Disp 28 (2000) 1440–1448* [1].

dependence. This poses practical problems for the prediction of drug-drug interactions as shown by an example with the antiarrhythmic dronedarone and treatment of stroke with rivaroxaban (see Box 6.3).

BOX 6.3

Unwelcome visitors.

Dronedarone is an antiarrhythmic used for the maintenance of sinus rhythm in patients with atrial fibrillation. Clinical trials have shown safety for up to 21 months after cardioversion to sinus rhythm. In experiments with standard CYP3A4 substrates, Dronedarone shows no CYP3A4 inhibition (i.e., no drug-drug interaction liability). However, when Rivaroxaban (used for stroke prevention in nonvalvular atrial fibrillation) is the substrate for CYP3A4, Dronedarone produces competitive inhibition of CYP3A4 with a KI of 64 μM. Thus, a combination treatment of Dronedarone and Rivaroxaban would be predicted to have serious drug-drug interactions interfering with the therapy with both drugs. In this sense, dronedarone becomes an "unwelcome visitor" to an ongoing treatment regimen of rivaroxaban.

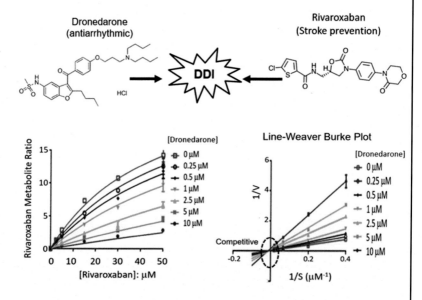

Source: Data redrawn from E.J.Y. Cheong, J.J.N. Goh, Y. Hong, G. Venkatesan. Application of static modeling in the prediction of in vivo drug–drug interactions between rivaroxaban and antiarrhythmic agents based on in vitro inhibition studies Drug Metab. Disp. 45 (2017) 260–268.

Reversible enzyme inhibition

The primary assumption for reversible enzyme inhibition is that the inhibitor binds to the enzyme through mass action but that the binding can be reversed upon washing the enzyme with inhibitor-free media, that

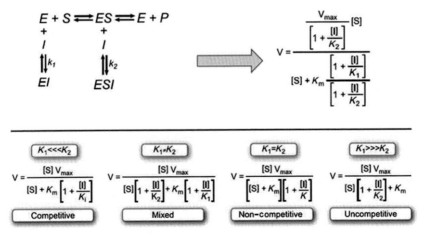

FIGURE 6.6 Schematic of the binding of inhibitors to various forms of the enzyme; either free enzyme [E] or the enzyme-substrate complex [ES]. The general equation for the inhibitor binding to the two forms of the enzyme is shown in the box to the right, with K_1 and K_2 describing interactions of inhibitor with E and ES respectively. Various relationships between K_1 and K_2 lead to four basic mechanisms of enzyme inhibition: competitive; mixed; noncompetitive, and uncompetitive (see text).

is, the inhibition is reversible. In general, there are two basic enzyme species to which an inhibitor could bind to produce enzyme inhibition; the enzyme not bound by substrate (E in Fig. 6.6) and the substrate-bound species (ES in Fig. 6.6). Combinations of affinities for these two species lead to the four general behaviors of enzyme inhibitors; competitive, noncompetitive, uncompetitive, and mixed (see Fig. 6.6). In order to increase the affinity of the inhibitor for the ES species:

Competitive inhibition

This is where the inhibitor competes for the substrate at the substrate binding site. An example of a competitive inhibitor is ritonavir, an HIV protease inhibitor. This antagonist contains three peptide bonds and resembles the protein substrate for HIV protease. Competitive inhibitors have virtually no affinity for the ES species since the substrate already occupies their binding site when bound ($K_1 <<< K_2$ in Fig. 6.6). Therefore, the inhibitor increases K_m but does not change V_{max}; the equation for enzyme velocity in the presence of a competitive inhibitor is shown in Fig. 6.6. The effect of a competitive antagonist on an enzyme velocity curve is shown in Fig. 6.7A and in the Lineweaver–Burk format in Fig. 6.7B. An example of competitive inhibition in a therapeutic setting is given in Box 6.4.

BOX 6.4

A Life-saving competition.

Methanol is extremely toxic due to central nervous system depression and the production of formate via the enzyme alcohol dehydrogenase. Formate is made from formaldehyde and is toxic to mitochondrial cytochrome c oxidase. This leads to symptoms of hypoxia, metabolic acidosis, and other metabolic disturbances. Treatment is through competitive inhibition of the enzymatic reaction using an excess of ethanol or fomepizole. These molecules compete for methanol at the active site of alcohol dehydrogenase and formaldehyde production is halted.

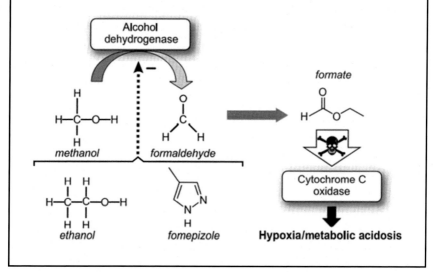

Mixed inhibition

This is where the inhibitor has affinity for both the E and ES forms but these affinities are not identical ($K_1 \neq K_2$; Fig. 6.6). In this type of inhibition, the inhibitor can bind to the ES form of the enzyme, but its affinity for the enzyme is altered when the substrate is bound. Under most circumstances, this type of inhibition is allosteric (see Chapter 5, Allosteric Drug Effects) in that the inhibitor binds to a site different from that of the substrate. Mixed inhibitors interfere with substrate binding (thus increasing K_m) and also hamper catalysis (decreasing V_{max}). The effect of a mixed antagonist on enzyme velocity is shown in Fig. 6.8A and in the Lineweaver–Burk format in Fig. 6.8B.

Reversible competitive

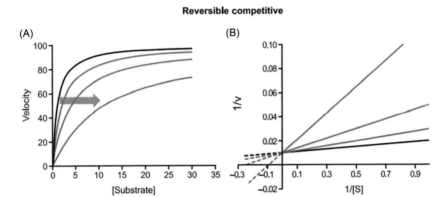

FIGURE 6.7　(A) Reversible competitive inhibition is characterized by an increase in the observed K_m for the substrate and no diminution of V_{max}. (B) The Lineweaver–Burk plots are of increasing slope (indicating increasing values of K_m) with higher levels of inhibitor, and intersect at the ordinate axis. The enzyme inhibitor has negligible affinity for ES since the substrate impedes binding to the ES species.

Mixed reversible

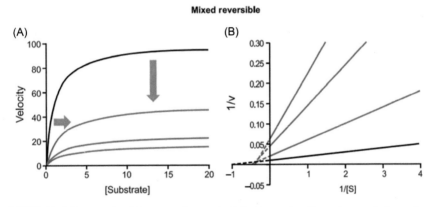

FIGURE 6.8　Mixed inhibition is characterized by increasing K_m values and decreasing apparent V_{max}. The enzyme inhibitor has an unequal affinity for E and ES. Panel A: Michaelis-Menten curves for enzyme activity. Panel B: Lineweaver-Burke plots of curves shown in panel A.

Noncompetitive inhibition

In this form of enzyme inhibition, the inhibitor has the same affinity for E and ES, does not affect the binding of the substrate ($K_1 = K_2$ in Fig. 6.6), but does reduce catalysis. Therefore, there is no effect on the K_m, but the V_{max} for the reaction is decreased; the equation for noncompetitive antagonism is shown in Fig. 6.6. The effect of a noncompetitive antagonist on enzyme velocity is shown in Fig. 6.9A and in the Lineweaver–Burk format in Fig. 6.9B. An example of a noncompetitive inhibitor for an enzyme is shown by the effects of efavirenz on HIV reverse transcriptase.

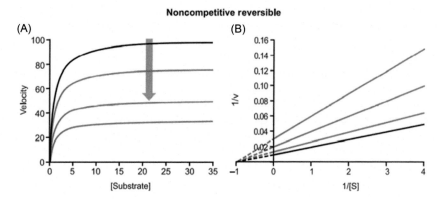

FIGURE 6.9   Noncompetitive inhibition is characterized by no change in the K_m value and a decrease in V_{max}. The enzyme inhibitor has an equal affinity for both E and ES. Panel A: Michaeilis-Menten curves for enzyme activity. Panel B: Lineweaver-Burke plots of curves shown in panel A.

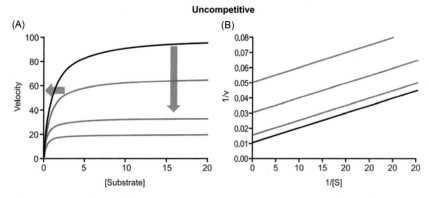

FIGURE 6.10   Uncompetitive inhibition is characterized by a decrease in the apparent K_m value and a decreased V_{max}. The Lineweaver—Burk plots are parallel and do not intersect. The enzyme inhibitor has negligible affinity for E but a high affinity for the enzyme—substrate complex (ES). Panel A: Michaeilis-Menten curves for enzyme activity. Panel B: Lineweaver-Burke plots of curves shown in panel A.

Uncompetitive inhibition

This is where the inhibitor binds only to the ES enzyme-substrate complex and not to the enzyme with no substrate bound ($K_1 >> > K_2$; Fig 6.65). Under these circumstances, V_{max} is decreased but the apparent K_m will decrease as well due to the selective binding of the inhibitor to the ES species. In essence the binding of the substrate creates the binding site for the inhibitor; therefore, the binding of the inhibitor is promoted by the presence of the substrate. The effect of an uncompetitive antagonist on enzyme velocity is shown in Fig. 6.10A and in

the Lineweaver–Burk format in Fig. 6.10B. A special case of uncompetitive inhibition is substrate inhibition whereby the substrate itself blocks
enzyme activity at high concentrations. This is caused by more than
one substrate molecule binding to the active site of the enzyme meant
for just one substrate molecule, for example, different parts of the substrate molecule bind to different parts of the enzyme-active site. Thus,
the counterpart for the inhibitor species in Fig. 6.6 is ESS. An example
of this type of effect is demonstrated by sucrose at the enzyme
invertase.

The equation for substrate inhibition is a variant of the equation for
uncompetitive inhibition:

$$V = \frac{[S]V_{max}}{[S]\left[1 + \frac{[S]}{K_S}\right] + K_m} \tag{6.4}$$

where K_S is the affinity of the substrate for the enzyme with another
substrate molecule already bound.

The mechanism of enzyme inhibition can be important since it may
define the relationship between the inhibitor concentrations needed to
produce blockade and the level of substrate present in the enzyme
compartment. For example, high substrate levels make a competitive
inhibitor less potent but an uncompetitive inhibitor more potent.
While a detailed analysis of the effects of inhibitors on enzyme activation curves (or an analysis of Lineweaver–Burk curves) can yield
information on the mechanism of inhibition, another relatively simple
approach is to quantify the relationship between the IC_{50} (molar concentration producing 50% inhibition of enzyme activity) and the K_i. Fig. 6.11
shows the relationship between the IC_{50} of the four types of inhibitors
and the level of substrate. The equations relating the IC_{50} and K_i are
given in Table 6.5.

Irreversible enzyme inhibition

Useful therapeutic effects can also be obtained from irreversible inhibition of enzyme function. These molecules do not dissociate (or dissociate extremely slowly) from the enzyme. An inhibitor can produce
essentially irreversible inhibition through the induction of a conformational change in the enzyme to form a highly stabilized complex. Such
"tight binding" inhibitors can be useful therapeutic agents since they
have K_i values typically less than 5 nM; only very low concentrations of
these are required for enzyme inhibition, thereby yielding considerable
selectivity. An example of such a tight-binding inhibitor is shown in

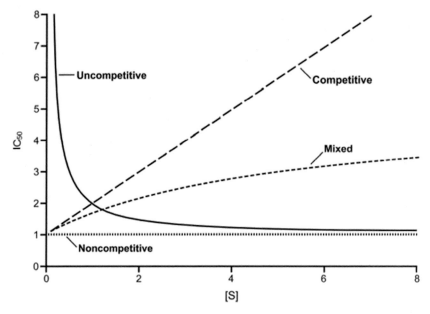

FIGURE 6.11 Relationships between IC_{50}s (molar concentrations producing 50% inhibition of an enzyme reaction run at a defined substrate concentration) and the substrate concentration. The potency of noncompetitive inhibitors is independent of substrate concentration, whereas a linear relationship defines competitive inhibition. A nonlinear relationship exists for mixed inhibitors (the extent of the nonlinearity depends on differences between K_1 and K_2). Uncompetitive inhibitors become more potent with increasing substrate concentration.

TABLE 6.5 Relationship between IC_{50} and K_i for various types of enzyme inhibition.

Description	IC_{50}/K_i relationship
Competitive inhibition	$K_i = IC_{50}/([1 + ([S])/K_m])$
Mixed inhibition	$K_i = IC_{50}/([K_m/K_1 + ([S])/K_2])$
Noncompetitive inhibition	$K_i = IC_{50}$
Uncompetitive inhibition	$K_i = IC_{50}/([1 + K_m/([S])])$

Fig. 6.12; Immucillin H blocks purine nucleoside phosphorylase irreversibly with extremely high potency.

Given sufficient time, an irreversible inhibitor will eventually inactivate all of the enzyme present until the velocity of the enzymes reaction

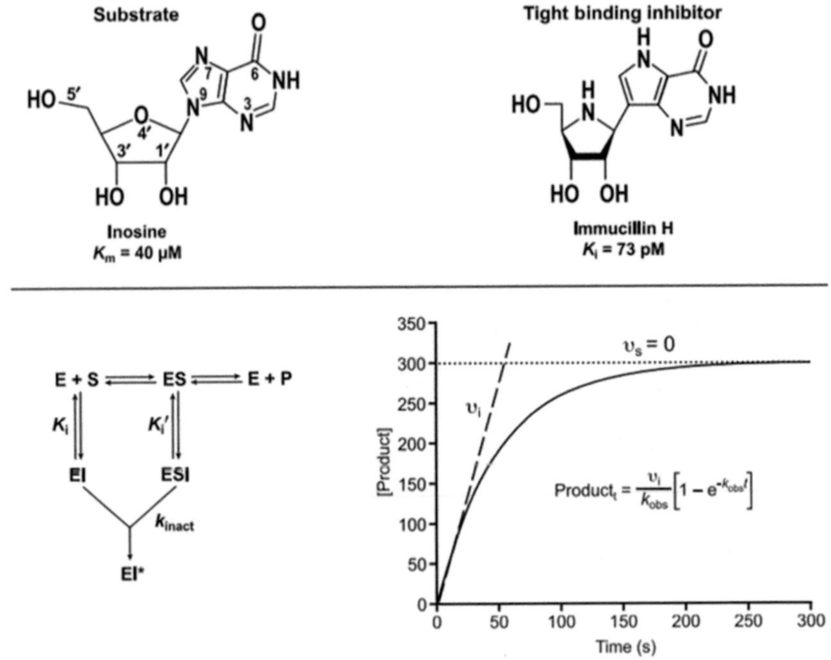

Substrate

Inosine
$K_m = 40\ \mu M$

Tight binding inhibitor

Immucillin H
$K_i = 73\ pM$

$$E + S \rightleftharpoons ES \rightleftharpoons E + P$$

FIGURE 6.12 Irreversible enzyme inhibition. Top panel: Example of a tight-binding inhibitor. The substrate for purine nucleoside phosphorylase is inosine; Immucillin H is an extremely potent and irreversible inhibitor although no covalent bond is formed. Bottom panels: The scheme for irreversible enzyme inhibition is shown on the left while a method for estimating the activity of an irreversible inhibitor is shown on the right. In this procedure, the kinetics of production of product, from a given concentration of substrate, are observed in the presence of an irreversible inhibitor. A tangent depicts v_i which is then used to estimate k_{obs}, a measure of inhibition. Values of k_{obs} for different substrate concentrations can be used to obtain a general parameter characterizing the activity of the irreversible inhibitor (see text).

is zero. Since, irreversible molecules do not come to equilibrium with their targets, the standard techniques to measure the potency of such molecules cannot be used; other methods are required. One example of this type of procedure is shown in Fig. 6.12. Specifically, this figure shows one approach whereby a concentration of irreversible inactivator is added to an enzyme preparation and the amount of product measured with time; it can be seen that eventually there is no further product formed as the enzyme becomes completely inactivated. The initial slope of this curve can yield a measure of the initial enzyme velocity V_i, which, for a one-step inactivation process, can be used to estimate a k_{obs} according to the equation:

$$[\text{Product}]_{time} = \frac{V_i}{k_{obs}}\left(1 - e^{-k_{obs}t}\right) \qquad (6.5)$$

A subsequent plot of various k_{obs} values with different concentrations of irreversible inhibitor yields a measure of $k_{obs}/[I]$ (from the slope of a regression of k_{obs} on [A]), which can be used to quantify irreversible inhibitor activity.

A common mechanism for irreversible enzyme blockade is alkylation where a covalent bond is formed with the protein (or one of its bound cofactors). An example of this type of effect is shown by the diisopropylfluorophosphonate alkylation of acetylcholinesterase. If an inhibitor forms a covalent bond, it usually means that a reactive species is involved, and this can lead to problems with specificity as a reactive species may alkylate a range of proteins in addition to the enzyme. One mechanism whereby an alkylating agent can be more specific is in the case of suicide substrates. These bind specifically to the active site and while bound are in a favorable orientation to alkylate; an example of such an agent is penicillin (see Box 6.2). The enzyme could also act on an initially nonreactive molecule to produce a reactive species, which then goes on to alkylate the enzyme; this is referred to as mechanism-based inhibition. This is often seen with hepatic cytochrome P450 enzymes designed to attack foreign molecules in the liver (see Chapter 7, Pharmacokinetics I: Permeation and Metabolism). Fig. 6.13 shows mechanism-based inhibition of CYP2C9 by erythromycin characterized by an inordinately long onset to steady-state effect. Usually in these cases, the only way to regenerate the enzyme activity is to promote synthesis of new enzyme.

There are certain circumstances where irreversible enzyme inhibition may still be acceptable for normal physiological function. Basically, it is a matter of the rate of new enzyme synthesis and the rate of increased enzyme degradation (through time-dependent inhibition). Specifically, the steady-state level of normal enzyme activity is given by an equilibrium between enzyme production; thus, the steady-state level of natural enzyme activity is given by $[E]_{ss} = k_{synth}/k_{degrad}$ where k_{synth} denotes the rate of production of new enzyme and k_{degrad} the rate of enzyme inhibition. A given drug degradation of enzyme activity (determined by k_{degrad}) defines a new physiological steady-state as $E_{ss} = k_{degrad}/(k_{degrad} + \lambda)$ where λ = the rate of enzyme-mediated degradation in the presence of a given concentration of the molecule. Therefore, it is a question of whether the rate of enzyme irreversible inhibition can significantly block the normal

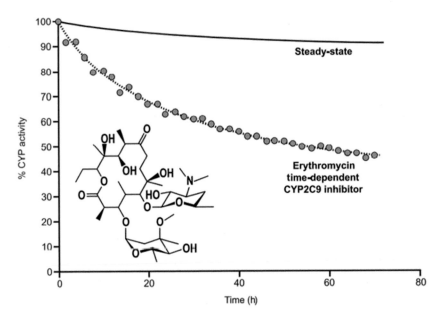

FIGURE 6.13 Time-dependent (mechanism-based) enzyme inhibition of cytochrome 2C9 by erythromycin. While a reversible inhibitor comes to equilibrium or steady-state within a few hours, time-dependent inhibition continues over an extremely long period as the inhibitor slowly (and irreversibly) binds to the enzyme and inactivates it. *Source: Data from D.F. McGinnity, A.J. Berry, J.R. Kenny, K. Grime, R.J. Riley, Evaluation of time-dependent cytochrome P450 inhibition using cultured human hepatocytes, Drug. Metab. Dispos. 34 (2006) 1130–1291 [2].*

rate of new enzyme inhibition. In general, noting that normal physiology is tuned to maximal efficiency, it would be expected that an irreversible enzyme inhibitor would significantly obstruct normal enzyme function and thus be an impediment to normal physiological function. A ratio "R" can be defined, which is the amount of enzyme under normal conditions divided by the amount of enzyme with time-dependent enzyme inhibition:

$$R = \frac{K_{degrad}}{k_{inact}\left[\frac{[I]/K_I}{[I]/K_I + 1}\right] + K_{degrad}} \tag{6.6}$$

where k_{inact} is the rate of irreversible enzyme inactivation, [I] the concentration of enzyme inhibitor, K_I the equilibrium dissociation constant of the inhibitor-enzyme complex and K_{degrad} the natural rate of enzyme degradation in the physiological system. It can be seen that if the rate of inactivation is slow or the rate of enzyme re-synthesis is high, then a time dependent enzyme inhibitor may not seriously affect enzyme levels (low value of R). In most cases, however, if a drug produces time-dependent inactivation of cytochrome P450 enzymes in the liver required for normal detoxification of substances, it cannot be used as a therapeutic agent.

Allosteric enzyme modulation

The interaction schemes for molecules with enzymes shown in Fig. 6.6 depict general maps of the interacting species but not the mechanisms by which they interact. Specifically, as pointed out for receptors, molecules can either interact orthosterically (steric hindrance of the enzyme-active site) or allosterically (binding to a separate site on the enzyme to affect substrate disposition through a conformational change in the protein). Historically, the study of allosterism is rooted in the study of allosteric enzyme effects (note Fig. 5.2 on negative feedback of enzyme cascades) and allosteric enzyme inhibitors (and activators) are well-known. Fig. 6.14 shows noncompetitive blockade of Ras-Raf-mitogen-activated protein kinase (MEK)1/2 by the allosteric cancer anti-tumor inhibitor AZD6244. An important therapeutic application of allosteric enzyme inhibitors is in the area of kinase inhibition for cancer chemotherapy. Traditional kinase inhibitors used in cancer therapy are orthosteric inhibitors of the ATP-binding site. However, the 518 human kinases show remarkable similarity in their ATP-binding domain and the majority of kinase inhibitors that utilize this site (so-called Type I inhibitors) have issues of lack of selectivity. In contrast, allosteric binding sites are less conserved across the kinome and are accessible

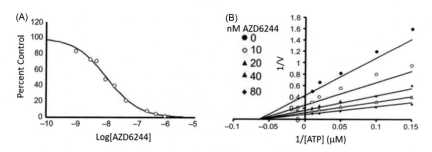

FIGURE 6.14 Inhibition of MEK1 activity by the allosteric inhibitor AZD6244 (panel A). The Lineweaver–Burk plots shown in panel B indicate a noncompetitive mode of blockade. *Source: Redrawn from D.F. McGinnity, A.J. Berry, J.R. Kenny, K. Grime, R.J. Riley, Evaluation of time-dependent cytochrome P450 inhibition using cultured human hepatocytes, Drug. Metab. Dispos. 34 (2006) 1130–1291 [2].*

through conformational changes in the protein leading to improved selectivity. In addition, allosteric inhibitors are unaffected by cellular ATP levels [3]. The most well-characterized allosteric MEK1 and MEK2 inhibitors, CI-1040 utilizes a separate binding pocket adjacent to the ATP-binding site (see Box 6.5). Allosteric molecules can have a wide range of activity on enzymes from inhibition to activation.

BOX 6.5

Tumors cannot compete with allosteric kinase inhibitors.

Kinases are enzymes that are intensively pursued as drug targets in a variety of diseases with a heavy emphasis on cancer [4]. Competitive kinase inhibitors, that is, those that must compete with the substrate ATP at the active enzyme catalytic site, lose activity in whole cell tumors due to the fact that there may be high concentrations of natural substrate in the cell—that is, see Box 6.4. However, allosteric enzyme inhibitors bind to their own site on the enzyme and thus may not be hindered by ATP binding. One of the most well-characterized allosteric kinase inhibitors blocks MEK1 and MEK2 through binding to a pocket adjacent to the ATP-binding site [5].

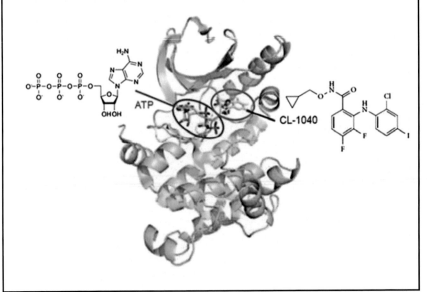

Enzyme activation

By definition, enzyme activators must be allosteric since they must allow the substrate to bind to the enzyme for the reaction to occur. In this regard, enzyme activators can be considered positive allosteric modulators (PAMs) are for receptors (see Chapter 5, Allosteric Drug Effects). Enzyme activation can be accelerated through biochemical modification of the enzyme (i.e., phosphorylation) or through low-molecular-weight positive modulators. Just as with agonists of receptors, it is theoretically possible to bind molecules to enzymes to increase catalysis (enzyme activators). These molecules must bind to a site other than the substrate binding site, otherwise substrate binding cannot occur. There are conditions where enzyme activators could be of benefit therapeutically. For instance, activators of glucokinase that increase the sensitivity of the enzyme to glucose could cause an increased insulin secretion and liver glycogen synthesis, and decreased liver glucose output in diabetes (see Fig. 6.15) [7]. Identification of enzyme activators requires correct configuration of the assay (e.g., low-substrate concentration) since most enzyme assays are designed to detect inhibitors. Box 6.6 shows the augmentation of acetylcholinesterase activity through an allosteric activator as a means to treat organophosphate poisoning.

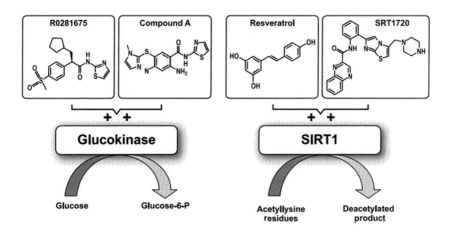

FIGURE 6.15 Enzyme activators. The production of glucose-6-phosphate from glucose is accelerated by RO281675 (data from Ref. [6]) and compound A, while Sirt1 production of deacylated products from acetyllysine residues is promoted by Resveratrol and SRT1720. Source: *Data from J.A. Zorn, J.A. Wells, Turning enzymes on with small molecules, Nat. Chem. Biol. 6 (2010) 179–188.*

BOX 6.6

Positive allosteric enzyme modulators for organophosphate poisoning.

Organophosphates and chemical nerve agents cause lethal toxicity through irreversible inhibition of the enzyme acetylcholinesterase (Acherase). Current therapy relies on pretreatment with a weak reversible Acherase inhibitor pyridostigmine bromide but since this agent is also an Acherase inhibitor, severe side effects can be seen with treatment. A novel approach to the treatment of organophosphate poisoning is to allosterically activate Acherase by binding to a separate site on the enzyme. This would have the effect of reactivating poisoned enzyme and alleviating the severe toxicity. One compound shown to do this is Cmpd II. As shown in the figure, this molecule increases the velocity of the Acherase hydrolysis of acetyl-thiocholine. This also translates to a beneficial diminution of Acherase blockade by organophosphate pesticides, such as Paraoxon where the IC_{50} value of Paraoxon of 20.4 nM is increased to 42.1 nM in the presence of Cmpd II. However, in keeping with allosteric probe dependence, this reduction does not extend to other organophosphate pesticides such as diisopropyl fluorophosphate and dicrophos [8].

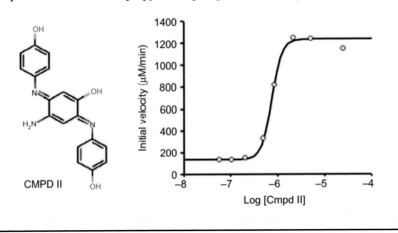

Intracellular effects of enzyme-active drugs

While enzymes can readily be assayed in biochemical assays where the concentration of substrate and inhibitor is known, most therapeutic enzyme inhibitors must access the enzyme in the cell. There are two elements important to assessing enzyme effects in cells; the level of endogenous basal enzyme activity and the concentrations of inhibitors that can access the enzyme in the cell. First to be considered is the level of basal enzyme activity, as this controls the observed consequences of enzyme inhibition in the therapeutic setting.

The inhibition of a pathologically-linked enzyme may not lead to excitation of a target protein, but may nevertheless lead to a thera-peutic effect. Endogenous basal activity can be very important to the inhibition of enzymes for therapeutic effect, since the magnitude of the observed effect depends directly on the endogenous tone of the system mediated by the enzyme. An example is the positive inotropic effect of PDE inhibitors in the treatment of CHF. In cardiac muscle, contractility is mediated by intracellular levels of cyclic AMP and these levels are tightly controlled by PDE-mediated hydrolysis. Therefore, blockade of PDE leads to a relaxation of this control and an excess of cyclic AMP; this leads to a positive stimulation of car-diac muscle. In the absence of basal cyclic AMP production in cardiac muscle, a PDE inhibitor will have no stimulant effect on the heart. It is useful to discuss the interplay between the basal activity of such systems and the observed response in vivo. One solution for the equation linking second messenger levels in cells and enzyme activ-ity is [9]:

$$
\begin{aligned}
\frac{[C_a]}{[K_m]} = \frac{1}{2} & \left(\frac{[C_b]}{[K_m]} - \frac{V_{max}}{K_t \cdot K_m} - \frac{[I]}{[K_i]} \right) \\
& + \frac{1}{2} \sqrt{ \left(1 + \frac{[I]}{K_i} + \frac{V_{max}}{K_t \cdot K_m} - \frac{[C_b]}{K_m} \right)^2 + \frac{[C_b]}{K_m} \left(1 + \frac{[I]}{K_i} \right) }
\end{aligned}
\tag{6.7}
$$

where $[C_b]$ and $[C_a]$ refer to the concentrations of cyclic AMP at the site of production (adenylate cyclase) and site of utilization (protein kinase), respectively, and K_t is an intracellular transfer rate constant between the two compartments. K_i is the equilibrium dissociation constant of the PDE-inhibitor enzyme complex, K_m is the concentration of cyclic AMP where hydrolysis is half-maximal, and V_{max} is the maximal rate of cyclic AMP hydrolysis.

This equation generally describes the effect of an enzyme inhibitor on free intracellular second messenger levels. It can be seen that a dif-ference in second messenger levels (leading to a physiological effect)

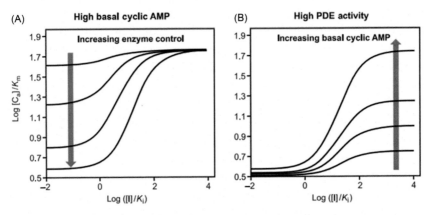

FIGURE 6.16 Effects of in vivo enzyme inhibition. (A) Dose-response curve of an enzyme inhibitor in systems where the ambient basal level of substrate is high. The range of curves result from various systems where the enzyme V_{max} is low (ordinate value is highest basal level of second messenger, $[C_a]/K_m = 1.64$) to high (ordinate value is basal $= 0.58$). Note: how the effects of the enzyme inhibitor are more pronounced in the system where the enzyme V_{max} is high, indicating that it is an important control of cellular second messenger levels. (B) Effects of an enzyme inhibitor for an enzyme of high activity in cells of varying levels of basal second messenger. Note: how the effects of enzyme inhibitor are more pronounced in systems with high levels of second messenger.

can be achieved, if there is a high production of second messenger that is reduced by a high level of enzyme activity. Fig. 6.16A shows the effect of basal enzyme activity on the observed dose-response curve to an enzyme inhibitor; it can be seen that if the enzyme activity is low (low level of V_{max}/K_tK_m) then the high-basal second messenger levels are not further increased by the enzyme inhibitor. In contrast, high values of V_{max}/K_tK_m lead to a wide range for the dose-response curve to the enzyme inhibitor. Similarly, Fig. 6.16B shows the effect of second messenger production in cells with high enzyme activity. Again, it can be seen that if basal second messenger levels are not high, there is little observed response to the enzyme inhibitor curve. These effects are important in the detection and quantitation of enzyme inhibition in cells. Box 6.7 shows how a subthreshold level of activation of cardiac β-adrenoceptors is required to produce direct effects of the PDE inhibitor Fenoximone; this mimics the observed in vivo effects of this drug where an ambient sympathetic tone (β-adrenoceptor activation) is present.

BOX 6.7

Enzyme blockade becomes relevant when the enzyme begins to work.

Elevated levels of the second messenger cyclic AMP increase myocardial contractility, but in normal physiology, the enzyme PDE keeps cellular cyclic AMP levels low. The PDE inhibitor fenoximone blocks PDE to cause elevated levels of cyclic AMP, resulting in positive myocardial contractility. This can be beneficial for a failing heart in CHF and fenoximone improves contractility in models of CHF in vivo. However, fenoximone has no effect in vitro until cyclic AMP is artificially elevated (through addition of subthreshold levels of catecholamines). This models the in vivo situation where natural sympathetic nervous system tone causes elevated cyclic AMP in heart muscle.

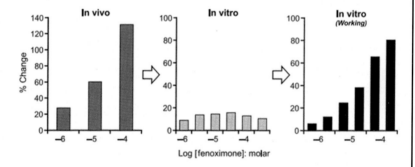

Source: *Data from: T.P. Kenakin, D.L. Scott, A method to assess concomitant cardiac phosphodiesterase inhibition and positive inotropy, J. Cardiovasc. Pharmacol. 10 (1987) 658–666 [9]; R.C. Dage, L.E. Roebel, C.P. Hsieh, D.L. Weiner, J.K. Woodward, The effects of MDL 17,043 on cardiac inotropy in the anaesthetized dog, J. Cardiovasc. Pharmacol. 4 (1982) 500–512 [10].*

There can be dissimulations between the concentration of inhibitor in the extracellular space (delivered by pharmacokinetics from the central compartment; see Chapter 7, Pharmacokinetics I: Permeation and Metabolism and Chapter 8, Pharmacokinetics II: Distribution and Multiple Dosing) and the actual concentration of the inhibitor at the enzyme. For example, if diffusion into the cell is slow and the clearance

6. Enzymes as drug targets

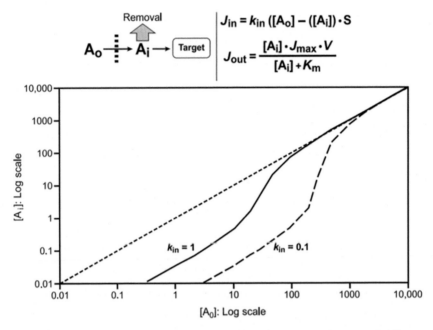

FIGURE 6.17 Drug concentration gradients under conditions of restricted diffusion. The bulk diffusion of enzyme inhibitor [A] (J_{in}) is driven by a concentration gradient and a diffusion constant k_{in}. It is assumed that the inhibitor is destroyed or otherwise diffuses out of the cell via a saturable process J_{out}. Depending on the rate of diffusion into the cell, there can be a deficit in the concentration of inhibitor inside the cell ([A_i]) compared to concentrations outside the cell ([A_o]), such that [A_i]/[A_o] < 1. This deficit can be overcome by high concentrations of inhibitor.

from the body is rapid, then the concentration in the cell available for enzyme inhibition may be chronically lower than the peak levels of the drug in the plasma. Fig. 6.17 shows the effect of restricted diffusion of an enzyme inhibitor into the cell. In the figure, [A_o] and [A_i] refer to the respective concentrations of inhibitors outside and inside the cell. It can be seen that as the rate constant for cell entry (k_{in}) diminishes, the deficit between the inside and the outside concentrations increases. While this deficit can be overcome by very high levels of inhibitor, there is a concentration range whereby extracellular drug levels are not reflected inside the cell; this would cause subsequent lower therapeutic inhibition for an intracellular enzyme. Box 6.8 gives an example of how the therapeutic effects of an anticancer drug are completely controlled by how well the drug can access the enzyme in the cell.

BOX 6.8

Intracellular transport trumps enzyme activity in whole cell enzyme inhibition.

Enzyme inhibitors must enter the cell to cause effects on intracellular enzymes. The anticancer benzoquinazoline folate analog 1843U89 is a potent noncompetitive inhibitor of thymidylate synthase ($K_i = 90$ pM). It gains access to the cell cytosol by being transported into the cell via the reduced folate carrier; the K_t for transport into human cells is 0.33 μM. While this compound is a potent inhibitor of cancer growth in human cells, it is 80- to 1300-fold less active as an anticancer compound in mouse. Subsequent studies have shown that 1843U89 is 80-fold less active as a substrate for transport into the cell in mouse L1210 versus human MOLT-4 cells. Thus, the inability to enter the tumor causes the striking difference in cellular activity of this compound.

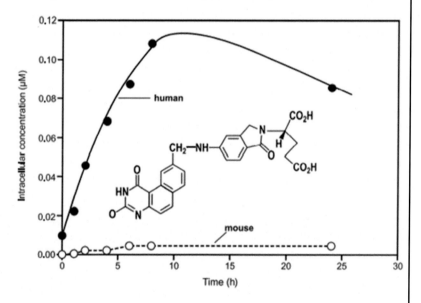

Source: *Data from: D.S. Duch, S. Banks, I.K. Dev, S.H. Dickerson, R. Ferone, L.S. Heath, et al., Biochemical and cellular pharmacology of 1843U89, a novel benzoquinazoline inhibitor of thymidylate synthase, Cancer Res. 53 (1993) 810–818 [11,12].*

Summary

- Enzymes are ubiquitous catalysts of biochemical reactions and as such furnish many potential drug targets.
- Even if a discovery target is not an enzyme, researchers need to be aware of enzyme kinetics as all drugs are subject to hepatic metabolism by Cytochrome P450 enzymes.
- The most common therapeutic approach to enzyme control is inhibition; there are four general classes of enzyme inhibition based on the relative affinity of the inhibitor for the enzyme and the enzyme-substrate complex.
- Competitive inhibition describes inhibitors that have exclusive affinity for the enzyme and compete for substrate binding.
- Mixed inhibitors bind to the enzyme and the enzyme-substrate complex with different affinity.
- Noncompetitive inhibitors bind equally well to the enzyme and the enzyme-substrate complex.
- Uncompetitive inhibitors bind only to the enzyme-substrate complex.
- These different inhibitory mechanisms yield different relationships between the potency of the inhibitor and the concentration of the substrate.
- Irreversible inhibitors can also be therapeutically useful; measuring their activity requires special techniques observing the kinetics of enzyme inhibition.
- The kinetics of enzyme inhibition are also important as reversible vs "time dependent" (irreversible) inhibition have different consequences.
- Although less common than inhibitors, enzyme activators can also be useful therapeutically.
- There are special considerations for the blockade of enzymes in cells in that concentrations may differ (from the extracellular medium). In addition, enzyme inhibitors may have no effect until the enzyme is active metabolically under in vivo conditions.

References

[1] D.M. Stresser, A.P. Blanchard, S.D. Turner, J.C.L. Erve, A.A. Dandeneau, V.P. Miller, Substrate-dependent modulation of CYP3A4 catalytic activity: analysis of 27 test compounds with four fluorometric substrates, Drug. Metab. Dispos. 28 (2000) 1440–1448.
[2] D.F. McGinnity, A.J. Berry, J.R. Kenny, K. Grime, R.J. Riley, Evaluation of time-dependent cytochrome P450 inhibition using cultured human hepatocytes, Drug. Metab. Dispos. 34 (2006) 1130–1291.
[3] J. Zhang, P.L. Yang, N.S. Gray, Targeting cancer with small molecule kinase inhibitors, Nat. Rev. Cancer 9 (2009) 28–39.

[4] J.F. Ohren, H. Chen, A. Pavlovsky, C. Whitehead, E. Zhang, P. Kuffa, Structures of human MAP kinase kinase 1 (MEK1) and MEK2 describe novel noncompetitive kinase inhibition, Nat. Struct. Biol. 11 (2004) 1192–1197.

[5] J. Zhang, P.L. Yang, N.S. Gray, Targeting cancer with small molecule kinase inhibitors, Nat. Rev. Cancer. 9 (2009) 28–39.

[6] M. Pal, Recent advances in glucokinase activators for the treatment of type 2 diabetes, Drug. Disc. Today 14 (2009) 784–792.

[7] R.R. Chapleau, C.A. McElroy, C.D. Ruark, E.J. Fleming, A.B. Ghering, J.J. Schlager, High-throughput screening for positive allosteric modulators identified potential therapeutics against acetylcholinesterase, Inhibition J. Biomol. Screen. 20 (2015) 1142–1149.

[8] T. Yeh, V. Marsh, B.A. Berant, J. Ballard, H. Colwel, R.J. Evans, Biological characterization of ARRY-142886 (AZD6244), a potent, highly selective mitogen-activated protein kinase kinase $1/2$ inhibitor, Clin. Cancer Res. 13 (2007) 1576–1583.

[9] J.A. Zorn, J.A. Wells, Turning enzymes on with small molecules, Nat. Chem. Biol. 6 (2010) 179–188.

[10] T.P. Kenakin, D.L. Scott, A method to assess concomitant cardiac phosphodiesterase inhibition and positive inotropy, J. Cardiovasc. Pharmacol. 10 (1987) 658–666.

[11] R.C. Dage, L.E. Roebel, C.P. Hsieh, D.L. Weiner, J.K. Woodward, The effects of MDL 17,043 on cardiac inotropy in the anaesthetized dog, J. Cardiovasc. Pharmacol. 4 (1982) 500–512.

[12] D.S. Duch, S. Banks, I.K. Dev, S.H. Dickerson, R. Ferone, L.S. Heath, Biochemical and cellular pharmacology of 1843U89, a novel benzoquinazoline inhibitor of thymidylate synthase, Cancer Res. 53 (1993) 810–818.

CHAPTER

7

Pharmacokinetics I: permeation and metabolism

By the end of this chapter, the reader should appreciate how the body is a balanced in vivo system of inflow (absorption) and outflow (clearance) of drugs, and how prospective drug molecules require a minimal set of physicochemical properties (referred to as "drug-like") to be able to cross biological membranes to gain entry into the body. In addition, readers will learn about how passive diffusion and transport processes control absorption, while metabolism and excretion govern

Pharmacology in Drug Discovery and Development
DOI: https://doi.org/10.1016/B978-0-443-14124-9.00008-2

the removal of drugs from the body. Finally, readers will see how in vitro metabolic assays can be used to estimate metabolic stability.

The importance of drug concentration

When testing drugs in vitro, the drug is confined to a known volume (i.e., well of a plate, test tube, etc.), therefore, the concentration of the drug is known. This is critical since all measures of drug activity (i.e., potency, efficacy, and affinity) are basically concentrations at which a defined drug effect is observed. Therefore, if a concentration of 1 μM is seen to produce a 50% inhibition of activity, then the IC_{50} is taken to be 1 μM; this is a characteristic value that would indicate a higher potency over another drug with an IC_{50} of 10 μM and a lower potency than one with an IC_{50} of 0.1 μM. The key to this type of system is accurate knowledge of the concentration. A useful way to view experiments is to define independent and dependent variables. Independent variables are what experimenters put into the experiment and what they are required to know; in this case, drug concentration. What comes out of an experiment is data in the form of dependent variables, that is, what the system being observed does with the independent variable to produce a system value, that is, potency. Independent variables have only random error whereas dependent variables have random plus system error.

In vitro data describing potency is not usually associated with a time because measurements are taken after a steady state or equilibrium has been attained. Fig. 7.1 shows the concentration of drug added to a closed vessel; the kinetics show an increase with time to a steady state after which the dependent variable attains a constant value, that is, it is a closed system. In contrast, in vivo systems are like a vessel with a hole in it; equilibrium for a single dose is not attained, and the level of fluid (e.g., concentration of drug) is very much dependent on the time that the measurement is taken, that is, they are open systems (see Fig. 7.1). Pharmacokinetics is the science of accurately determining the concentration of drug in the body and devising methods of attaining steady-state levels of drug for therapy through repeat dosing. Fig. 7.2 shows how giving repeated doses of a drug at regular intervals can achieve a steady-state level of drug in vivo. While a constant steady-state concentration of a drug can often be attained in vivo with repeated dosing, it should still be recognized that this is still a nonequilibrium system, and that the steady state depends upon both the rate of entry and the rate of exit of the drug. Changes in either of these will subsequently alter the steady-state level of drug in the body. Fig. 7.2 shows how an increase in the rate of entry of drug into the body leads to an increased steady-state, while a decrease in the rate of entry leads to a

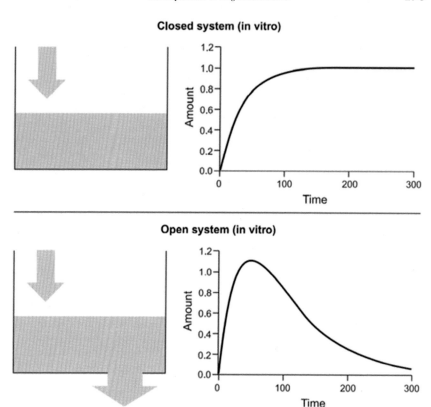

FIGURE 7.1 Model systems for drug delivery in vitro (top panel) and in vivo (bottom panel). The volume of an in vitro system is fixed; therefore, the kinetics can be likened to filling a cup. The top right panel shows the change in fluid level with time as the vessel is filled; this level models the change in concentration of a system in vitro upon the addition of a drug. In this type of system, the concentration reaches a steady-state level. The bottom panel models an in vivo system where a steady state is not attained (vessel with a hole in it). Under these circumstances, the concentration depends on the time the measurements are taken (see text).

corresponding decrease in the steady state. Fig. 7.3 shows how the rate of exit of the drug correspondingly affects steady-state levels. Thus, an increased rate of exit leads to a reduced steady state while a decrease in the rate of exit leads to an increased steady-state level. This chapter will discuss the various in vivo processes that control the rate of entry and exit of a drug from the body and the use of this knowledge to attain a therapeutically useful steady-state level.

Fig. 7.4 shows a schematic of the various processes that affect the entry into and exit the body. It is worth considering these separately as a prelude to understanding how they combine to affect in vivo drug concentration. An acronym (ADME) is often used to describe the

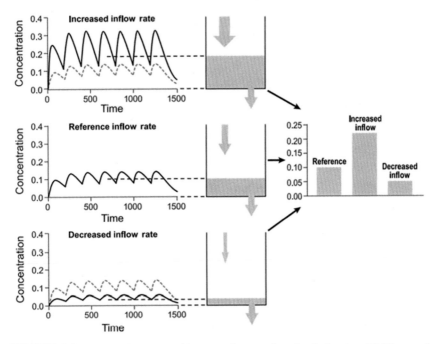

FIGURE 7.2 Repeat dosing to achieve steady-state drug levels in vivo. Middle panel shows how repeating a single dose of drug in an in vivo system can lead to a sustained level of drug after a prescribed number of doses depending on the frequency and timing of the dose (vide infra). The in vivo system is still not an equilibrium system in that it is modeled by filling a cup with a hole in it. Therefore, changes either in the rate of flow into the cup or out of the cup result in a change in the steady-state level of fluid in the cup. The top panel shows how an increase in the rate of flow into the vessel causes an increased steady-state level. The lower panel shows how a decrease in the rate of inflow causes a decrease in the steady-state level.

interaction of a molecule with these processes: absorption, distribution, metabolism, and excretion. Clearly, drugs require adequate ADME properties to be therapeutically useful; Box 7.1 shows how inferior pharmacokinetics can preclude otherwise favorable in vitro activity.

Drugs require three basic properties: primary activity at the therapeutic target; favorable ADME behavior to enter and stay in the body to produce an effect and a safety margin such that the drug causes no harm (Fig. 7.5). Having the correct chemical structure to confer favorable ADME properties for in vivo drug availability often involves separate structure-activity relationships than those required for primary therapeutic activity. The same is true for drug safety, that is, eliminating any structural feature of the molecule that enables it to interact with a system in the body to cause harm (see Chapter 10, Safety Pharmacology). An illustration of how to separate these structure-activity relationships can be is

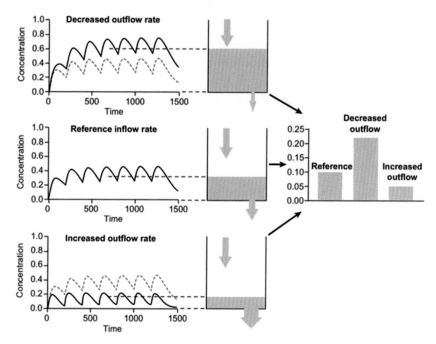

FIGURE 7.3   As shown in Fig. 7.2, repeated dosing in an in vivo system can lead to the attainment of a steady state that depends on the relative rates of entry and exit from the system. The top panel shows how a decreased rate of exit can lead to an increased steady-state level, while the bottom panel shows how an increase in the rate of exit leads to a decrease in the steady-state level.

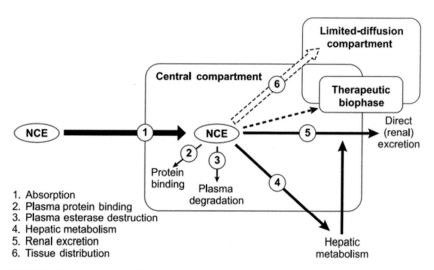

1. Absorption
2. Plasma protein binding
3. Plasma esterase destruction
4. Hepatic metabolism
5. Renal excretion
6. Tissue distribution

FIGURE 7.4   Schematic diagram of the various processes controlling the steady-state concentration of drug (labeled NCE for "new drug entity") introduced into the body. Measurements are made from a reference region referred to as the central compartment; this is usually the systemic circulation.

BOX 7.1

The practical importance of pharmacokinetics.

Inadequate ADME properties can be devastating to otherwise good drug activity; shown below are two antitumor molecules, one five times more potent than the other. The poor pharmacokinetic properties of the more potent compound make it far less active in vivo [1]. Several iterations may be required before a suitable drug candidate profile is achieved. While the first histamine H2 antagonist for ulcer treatment, burimamide, had primary target activity, it required further work to develop metiamide (target active but an inadequate safety profile) and finally cimetidine (target active, safe, and acceptable ADME properties) to achieve drug status. Pharmacokinetic problems led to a rate of 40% failure in drug development in 1991. Access to economical in vitro ADME assays led to a decrease in the failure rate to 10% in 2000 and <1% by 2008 [2].

$IC_{50} = 0.004$ nm   →Fivefold ↓ in potency $IC_{50} = 0.021$ nM

Very weak in vivo activity
Low solubility

High active in vivo
High solubility

---

shown in Fig. 7.6. It can be seen from this figure that structural changes that have little effect on the primary activity (in this case inhibition of insulin-like growth factor receptor-1) produce a two to three orders of magnitude change in a debilitating effect on cytochrome P450 enzyme inhibition that could cause a damaging drug-drug interaction (DDI) (vide infra) [3].

There is a general set of physicochemical properties common to the majority of therapeutically successful drugs; these are referred to as "drug-like" properties. Drug discovery and development common experience has shown that proactive efforts to incorporate certain drug-like properties into prospective drug candidates greatly reduce late-stage attrition in the development process (see Box 7.2). It is worth considering some of the most common drug-like activities in this light.

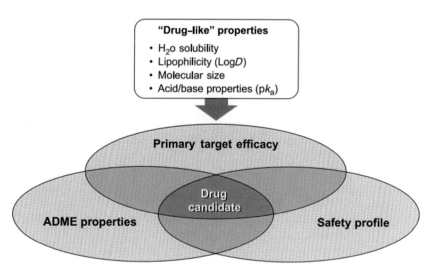

FIGURE 7.5 Four important elements of chemical structure for drugs. Overall, drugs require a set of physicochemical properties that allow them to solubilize in aqueous media, but also to cross lipid membranes. In addition, the three main activities that a molecule needs to have to be a therapeutic entity are activity at the primary target, the pharmacokinetic properties to enter the body and be present at the target for a sufficient time to produce effect, and the ability to not cause harm to the host. These three main activities may have different structure-activity relationships.

New terminology

The following new terms will be introduced in this chapter:

- *ADME*: Acronym for absorption, distribution, metabolism, and excretion, four primary elements of pharmacokinetics.
- *Antedrug*: Molecule that is itself an active drug but is also unstable, such that as it is absorbed into the body, it is metabolized into an inactive compound.
- *Bioavailability*: This parameter quantifies the amount of drug that is available for physiological action in the central compartment after absorption.
- *Central compartment*: The main circulation (bloodstream) from where pharmacokinetic sampling of drug levels is taken.
- *Clearance*: The removal of drug from the body in units of volume per unit time (e.g., mL/min).
- *Dependent variable*: Experimental observation taken from a system that has taken an independent variable and yielded a system response.
- *Drug-drug interaction*: When one drug interferes with the pharmacokinetics of another drug in the body to produce an adverse effect.

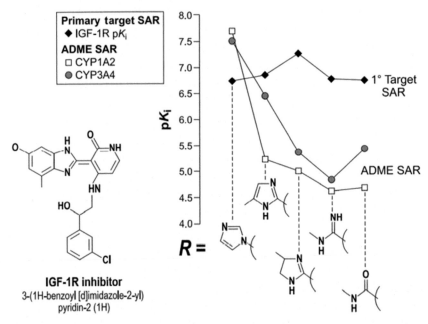

FIGURE 7.6 Analogs of an insulin growth factor receptor antagonist showing how changes in the nature of the R group lead to striking changes in the activity of the molecule at cytochrome P450 enzymes CYP1A2 and CYP3A4 (that would lead to drug-drug interactions (DDIs); *vide infra*) but relatively no change in the primary IGF-1R activity. Source: *Data redrawn from U. Velaparthi, P. Liu, B. Balasubramanian, J. Carboni, R. Attar, M. Gottardis, et al., Imidazole moiety replacements in the 3-(1H-benzo[d]imidazol-2-yl)pyridin-2 (1H)-one inhibitors of insulin-like growth factor receptor-1 (IGF-1R) to improve cytochrome P450 profile, Bioorg. Med. Chem. Lett. 17 (2007) 3072–3076.*

- *Drug-like*: The physicochemical properties of molecules that cause them to be successful drugs in vivo.
- *Enzyme induction*: The reaction of the liver to pharmacokinetic stress such that levels of metabolic enzyme activity increase either through activation of gene expression, stabilization of mRNA or PXR activation.
- *First pass effect*: The metabolic gauntlet for drugs taken orally whereby they must first be absorbed through the gastrointestinal lumen and then immediately pass through the liver via the portal vein to be metabolized.
- *Flip flop pharmacokinetics*: A characteristic mismatch of the elimination rates of extended-release preparations and iv preparations that is caused when the rate of absorption is slower than the rate of elimination
- *Independent variable*: The experimental quantity (usually drug dose or concentration) known by the experimenter that is processed by the system to yield the dependent variable.

BOX 7.2

Introducing ADME properties: the sooner the better.

Prior to 1990, a common practice in drug discovery was to optimize primary target activity with the idea of modifying structures for ADME activity later in the process. This can be problematic since the molecular structure may be such that any changes could lead to a loss of activity; that is, there would be insufficient places in the chemical scaffold to modify ADME properties without compromising the original activity. This is illustrated by a sample of drugs shown below, where it can be seen that the original lead molecule obtained from the screening process is extraordinarily similar to the final drug. This supports the notion of having molecules in screening libraries that already have favorable ADME properties.

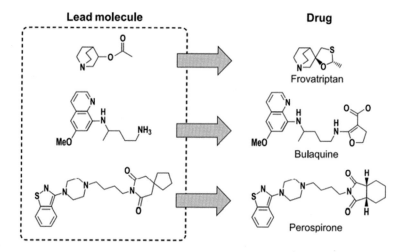

Source: *Data from J.R. Proudfoot, Drugs, leads, and drug-likeness: an analysis of some recently launched drugs, Bioorg. Med. Chem. Lett. 12 (2002) 1647–1650.*

- *In vitro system*: Latin for "within the glass," this term refers to an experiment done in a controlled environment. For pharmacology, it is when experiments are done in contained vessels and where concentration is known (a closed system).
- *In vivo system*: "Within a living organism," this term refers to experiments done in the whole body (an open system).

- *Lipophilicity*: The ability of a molecule to dissolve in lipids or organic solvents, such as octanol or heptane, as opposed to water.
- *LogP (LogD)*: Logarithm of the ratio of the solubility of a compound in organic medium versus aqueous medium. cLogP is calculated and mLogP is measured. LogD takes into account ionized species in the aqueous medium and must be reported with a distinct pH value.
- *MAD*: "Maximal absorbable dose" is the maximum amount of drug that can be expected to be absorbed from the GI tract when a compound is given orally.
- *Mechanism-based inhibition (also time-dependent inhibition)*: Blockade of an enzyme that is essentially irreversible. The onset time for full blockade is prolonged and new enzyme activity can only be obtained through synthesis of new enzyme.
- *PAMPA*: "Parallel artificial membrane permeation assay" consisting of a synthetic hexadecane lipid membrane layered over a screen to allow measurement of molecules traversing the membrane via bulk lipid diffusion.
- *Permeation (Papp)*: The rate of transfer of a molecule across a membrane (usually expressed in cm/seconds).
- *pK_a*: Negative logarithm of equilibrium equation describing relative amounts of a molecule in the acid/base form over the unionized form.
- *Prodrug*: Molecule that itself is not biologically active but is optimized to be absorbed into the body. Once the molecule is absorbed, biological, or chemical processes transform the prodrug into the active drug.
- *$t_{1/2}$*: The time required for the amount of substance, decaying as a result of an exponential process, to decrease to half of its initial value.

"Drug-Like" properties of molecules

The physicochemical properties of molecules that are important to their function as drugs can be summarized under the following headings:

- Water solubility;
- Lipophilicity;
- pK_a and acid/base properties;
- molecular weight.

It is worth considering these separately.

Water solubility

A molecule *must* dissolve in water before it can interact with any process in the body, including passage through lipid membranes. Molecules can have a wide range of solubility in water and this can greatly affect how well they are absorbed and metabolized, how they distribute through the body compartments, and how they are excreted. An indication of how important water solubility is can be determined from consideration of maximal absorbable dose (MAD) values. This is basically the maximal amount of drug that can be absorbed orally if the small intestine (the site for oral drug absorption) were saturated with the drug (i.e., the maximum amount dissolved in water) for 4.5 hours (the transit time for intestinal contents). The MAD is given by:

$$MAD = S \times K_{ab} \times SIWV \times SITT \tag{7.1}$$

where S is H_2O solubility in mg/mL at pH 6.5, K_{ab} is the transintestinal absorption rate constant per minutes, SIWV is the small intestine water volume (≈ 250 mL), and SITT is the small intestine transit time (≈ 4.5 hours). Calculation of the MAD can be revealing. For example, if a required therapeutic level of a drug were 0.5 mg/kg, then 35 mg would need to be absorbed for a 70 kg patient. If a given drug has an absorption rate constant from the intestine of 0.03/minutes and a low solubility (0.001 mg/mL), the MAD would only be 2 mg, well below that needed for any effect. For cases of low absorption, solubility may be much more amenable to change than intestinal absorption. The latter value generally can effectively be increased by a factor of 50 (from 0.001 to 0.05/minutes) through medicinal chemistry, whereas solubility can change by five orders of magnitude (0.001 to 100 mg/mL). In the previous example, chemical modification to increase water solubility to a value of 0.02 mg/mL would put the drug in the therapeutic range (MAD = 40 mg). A high-water solubility for a drug molecule is 85% solubility at pH values from 1 to 7.5 occurring in less than 30 minutes.

Lipophilicity

This is the degree to which the drug molecule will dissolve in organic media; it is a surrogate for how well the drug will dissolve in biological lipid membranes. This can be estimated through LogP or LogD values, which can, in turn, be measured or calculated through indices associated with chemical groups on the molecule. LogP values are logarithms of the relative concentration of the molecule dissolved in an organic medium, such as octanol or heptane versus that dissolved in water. Thus, a LogP value of 0.5 indicates a fairly water-soluble molecule with a ratio of 3.16—1 for octanol to water. LogP values >3 indicate highly lipid-soluble molecules (ratio octanol to water of >1000 to 1). LogD values are the same as LogP values except, unlike the latter, they also include the ionic species. For this reason, they must be reported with a given pH value, as the ionization of molecules can change at different pH values (vide infra). The dependence of cellular absorption on LogP or LogD values illustrates the particular dichotomous behavior drug molecules must have toward aqueous and organic media, that is, drugs must dissolve in water but also in lipid to interact with biological systems and cross membranes; this will be considered further in the discussion of drug absorption. A drug-like value for LogP ranges from $0.5 < LogP < 3$. LogP and LogD values are widely used in the structure-activity analyses of ADME properties, since they are readily available for molecules and can be correlated with a wide range of ADME processes. Of a sample of 1791 approved drugs, the mean LogP value is 2.5 [4].

Acid/base properties

Molecules can function as acids or bases in aqueous media depending on the ability of various chemical groups to lose or gain hydrogen ions. The ease with which this occurs depends on the pH of the medium. The relationship between the propensity of a molecule to be in an acidic or basic state and the pH is given by the Henderson—Hasslebach equation:

$$pK_a = pH + Log([acidform]/[baseform]) \qquad (7.2)$$

Where pK_a refers to the $-$logarithm of the K_a, which is a dissociation constant of a molecular species HB such that $K_a = [H^+][B]/[HB]$ (B is the conjugate base of the molecule HB). The important point to note is that the pK_a of a given molecule can dictate the relative number of ionic species in the aqueous medium. Since, ions do not cross lipid barriers through bulk diffusion, this can affect drug absorption. For example, the decongestant phenylpropanolamine has a pK_a of 9.4, which indicates that it essentially exists in the charged conjugate acid form throughout all of the physiological range of pH (1.5—7.8). The population of known drugs have a huge range of pK_a from 1 (dapsone) to nearly 14 (caffeine). The pK_a is mainly used to assess drug absorption and distribution in pharmacokinetic studies.

Molecular weight

Extremely large molecules do not cross plasma-lipid membranes well; therefore, a molecular weight <350 is a good target for drug-like activity. Of a sample of all marketed drugs up to 1995, the median molecular weight is 350. However, there are classes of drug that seem to require greater mass, for example, HIV protease and renin inhibitors have a median molecular weight of 680—700.

In general, the physicochemical properties of a molecule should be within certain ranges for drug-like activity but exceptions to these rules can be found in every category (see Box 7.3). A frequently used guideline is the so-called "rule of 5" reported by Lipinski and colleagues [7,8]. From an analysis of 2245 drug-like compounds, it was observed that 89% had a molecular weight <550, only 10% had a calculated LogP > 5.0, only 8% had a sum of OH and NH (hydrogen bond donors) groups >5, and only 12% had the sum of N and O atoms (hydrogen bond acceptors) >10. From these facts came a set of four rules involving the number 5 suggesting that poor absorption or permeation would be more likely from molecules that had:

- > 5 H-bond donors;
- > 10 hydrogen bond acceptors;
- > 500 molecular weight;
- > 5 calculated LogP.

Once a molecule that has been synthesized shows primary therapeutic target activity in the appropriate in vitro systems and does not greatly violate drug-like property rules, it can be tested in vivo; under these conditions it must enter the human body to reach the therapeutic target organ and remain in the target compartment long enough to produce therapeutic activity. The first step in this process is absorption.

Drug absorption

All drugs must cross cell lipid bilayer membranes to reach their site of action in the body. The rate at which they do this, coupled with the rate at which they are removed from the compartment into which they diffuse, dictates the overall concentration in the compartment (as shown in Figs. 7.2 and 7.3). One of the most important mechanisms to enable passage through membranes is bulk diffusion. Fig. 7.7 shows three possible outcomes for a molecule interacting with a cell membrane: the molecule may or may not pass through the membrane, or it may dissolve and stay in the membrane. The relative propensity of the molecule to dissolve in water and lipid dictates which of these will occur; as discussed previously, a useful measure of water to lipid solubility is the LogP or LogD value for the molecule. If a molecule is highly soluble in water (LogP ≤ 0.5), it will not penetrate lipid membranes well (Fig. 7.7 region A). A molecule with solubility both in water and lipid (0.5 < LogP < 3.0; Fig. 7.7 region B) may cross lipid membranes while an extremely lipid-soluble molecule (LogP > 3) may dissolve in the lipid membrane and stay there (Fig. 7.7 region C). Bulk diffusion is driven by a concentration gradient, thus, there will be a flow of molecules from the region of high

BOX 7.3

Water versus lipid solubility of drugs.

Guidelines for drug absorption can be derived from solubility and LogP data, but there are exceptions. For instance, azithromycin has an extremely low transintestinal absorption rate constant ($K_{ab} = 0.001/$ min) normally predictive of very poor absorption. However, the extraordinarily high solubility of this molecule (> 50 mg/mL) allows it to have a very high MAD of 3.75 g [5].

Usually, exceedingly high LogP values are associated with lack of membrane permeation due to the fact that the molecules may lodge in the lipid membrane and not traverse the cell (i.e., dihydropyridines). High LogP values are also associated with nonspecific activity and undesirable drug profiles. However, torcetrapib, a drug for dyslipidemia targeting cholesterol ester transfer protein, has a cLogP of 8.2. In this case, the natural substrates for this target are cholesterol esters (cLogP = 18) thus, the high LogP for torcetrapib is a requirement for activity [6].

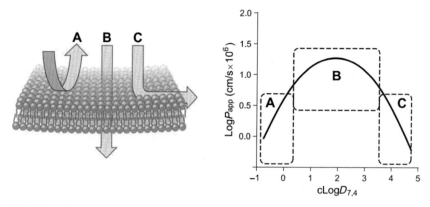

FIGURE 7.7 Diffusion through lipid membranes. Region A contains compounds of low LogP values (highly water-soluble). These may not penetrate lipid membranes and remain in the aqueous phase. Region B contains molecules that dissolve both in water and lipid (0.5 < LogP < 3.0) and thus may cross lipid membranes. Highly lipid-soluble compounds (region C; LogP > 3) may dissolve in the membrane and not emerge (i.e., dihydropyridines). Graph on right shows the relationship between permeation and $cLogD_{7.4}$.

concentration (i.e., outside the cell) to a region of low concentration (inside the cell and/or beyond the cell layer barrier). A system has been devised that considers how well molecules permeate lipid membranes and also their water solubility. Termed the BCS system, it generally predicts how well molecules will be absorbed (see Box 7.4).

In addition to bulk diffusion, cells may cross cell membranes through a transport process, such as:

- *Facilitated diffusion*: An oscillating carrier protein shuttles molecules across the membrane. These processes are concentration-gradient driven and do not require energy. They generally transport sugars and other nutrients and are not especially relevant to drugs.
- *Active transport*: Passage across the membrane is mediated by a saturable transport process that requires energy. These can operate against a concentration gradient and are important in the liver, kidney, gut epithelium, and blood-brain barrier (vide infra). Importantly, they can operate to take molecules both inside and outside of the cell.

Fig. 7.8 shows three important mechanisms for molecular transfer across cell lipid membranes; bulk diffusion, transport into the cell (influx) and transport out of the cell (efflux). In many cases, all three of these may be operable for drug entry into the cell and beyond a cellular barrier such as the intestinal tract. It is important to note that, since the transport processes are saturable and bulk diffusion is not, the overall rate of uptake of a molecule into the cell can be concentration-dependent. This means that,

BOX 7.4

The biopharmaceutics classification system (BCS).

The BCS system ranks molecules in terms of solubility and permeability. For Class 1 molecules (ideal for oral drugs) the rate of dissolution limits absorption. Class 2 molecules typically require formulation since solubility limits absorption. For Class 3 molecules, permeability limits absorption; in these cases, a prodrug strategy is often employed. While LogP values can be useful guidelines for solubility, wide variations can be observed. For example, in spite of a 21,000-folds difference in LogP values for clazozimine (LogP = 5.39) and levonorgestrel (LogP = 0.06), they have equal water solubilities (0.01 mg/mL) [9].

	High solubility	Low solubility
High permeability	Class 1 (amphiphilic) Nortriptyline Diltiazem Captopril Labetolol Enalapril Propranolol Metoprolol	Class 2 (lipophilic) Phenytoin diclofenac Naproxen Piroxicam Carbamazepine Flurbiprofen
Low permeability	Class 3 (hydrophilic) Cimetidine Atenolol Ranitidine Nadolol Femotidine	Class 4 Hydrochlorthiazide Furosemide Ketoprofen Terfenadine

depending on where the process is being viewed (i.e., GI tract versus therapeutic cell in the central compartment), diffusion, influx, and efflux can be of varying importance. Efflux processes (such as P-gp, p-glycoprotein transport) shuttle molecules that have already entered the cell and transport them out of the cell again; they are designed to protect cells from foreign chemicals. As shown in Fig. 7.8, an efflux process can effectively stop entry into the cell at low concentrations (see curve for observed absorption). However, if the molecule diffuses through lipid membranes, then high concentrations that saturate the efflux process can still enter cells. Similarly, if a drug is transported into the cell, then lower doses may rely more on this mechanism than on bulk diffusion. This may be important for low concentrations of drug that are transported into hepatic cells for degradation.

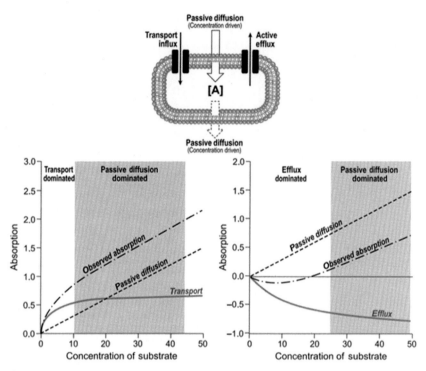

FIGURE 7.8 Mechanisms of entry into and through cells. Molecule A may enter the cell through bulk diffusion through the lipid membrane and/or an influx through a transport carrier. It can leave the cell through bulk diffusion (although this is concentration driven and thus the flow will be to the region of lower concentration) or an efflux carrier. The efflux carrier can proceed against a concentration gradient; thus, it serves as a barrier to absorption while diffusion promotes absorption. Influx and efflux mechanisms are saturable with respect to concentration (curved Michaelis—Menten-like curves) while diffusion is not (straight line). Bottom panels show how overall transfer of molecules through cells is the sum of diffusion and influx-efflux. It can be seen that low concentrations are more subject to transport processes, making overall entry dependent on concentration. It can also be seen that low concentrations may be dominated by efflux processes, but that these can be overcome through bulk diffusion of higher concentrations.

On a more general note, molecules must not only enter cells but must also cross into and back out of cells in a vectorial manner to gain access to therapeutically relevant compartments in the body. A useful model of this larger scale absorption is the transfer of molecules from the lumen of the GI tract to the bloodstream. Fig. 7.9 shows a range of operative processes when cells cross the GI epithelial cell layer to gain access to the central compartment. In addition to bulk diffusion and influx, and battling efflux processes, molecules may be destroyed by metabolic enzymes as they try to cross the epithelial cell layer. Notably, the metabolic enzyme cytochrome P450 type 3A4, an extremely common

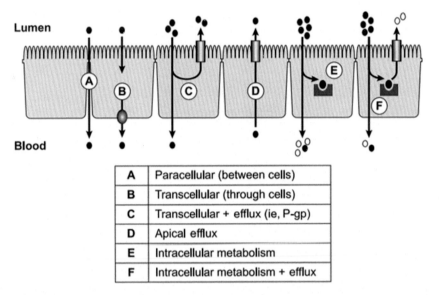

A	Paracellular (between cells)
B	Transcellular (through cells)
C	Transcellular + efflux (ie, P-gp)
D	Apical efflux
E	Intracellular metabolism
F	Intracellular metabolism + efflux

FIGURE 7.9   Processes operative as molecules cross cell layers to gain access to the central compartment through epithelial cells from the lumen of the gastrointestinal tract. (A) Molecules may pass through small openings between cells (8–10 angstroms). (B) Cross the cell membrane through bulk diffusion or an influx transport process or both. (C) Cross through membranes via diffusion and influx but are also subject to apical efflux (i.e., P-gp). (D) Bulk diffusion can also cause reverse passage of drug from the central compartment to lumen (minor). (E) Molecules enter the cell but then are metabolized. (F) Molecules enter the cell, are metabolized and also are removed from the cell through active efflux.

metabolizing enzyme for drug molecules (vide infra), is present in these cells and can notably deplete the concentration of drug as it passes from the lumen into the bloodstream. The most formidable barrier to lumen–bloodstream absorption is a combination of metabolic degradation and active efflux from the cell (process F in Fig. 7.9).

There are very useful in vitro model systems that can be used to measure the ability of molecules to pass through membranes (measured as permeation values [P_{app}] with units of rate $\times 10^{-5}$ cm/s). For passive lipid membrane diffusion, the rate of passage through a phospholipid coated filter membrane (referred to as PAMPA for Parallel Artificial Membrane Permeation Assay) is measured. Permeation through biological membranes can also be measured in vitro by-passing molecules through a layer of cells designed to model the gastrointestinal tract. The most commonly used cells are Caco-2 cells (human colonic adenocarcinoma cells). These preparations allow molecules to pass through the lipid membrane by bulk diffusion as well as through influx transport and also to encounter efflux transport processes, such as P-gp. Comparison of permeation values in PAMPA and Caco-2 assays can be used to determine whether molecules primarily cross membranes through bulk diffusion or if they are substrates of either active influx or active efflux processes (see Fig. 7.10). Similarly, the bidirectional permeation across CaCo-2 cells can be used to detect efflux mechanisms, such as P-gp. In this case, the P_{app} for transfer from the basal to the apical side (inside to outside) will be greater than P_{app} values for diffusion from the apical to the basal side (outside to inside). If this difference is eliminated by efflux transporter inhibitors (such as verapamil for P-gp) then activity of an efflux transporter is confirmed. While CaCo-2 cells have proven extremely serviceable in ADME permeation studies, there are exceptions to their predictive value. For example, β-lactam antibio-

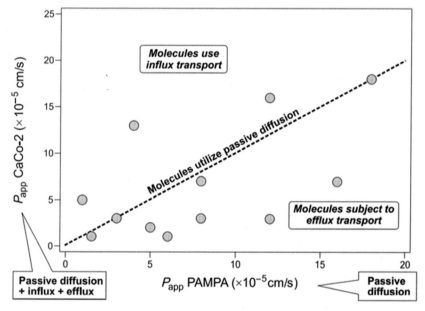

FIGURE 7.10 Differences in permeation values for compounds in a passive diffusion assay (abscissa) and a biological membrane assay (ordinates). If P_{app} values are the same in each assay, then the presence of influx or efflux does not alter permeation, supporting the view that passive diffusion is the primary mechanism. If P_{app} in parallel artificial membrane permeation assay (PAMPA) is greater than CaCo-2, then a retarding efflux in the biological membrane is suggested. Similarly, if P_{app} in CaCo-1 is greater than PAMPA, then the presence of an assisting influx transporter in the biological membrane is suggested.

tics (cephalexin, amoxicillin) and ACE inhibitors are good substrates for peptide transporters and have poor permeability in Caco-2 cells, yet these drugs are completely absorbed in vivo in humans.

Drug absorption is important for the entry of molecules into cells for therapy and also for entry into the body, especially via the oral route of administration. This latter important process is greatly affected by drug metabolism, so it will be considered later in this chapter after metabolism has been discussed. An important variable in drug absorption is the route of administration and this can be manipulated for therapeutic advantage. There are generally three routes of administration:

- Parenteral: This route pieces an outer protective boundary of the body (i.e., skin). Examples of parenteral administration are intravenous, intramuscular (vaccines, antibiotics, and psychoactive drugs), subcutaneous (insulin), intrathecal (anesthesia, chemotherapy).
- Enteral: This is oral and/or rectal delivery.
- Topical: This route requires penetration of a boundary exposed to the environment. Examples of topical administration are inhalation (bronchodilators for treatment of asthma), skin (epicutaneous, topic antiinflammatory drugs), eye drops (antibiotics), ear drops (antibiotics, otitis treatments), intranasal (decongestants), and vaginal (estrogen, antibiotics).

There can be several reasons for choosing a particular route of drug administration. For instance, it may be a necessity, as in the case of nitroglycerin in the treatment of cardiac angina. The treatment must reach the heart quickly without being broken down in the body; via the oral route, nitroglycerin is nearly completely destroyed as it passes through the liver, thus it does not reach the heart in any appreciable concentration. However, taken sublingually, it is readily absorbed and immediately travels via the venae cava to the heart—see Box 7.5.

The speed of drug absorption can be affected by the route of administration. Fig. 7.11 shows the absorption of the antimigraine treatment Rizatriptan. To alleviate a migraine attack, it can be taken via inhalation, where it can be seen that a serum level of nearly 400 ng/mL can be attained within 5 minutes. In contrast, as a maintenance treatment to prevent a migraine attack, it can be taken subcutaneously where a lower serum level (40 ng/mL) can be sustained over at least 45 minutes [10] The route of absorption is an important determinant of optimizing the location of drug application and also of safety. For instance, β_2-adrenoceptor agonist bronchodilators are given via aerosol, where the maximum concentration is delivered to the airways and bronchi, where they

BOX 7.5

Nitroglycerin's highway to the heart.

Angina is a serious disease whereby the energy demands of the heart exceed the energy that can be made available through occluded coronary arteries. The result is crushing chest pain and a debilitating compromise of myocardial contractility. Once an attack of angina occurs, it is crucial to deliver the coronary vasodilator nitroglycerin directly to the coronary arteries to produce vasorelaxation and concomitantly increase oxygen supply to myocardial muscle. However, the oral route of absorption is not fast enough to produce relief of pain and moreover, nitroglycerin is nearly completely destroyed by the liver in the first-pass effect. In contrast, sublingual administration produces a rapid absorption and no metabolic impediment to accessibility to the heart as the blood supply from the sublingual area directly flows into the venae cava and subsequently to the myocardial muscle.

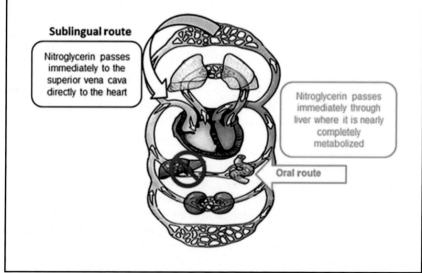

Sublingual route

Nitroglycerin passes immediately to the superior vena cava directly to the heart

Nitroglycerin passes immediately through liver where it is nearly completely metabolized

Oral route

are needed. The agonist then dilutes into the bloodstream and reaches the heart, where debilitating tachycardia can ensue, in a much lower concentration.

Table 7.1 shows the various common routes of drug administration and some of their salient features. With the exception of parenteral

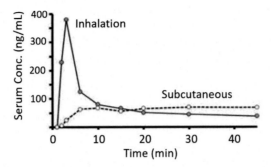

FIGURE 7.11   Absorption of the antimigraine drug Rizatriptan taken via inhalation (gray-filled circles solid line) and subcutaneously (open circles, dotted line). It can be seen that both the speed of absorption and the level of drug absorbed vary considerably with route of administration. *Source: Data redrawn from T. Otulana, J. Thipphawong, Systemic delivery of small molecules: product development issues focused on pain therapeutics. Respir. Drug Deliv. VIII (2002) 97–104.*

administration directly into the bloodstream, absorption is an important element of available drug levels.

There are certain physicochemical molecular properties that are important for drug absorption (correct LogP, molecular size, etc.) and there are some situations where the structure-activity relationships required for primary drug activity cannot be reconciled with those required for absorption. Under these circumstances, a prodrug of the active drug molecule may need to be used in vivo. A prodrug is a metabolically unstable derivative of the active drug that is itself well absorbed but degrades to the active drug in the central compartment after absorption (see Fig. 7.12 and Box 7.6).

Some commonly used drugs that actually are administered as prodrugs are Enalapril (esterase release of active moiety enalaprilat for hypertension), Valaciclovir (esterase release of acyclovir for herpes), and Levodopa (DOPA decarboxylase-mediated release of dopamine for Parkinson's disease). In addition to aiding drug absorption, prodrugs are used as a strategy for improved lipophilicity, aqueous solubility, parenteral administration, improved ophthalmic and dermal delivery and exploitation of exploit carrier-mediated absorption. Fig. 7.13 shows some common chemical linkers used to construct prodrugs; these are covalently linked through bioreversible groups that are chemically or enzymatically labile and some examples of prodrugs utilizing these strategies. In general, good prodrugs have nontoxic hetero-aromatic pro-moieties and yield parent drugs with high recovery ratios. A variation of this theme is an antedrug which is a molecule that has limited distribution and absorption properties due to the fact that it degrades to a nonabsorbable and/or inactive derivative

TABLE 7.1 Routes of administration for drugs.

Route	Advantages	Disadvantages
Parenteral		
Intravenous	• Rapid attainment of concentration • Precise delivery of dosage • Easy to titrate dose	• High initial concentration: toxicity • Invasive: risk of infection • Requires skill
Subcutaneous	• Prompt absorption from aqueous • Little training needed • Avoid harsh GI environment • Can be used for suspensions	• Cannot be used for large volumes • Potential pain/tissue damage • Variable absorption
Enteral		
Oral	• Convenient (storage/portability) • Economical/noninvasive/safe • Requires no training	• Delivery can be erratic • Depends on patient compliance • Drugs degrade in GI environment • First pass effect
Sublingual	• Rapid onset • Avoids first pass	• Few drugs adequately absorbed • Patients must avoid swallowing • Difficult compliance
Pulmonary	• Easy to titrate dose/rapid onset • Local effect/minimizes toxic effects	• Requires coordination • Lung disease limits • Variable delivery
Topical	• Minimize side-effects • Avoids first pass effect	• Cosmetically unappealing • Erratic absorption

after leaving the active therapeutic compartment (Fig. 7.12). Some examples of antedrugs are given in Box 7.7.

Absorption of biologics

The absorption of molecules through cell lipid membranes involves physiochemical properties associating the cell membrane and the molecule. However, if the drug is a biologic (i.e., protein, peptide, antibody, nucleotide-congener) then the standard lipid-soluble model of drug absorption may not be applicable. In general, the pharmacokinetics of biologic molecules is characterized by (1) slow rate of absorption, (2) confined distribution, and (3) mechanisms of metabolism and excretion that are different from those of small molecules. The large size of biologics (some molecular weights exceeding 100 kD) and susceptibility to degradation pose special

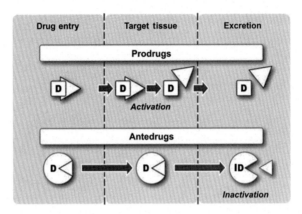

FIGURE 7.12   Two strategies for controlling drug absorption. *Prodrugs* are derivatives of an active drug that are well absorbed. Once in the therapeutic compartment they are degraded to the active drug. *Antedrugs* are unstable active drugs that reach the therapeutic compartment and are then degraded to inactive products before they distribute further in the body.

problems for the therapeutic administration of biologics. Size leads to greatly reduced permeability across barriers, such as skin, mucosal membranes, and cell membranes while various enzymatic barriers also are present as the biologic moves from the site of administration to the site of action. The absorption of biologics can determine therapeutic effectiveness. In general, issues range from poor bioavailability, rapid degradation, short half-life (median levels of ≈ 5.3 minutes), and high levels of clearance.

In some cases, short half times are beneficial as in the transient effects of oxytocin used to induce labor and strengthen contractions. However, where needed, biologics have been modified by a number of strategies to improve pharmacokinetic properties including: (1) mutation of one or more amino acids (creating a protein analog as has been extensively with insulin) and (2) acylation/pegylation (reducing metabolism and immunogenicity). In terms of administration, obviously the most direct method for presentation of a biologic to an in vivo system is injection. This method has the advantage of high reproducibility and 100% bioavailability; possible disadvantages are pain at the site of injection, and requirement of medical personnel. An innovation for this method is jet injection. This has the advantage of being needle-free and leads to rapid systemic absorption; also, it does not require modifications of injector designs. Possible disadvantages are that this method can cause inconsistent delivery of drugs, occasional pain, and bruising. An extension of this technique is depot injections, whereby larger doses of drug, perhaps modified to reduce the rate of absorption, are given as an injection.

BOX 7.6

Prodrugs: strategies for drug delivery.

There are cases where valuable drug therapy cannot be delivered to the organ where it is required. Also, there are some compartments of the body that have restricted access (i.e., cerebrospinal, endolymph, synovial, and pleural fluid). One of these is the eye, which, in addition to providing an aqueous outward flow that prevents entry, also requires drugs to cross the cornea. A useful molecule to lower the elevated pressure in the eye in glaucoma is the natural hormone epinephrine. However, this molecule does not cross the cornea, making the administration of epinephrine in glaucoma a problem. The diester dipivalylepinephrine crosses the cornea readily and when this molecule enters the eye, esterases release the active epinephrine molecule. Prodrugs can also be used to limit side-effects, a strategy often used for drugs administered by aerosol in the lung, where the surface area for absorption in humans is the size of a tennis court. This method of delivery is rapid, avoids first pass degradation in the liver, presents the drug in a high concentration at the organ for treatment (i.e., bronchioles), and then diffuses in much lower concentrations at organs where safety may be an issue (i.e., the heart).

Cornea

Dipivalylepinephrine

Esterase

Epinephrine

For example degarelix, a synthetic derivative of GnRH that blocks endogenous receptors in the pituitary gland for prostate cancer, is slowly released from a depot injection to give half times ranging from 42 to 70 days [11]. This approach can be applied with a wide variety of formulations that avoid reconstitution and can be prepared for weekly, monthly, quarterly or semiannual doses. However, this technology, which can produce a fairly continuous release of drug into the blood,

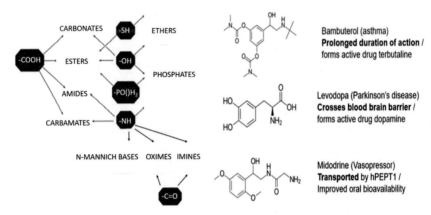

FIGURE 7.13 Chemical linkers providing biologically labile groups for degradation to parent compounds for prodrugs. This strategy can be used for a variety of applications including increased absorption and duration of action. This strategy has been used for Bambuterol (increased duration of action), Levodopa (increased blood brain barrier permeation), and Midrodine (improved oral bioavailability). Source: *Data redrawn from J. Rautio, H. Kumpulainen, T. Heimbach, R. Oliyai, D. Oh, T. Jarvinen, J. Savolainen, Prodrugs: design and clinical applications. Nat Rev Drug Disc.7 (2008) 255—270.*

can demonstrate "flip-flop" kinetics to confound absorption and elimination pharmacokinetics. This effect can be seen with controlled, extended, and sustained-release formulations, gels, film prodrugs, liposomes, micelles, and polymeric nanoparticles (see Fig. 7.14).

Subcutaneous injections can be a viable route of administration for biologics. These have the advantage of avoiding first-pass metabolism and they can be self-administered. However, the injection can be painful and there may be limited space for injectable volumes (<1.5–2 mL). Improved dispersion and tissue permeability can be enhanced by using hyaluronidases (natural enzymes found in mammalian tissue, to digest hyaluronan, a major component the subcutaneous extracellular matrix). Microparticles can be used to control release for long-term delivery (1 week or longer) and these can be administered by intramuscular or subcutaneous injection. Even smaller particles can be employed in the form of nanoparticles. These can be used for the delivery of cytokines for tumor immunotherapy where delivery depends on the small size of the particles to enhance permeation and retention in tumors. This technology has been advanced with pegylation (prolonged circulation of nanoparticle enhancers to allow deep tumor penetration).

Another technology for the absorption of biologics is transdermal delivery. This has the advantages of being painless (high patient compliance), providing sustained effect, allowing active control and discontinuation of delivery, being noninvasive, and allowing self-administration

---

BOX 7.7

Antedrugs as "Hit and Run" therapy.

Antedrugs are molecules with pharmacologic activity that is expressed where the drug is deposited but then disappears as the drug leaves the therapeutic receptor compartment. This prevents drugs, that may have harmful effects in other regions of the body, from expressing those effects. For example, glucocorticoids can provide therapeutic alleviation of inflammation on the skin but when absorbed into the body, can also produce debilitating adrenal insufficiency, fluid and electrolyte abnormalities, hypertension and hyperglycemia. Glucocorticoid analogs that degrade to an inactive species upon absorption beyond the skin prevent these effects from occurring. Another scenario for antedrug strategies is bronchodilators for asthma. β-Adrenoceptor bronchodilators open constricted airways in the lung but if allowed to diffuse throughout the body, can also cause harmful cardiac effects. The fact that 90% of all inhaled drugs are actually swallowed and go into the GI tract provides a convenient way to antedrug bronchodilators. Specifically, using structures that are rapidly destroyed by the liver prevents whole body harmful effects; CYP2D6 is an effective eliminator of β-bronchodilator molecules.

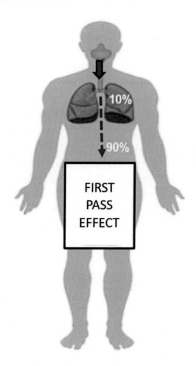

FIRST
PASS
EFFECT

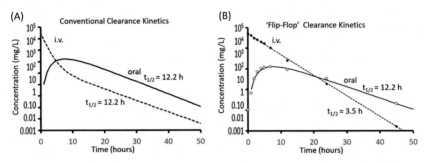

FIGURE 7.14   Clearance kinetics of drugs given via the iv and oral route. (A) Conventional clearance kinetics dictate that the rate of elimination (and $t_{1/2}$) for elimination should be the same. (B) If the rate of absorption is much slower than the rate of elimination, then "flip-flop" clearance kinetics are observed whereby the $t_{1/2}$ for elimination after iv administration is $<t_{1/2}$ for elimination after oral absorption. Data in panel B is for levovirin, a nucleoside DNA/RNA antiviral. Source: *Redrawn from C.-C. Lin, T. Luu, D. Lourenco, L.-T. Yeh, J.Y.N. Lau, Absorption, pharmacokinetics and excretion of levovirin in rats, dogs and Cynomolgus monkeys. J. Antimicrob. Chemother. 51 (2003) 93–99.*

to avoid first-pass metabolism A possible disadvantage of this technique is that it may provide a low bioavailability and some devices can be expensive. Biologics can be administered as microparticles, intramuscular or subcutaneous injections; these have the advantage of producing controlled release for long term delivery (1 week or longer). A further variation involves biologics as nanoparticles composed of polymers, lipids and dendrimers; these are used as carriers for targeted delivery (i.e., cytokines) for tumor immunotherapy. The small size of the particles give enhanced permeation and facilitates retention in tumors. Nanoparticles have been applied to the problem of oral absorption (absorption through the intestinal epithelium).

Biologics also can be administered via the pulmonary system through inhalation. The lungs have a large surface area for absorption to allow rapid and high bioavailability; in addition, this route of administration avoids first-pass metabolism. However, this method requires patient training and has a high rate of variability in dosing (depending on inhaler technique).

Oral delivery also has been explored for biologics; this has the advantage of high patient compliance and being noninvasive and easy to use (can be self-administered). However, the biologic enters a harsh chemical environment that causes it to be degraded by first-pass metabolism. Also, the biologic encounters epithelial cells, mucus, bacteria, acid, enzymes, and proteases as barriers to absorption. Proteins are quickly digested and inactivated by the enzymes designed to break down amide bonds and this can cause low bioavailability. In addition, the GI tract is dynamic (normal transit time to traverse the GI tract is approximately 3–3.5 hours) thus absorption must be relatively rapid to allow sufficient biologic to

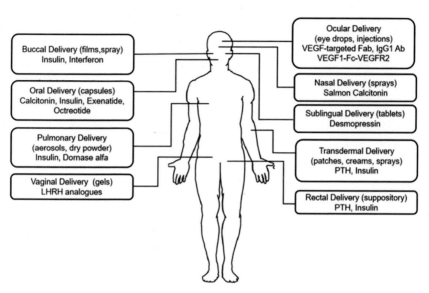

FIGURE 7.15 Diagrammatic representation of the various routes of administration for biologics.

enter the body. This can be a problem as biologic absorption is notoriously slow thereby limiting this process. Oral absorption with nanoparticles that are absorbed through the intestinal epithelium and mucoadhesive with devices, have been explored for insulin and calcitonin. The various routes of administration for biologics are summarized in Fig. 7.15.

Drug metabolism

Foreign chemicals are destroyed by metabolic enzymes present in numerous regions of the body including the lungs, intestinal. and nasal mucosa, brain, plasma, kidney, and the liver. In general, however, the most important organ in the body for protection from foreign chemicals is the liver. This organ directly receives chemicals ingested by the oral route and acts as a cyclic filter of chemicals introduced by other means (parenterally, topically, or via aerosol). It is designed to destroy all chemicals foreign to the body and does so through an extensive collection of degradative enzymes. There are two general classes of metabolic reactions present in the liver known as Phase 1 (functionalization) and Phase 2 (conjugation) reactions. Phase 1 reactions introduce or expose functional groups into the molecule which can then be linked to functional groups by Phase 2 enzymes to yield highly polar (and usually

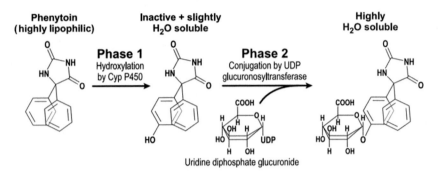

FIGURE 7.16 The metabolism of Phenytoin, an anticonvulsant used for the treatment of seizures. Phase 1 hydroxylation converts the lipophilic active drug into a more water-soluble inactive hydroxylated product, which then undergoes Phase 2 metabolism to a highly soluble and readily excretable product through conjugation with uridine diphosphate glucuronide.

inactive) metabolites that are rapidly excreted by the renal system. An example of this process for the drug Phenytoin is shown in Fig. 7.16.

Phase 1 reactions are mainly carried out by a class of enzymes known as cytochrome P450s (CYPs). The 63 gene family of cytochrome P450 enzymes makes up the bulk of the metabolizing function of the liver. They are membrane-bound enzymes in the endoplasmic reticulum that have an amazing diversity in the types of substrates they can attack (see Box 7.8); they generally insert a molecule of oxygen into their substrates.

There are a number of possible outcomes for these reactions:

- Active drug → inactive metabolite (most common); for example, hydroxylation of phenobarbital to hydroxyphenobarbital.
- Active drug → active metabolite; for example, acetylation of procainamide to N-acetylprocainamide.
- Inactive drug → active metabolite; for example, demethylation of codeine to morphine.
- Active drug → reactive metabolite; for example, acetaminophen → reactive metabolite.

Of the choices above, the formation of reactive metabolites is the most damaging since this can produce lasting harm to the body (vide infra).

Hepatic enzymes (notably cytochrome P450 enzymes) are numerous and the liver has them in variable quantities that may adjust in accordance with the metabolic stress experienced by the organ. In practical terms, there are certain main CYPs that do much of the metabolizing of most drugs. Thus, the most prevalent forms of CYPs in the human liver are CYP3A4/5/7, CYP2D6, CYP2C8/9/18, CYP3E1, CYP2A6, and CYP1A1/2. Approximately 80% of known drugs are metabolized by CYP3A4, CYP2D6, CYP2C19, CYP2A6, CYP2E1, CYP1A2, and

---

BOX 7.8

The amazing range of CYP3A4.

Most enzymes are optimized for a given substrate to preserve the fidelity of cellular signaling. Cytochrome P450s, however, have a huge range of possible substrates to best equip them to metabolize diverse foreign chemicals. Below are a few of the known substrates for CYP3A4. Circles denote the site of CYP3A4 metabolism.

CYP2C8–10. Some of these are more variable (both in quantity and genetics) than others and this can lead to more pharmacokinetic variability in drug studies for the drugs involved. For example, in random samples of human liver, there can be a variation of over 500-fold in the quantity of CYP2D6. In addition, there can be considerable genetic variability leading to functional polymorphism (notably for CYP2A6, CYP2C9, CYP2C19, and CYP2D6). For example, polymorphisms in CYP2C19 affect 20% of all Asians and 3% of Caucasians, leading to Japanese/Chinese susceptibility to ethanol effects. An example of variation in the metabolism of isoniazid through gene polymorphism is shown in Box 7.9.

Before further discussion of drug metabolism, it is important to consider the form of the drug being metabolized once it enters the central compartment. Once the drug enters the general circulation, there are

BOX 7.9

People are different.

The liver is a dynamic organ and can adjust the gene expression of enzymes when stressed. Moreover, humans are extremely variable in terms of the types and amounts of hepatic enzymes they possess and for a given patient, enzyme profiles can change with disease, age, and habits such as cigarette smoking and even consuming charcoal grilled meats. However, a more stable differentiation in hepatic gene makeup can be found between patients due to gene polymorphism. An example of where this is operative in the absorption of isoniazid in 267 patients. The clear bimodal distribution reflects two populations where the second distribution to the right of the first one indicates patients with reduced N-acetyltransferase activity (and subsequent increase isoniazid absorption).

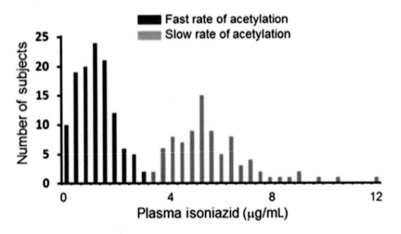

Source: Data redrawn from R. Weinshilboun, Genomic Medicine: inheritance and drug response. New Eng. J. Med. 348 (2003) 529–537 [12].

processes that can compromise free drug concentration. One of the most important of these is plasma protein binding. Human plasma contains more than 60 proteins, some of which can bind small drug molecules. These proteins are of three general types: albumin (binding anionic drugs); α1-acid glycoprotein (binding cationic drugs); and lipoproteins. Plasma protein binding can function as a buffer between the drug and physiological processes. Thus, a protein-bound drug cannot be metabolized by the hepatic system, be functionally active at the target site for therapy, or be filtered by the glomerulus of the kidney to take part in renal clearance. Plasma protein binding is relevant to metabolism because Gs protein-bound drug cannot be metabolized. Therefore, when considering the concentration of drug that can be metabolized, a fraction f_u is used which simply denotes the fraction not bound by plasma protein.

Fig. 7.17 shows some possible outcomes of hepatic metabolism of a molecule. In contrast to the production of an inactive metabolite, a metabolic creation of an active molecule can lead to complications. In some cases, the effect could be beneficial and the parent drug may take on the role of a prodrug. This may assist in the duration of action and therapeutic utility. If the rate of formation of the metabolite is rate limiting and the metabolite has a rate of clearance greater than the parent, then the pharmacokinetics of the parent are of particular importance. If, however, the rate of clearance of a metabolite is lower than that of the parent, then separate pharmacokinetic consideration of the metabolite must be taken in vivo. For example, hydroxyhexamide, the active metabolite of the antidiabetic drug acetohexamide, has a much slower rate of clearance than the parent. Repeat dosing with acetohexamide thus can cause accumulation of hydroxyhexamide unless the activity of this secondary molecule is considered in the dosing regimen of the parent [13].

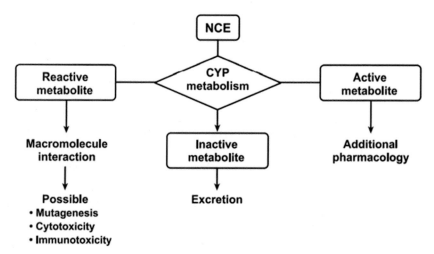

FIGURE 7.17   Possible outcomes of hepatic metabolism. A molecule could be subjected to Phase 1 metabolism to produce an inactive metabolite which then may be excreted at that point or further converted through Phase 2 metabolism to a more polar metabolite to be subsequently excreted by the renal system. This process could also yield a pharmacologically active metabolite, which could produce responses in its own right. Finally, a chemically reactive metabolite may be made which then irreversibly interacts with proteins and/or DNA to produce toxicity or mutagenicity.

Hepatic metabolism also has the capability of producing a reactive molecule, that is, a molecule that can chemically react with proteins and/or DNA to cause irreversible modification. These effects can lead to mutagenesis and cyto- and immunotoxicity. For example, the production of procarcinogens has been observed from the action of CYP1A1 on polycyclic aromatic hydrocarbons, CYP1A2 on heteropolycyclic amines, CYP3E1 on chloroform and methylene chloride, and CYP3A4 on estradiol and aflatoxin B1. The production of reactive chemical groups such as epoxides and nitrenium ions can lead to these effects as well. If this is encountered in a discovery or development program, it must be addressed chemically as it is unacceptable in a drug candidate profile.

Phase 2 reactions generally add a highly water-soluble group onto a hydroxyl (or other suitable) group on the molecule (see Fig. 7.16). Thus, conjugates can be made with glucuronic acid, sulfonates, glutathione and amino acids in reactions resulting in glucuronidation, sulfation, methylation, acetylation, and mercapture formation. While Phase 2 reactions generally precede Phase 1 reactions, there are exceptions to this rule.

It is clear that hepatic degradation can be a major obstacle to attaining a stable steady-state drug concentration in the body for therapeutic use. Because of this, molecules are tested in vitro in hepatic enzyme preparations at an early stage of drug development to identify possible problematic chemical scaffolds. There are three major in vitro preparations of human liver enzymes utilized for this: microsomes, S9 fraction, and hepatocytes. Liver microsomes are homogenized liver fragments partially purified through centrifugation. They can be prepared in large quantities and frozen, leading to a convenient and stable assay system. Microsomes primarily contain Phase 1 enzyme activity. Test molecules are incubated with microsomes in vitro and the half time ($t_{1/2}$) for disappearance of compound is used to estimate the stability of the compound in the assay. The $t_{1/2}$ is the time required for the concentration of parent to be reduced to $1/2$ of its value. For example, if one compound has a $t_{1/2}$ of 35 minutes and another of 5 minutes, then it is clear that the second compound is much less stable in the microsome preparation, that is, it is a better substrate for Phase 1 metabolic reactions. If it is assumed that the disappearance of the compounds can be estimated by a first order decay, then a single timepoint can be used as a measure of stability. Fig. 7.18 shows the degradation of a set of compounds in a microsome assay with an arrow near the percentage of compound remaining at 60 minutes. This single value then represents the stability of the compounds, that is, a compound with 80% remaining after 60 minutes is more stable (and a poorer substrate for Phase 1 reactions) than a compound with a value of 15% remaining at 60 minutes. If the quantity of enzyme is known for the assay, then the data can be scaled to predict in vivo removal of

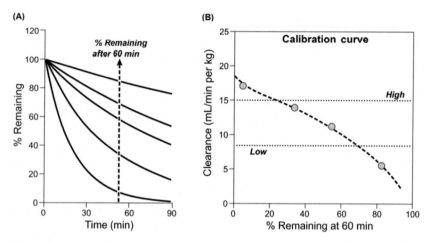

FIGURE 7.18 Estimation of compound stability in liver microsomes. (A) Degradation of a series of compounds in a microsomal assay; five compounds of varying stability are shown. A measure of stability can be obtained from a single value of percentage of parent compound remaining after 60 minutes in the assay. A select range of compounds can be studied in detail to obtain predicted clearance values from values of the percentage of remaining parent. This can furnish a calibration curve (shown in panel (B)). With this curve, large numbers of compounds can be assessed for stability at 60 minutes to estimate clearance.

compound by hepatic degradation. This is termed "clearance" and it is one of the most important parameters in pharmacokinetics. It will be specifically discussed in a later section of this chapter, but for the purposes of this present discussion it is used to extrapolate the in vitro stability of the compound to what might be expected to be a clinical parameter in vivo. Thus, an unstable compound would be predicted to have a high clearance (high rate of removal) and a stable compound a lower clearance. These correlations are not absolute as the in vitro microsome assay gives a partial answer, that is, Phase 2 metabolism, transport into the hepatic cell, protein binding and clearance by other routes, such as, renal, are not considered. However, as an early indicator of pharmacokinetic problems, microsomes give a reasonable prediction of possible problems to come later in drug testing. Fig. 7.18B shows a calibration curve of scaled values relating the percentage of compound remaining in the microsome assay and the predicted in vivo clearance. Once this is in place, the stability of hundreds of compounds can be tested at a given timepoint for a rapid estimate of predicted clearance.

In general, microsomes form the first line of hepatic in vitro testing. However, there are two other in vitro hepatic preparations used for the analysis described above. An assay utilizing a differentially centrifuged sample of microsomes termed the S9 fraction contains some Phase 2 enzymes and yields more information. Another assay utilizes hepatocytes. These are liver cells that contain the natural ratio of Phase 1 to Phase 2 enzymes and also have the added property of having the physiological transport systems (both into and out of the cell) in place to govern access of the compound to the hepatic system. While more physiological, this assay is somewhat more complex and is not as robust as microsomes or S9. In addition, it can be argued that most new drug entities do not have the functional groups required for Phase 2 metabolism (Phase 1 processes put them there) and that Phase 1 metabolism is usually rate limiting and the more important process. There can be dissimulations between data obtained from microsomes versus hepatocytes relating to access of the compounds to the enzymes. Specifically, microsomes may underestimate stability by exposing the compounds to enzymes they may never see in vivo (if they are not substrates of the transport process that pump them into the liver cell). Alternatively, they may overestimate stability of a compound, that is actively pumped into the liver cell and thus is at a lower concentration in microsomal preparations. In any case, the scaling procedure described for microsomes above which relates in vitro stability to clearance can still be undertaken. Once the compound stability is determined in a mixture of CYPs, the responsible enzymes can be identified through the use of specific inhibitors; a list of common inhibitors of various CYPs is shown in Table 7.2. As an example, if 5 µM of Furylline blocks a microsomal degradation of a given compound, this would suggest that CYP1A2 is involved. Further detailed kinetic analysis of CYP activity can also be done with purified recombinant preparations of various CYPs.

TABLE 7.2   Some common inhibitors of cytochrome P450 enzymes.

CYP	Inhibitor	K_i (µM)
1A2	Furylline	0.6−0.73
2A6	Tranylcypromine	0.02−0.2
Methoxsalen	0.01−0.2	
2B6	Sertraline	3.2
Clopidogrel	0.5	
2C8	Quercetin	1.1
2C9	Sulfaphenazole	0.3
2C19	Ticlopidine	1.2
2D6	Quinadine	0.027−0.4
2E1	Clomethiazole	12
3A4/5	Ketoconazole	0.0037−0.18

While the diminution of drug concentration by hepatic metabolism is an important consideration, the metabolic products of this process can be equally important. In fact, understanding the metabolism of a drug in vivo requires the quantification of levels of and pharmacology of every metabolic product. Most of these products are produced by hepatic metabolism and many through the Cytochrome P450 enzyme system (i.e., see Table 6.3). Fig. 7.19 shows the complete metabolic profile for the HIV entry inhibitor drug maraviroc; these profiles (known as "mass conservation" profiles) illustrate the complete metabolic history of a drug as it progresses through the in vivo system. They are obtained through studying the metabolism in hepatocytes and then applying a combination of high-pressure liquid chromatography and mass spectrometry to identify the products.

Fig. 7.20 shows a mass conservation study for the cardiac myosin activator (designed for the treatment of congestive heart failure), omecamtiv mecarbil. It can be seen that of the 93.5% drug entering the central compartment, 11.5% is excreted unchanged and the rest metabolized.

Up to this point, the discussion has centered on what the liver can do to the drug; it is equally important to know what the drug can do to the liver. As mentioned earlier, the liver is the first line of defense against foreign chemicals. As such, it receives high concentrations of exogenous xenobiotics, which could compromise the normal hepatic function. If this occurs due to drug treatment, serious health problems could result. Moreover, frequently patients are on multiple regimens of more than

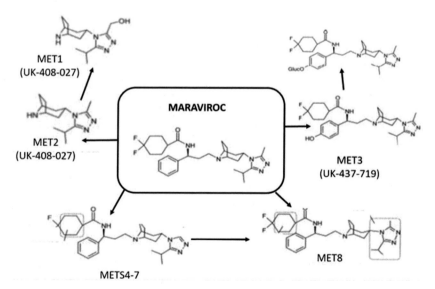

FIGURE 7.19 The metabolic profile of the HIV-entry inhibitor drug maraviroc. Mass Conservation studies illustrate the compounds made by hepatic metabolic enzymes and their relative quantity in various species.

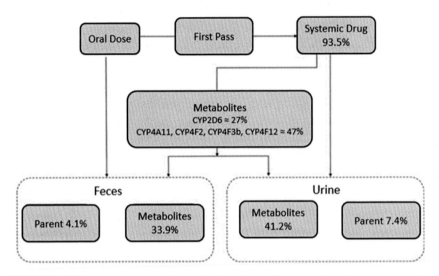

FIGURE 7.20 Mass conservation study for the cardiac myosin activator omecamtiv mecarbil. *Source: Redrawn from A. Trivedi, J. Wahlstrom, M. Mackowski, S. Dutta, E. Lee, Pharmacokinetics, disposition, and biotransformation of [14 C]omecamtiv mecarbil in healthy male subjects after a single intravenous or oral dose. Drug Metab. Disp. 49 (2021) 619−628.*

one drug and those treatments will have been titrated to the patient for safe therapy. Thus, the patient can be considered a steady-state system where the rate of entry and exit of these drugs have been optimized to achieve a steady-state therapeutic level of drug. Therefore, anything that perturbs that steady state may cause harm, either by allowing the minimum concentration to fall below therapeutic levels or by elevating concentrations into a toxic range. If this is caused by the introduction of another drug, this is referred to as a DDI. It has been estimated that DDIs leading to toxicities are among the most prevalent causes of death in the United States, resulting in over 100,000 deaths a year. Determining the proclivity of a new drug entity to cause such interactions is a major function of the development process. One of the most common causes of DDI is common activity at the hepatic system.

There are two ways in which one drug (considered here as the perpetrator) can affect the hepatic metabolism of another drug (considered as the victim). One is by functioning as a substrate for the same CYP as the victim (thereby reducing the metabolism of the victim). For example the antidiabetic drug metformin increases exposure to the antifungal itraconazole by 167% as both drugs are substrates for CYP3A1/2 [14]. Many drugs are cosubstrates for a common cytochrome enzyme and this can lead to DDIs. A particularly interesting common effect is seen with caffeine which is solely metabolized by CYP1A2 and thus can interfere with the metabolism of a wide range of drugs—see Box 7.10.

BOX 7.10

Monopolization of Cyp1A2 by caffeine can lead to drug–drug interactions (DDIs).

DDIs can be prominent for drugs that are metabolized by single mechanisms. For example, caffeine is nearly completely (97%) metabolized by the cytochrome P450 enzyme CYP1A2 to the extent that it is used as a physiological probe of CYP1A2 function. High concentrations of caffeine in the bloodstream can monopolize this enzyme leading to interactions with other drugs that require it to be cleared. This cointeraction at the CYP1A2 enzyme with other drugs can lead to toxic drug-drug interactions with a number of drugs including some selective serotonin reuptake inhibitors such as fluvoxamine used in the treatment of obsessive-compulsive disorder and severe depression, antiarrhythmics, such as mexiletine, the antipsychotic clozapine, the bronchodilators furafylline and theophylline, and the quinolone antibiotic enoxacin [13,14].

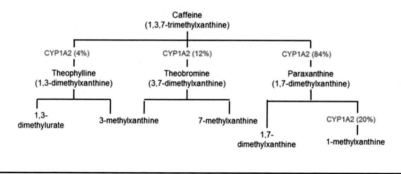

Another way in which hepatic DDIs can occur is if the perpetrator functions as a CYP inhibitor. This type of effect is separated into two types of activity. The first is a simple reversible inhibition which may or may not be debilitating; the point is that it subsides when the drug is removed by clearance and the enzyme activity returns. A second, and more serious, type of inhibition is termed "mechanism-based" (also referred to as "time-dependent"—see Fig. 6.9). This is an essentially irreversible inhibition of the enzyme characterized by an extremely long onset of effect and no recovery upon removal of the perpetrator. Thus, CYP is essentially poisoned and normal CYP activity can only be regained with new synthesis of enzyme. An example of such interactions is the effect of psoralens from grapefruit juice (see Box 7.11). The five major CYPs (CYP1A2, 2C9, 2C19, 2D6, and 3A4) are targeted for testing

BOX 7.11

The unexpected effects of grapefruit juice in clinical trials.

Grapefruit juice was often used as a vehicle for drugs and placebos in double-blind clinical trials, since the strong bitter taste masked the taste of drugs. This preserved the double-blind nature of the trial. However, grapefruit juice contains psoralens, which produce "suicide inhibition" of CYP3A4 (a reactive intermediate forms a covalent bond to irreversibly inactivate the enzyme). This causes large increases in blood levels of drugs that are metabolized by CYP3A4, notably lovastatin (see below data from [15]). Untoward reactions from this effect have been noted for midazolam, triazolam, and buspirone (impaired CNS function), and felodipine (hypotension).

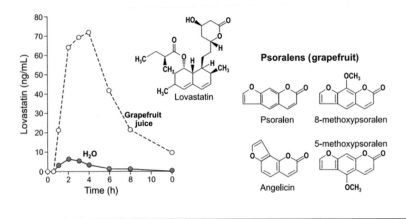

for DDIs and when this activity is observed, it must be eliminated from the candidate molecule through chemical modification. Just as with the cosubstrate mechanisms, blockade of CYP activity can lead to serious DDIs. For instance, potentially fatal levels of the antihistamine terfenadine can be produced by inadvertent inhibition of CYP3A4. This is a particularly serious effect leading to fatal cardiac arrhythmias from a condition known as *Torsades des pointes*; this activity caused the recall of Terfenadine from the market.

As noted previously, the liver is a reactive organ, which can elevate its function in response to stress. This can also occur in response to drugs and many are known to actively induce CYP enzyme synthesis and activity; this effect is termed "enzyme induction." Enzyme synthesis is initiated within 24 hours of exposure and increases over 3–5 days.

The effect decreases over 1–3 weeks after the inducing agent is discontinued. Induction can occur through increased transcription of CYP genes through receptor-dependent mechanisms (PXR receptors) or stabilization of mRNA. Enzyme induction can seriously affect drug therapy. For instance, the already low oral bioavailability of the antihypertensive felodipine (15%) is reduced to near zero levels when administered with liver enzyme-inducing anticonvulsants—see Fig. 7.21. However, as a general pharmacokinetic problem, it is (like plasma protein binding) not clear how it should be dealt with in early development. This is because it usually occurs at high doses (although some PXR effects can be seen at low doses) and it is extremely species-dependent. This latter fact makes it difficult to use animal models to predict how important the effect will be in humans. Enzyme induction can be determined in vitro through exposure of hepatocytes in cell culture over a prolonged period, homogenization of the cells to produce microsomes, and observing any possible increase in enzyme activity or mRNA.

It can be seen how in vitro hepatic assays can be used to estimate drug metabolism, DDIs, and liver enzyme induction. Fig. 7.22 shows a decision tree illustrating a logical pathway for the testing of new molecules to assess their interaction with the hepatic system. In general, it is important to test new chemical entities (NCEs) in vitro, because this may allow the detection of reactive intermediates, the identification of major metabolite(s) (which could then be synthesized and tested for activity), and the collection of data could aid in the selection of species for toxicological testing, (which, in turn, would cover all human metabolites formed). In addition, metabolites formed only in humans could

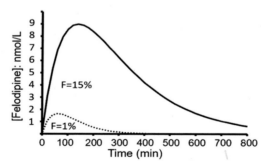

FIGURE 7.21   Felodipine, a dihydropyridine calcium antagonist used for hypertension, undergoes extensive first-pass hepatic metabolism giving an oral bioavailability of 15%. In 10 patients who with microsomal enzyme induction due to chronic anticonvulsant therapy showed a large reduction in bioavailability (from 15% to 1%) compared to 12 normal volunteers matched for age and sex. Source: *Data redrawn from S. Capewell, J.A.J.H. Critchley, S. Freestone, A. Pottage, L.F. Prescott, Reduced felodipine bioavailability in patients taking anticonvulsants. Lancet 332 (1988) 480–482.*

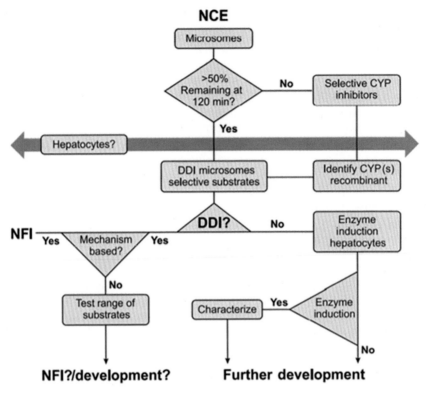

FIGURE 7.22 Decision tree for the study of hepatic effects of new chemical entities (NCEs). An assessment of stability in microsomes indicates whether the compound is a substrate for CYPs; if this is the case, then the CYPs can be identified through selective inhibitors or studied with recombinant enzymes. Irrespective of the outcome of this first step, the NCE must be assessed for possible proclivity to cause drug-drug interactions (DDIs). If CYP inhibition is observed, then it must be determined whether it is mechanism-based. If so, development is halted. If not, it may still be unclear if the DDI should preclude further development. If no DDI are observed, the compound must still be tested for enzyme induction.

be detected; if this occurs, this identifies molecules that would be more costly to develop since there would be no animal species to test for relevant toxicology.

Oral bioavailability

One of the most common routes of drug administration is via the oral route and oral bioavailability poses special problems in pharmacokinetics. This is because the drug must be absorbed through the GI tract wall

(A)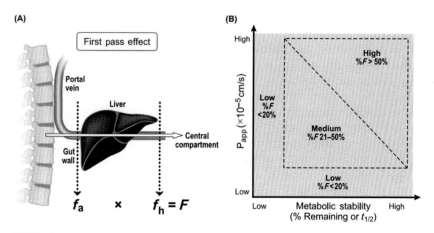

FIGURE 7.23   Oral bioavailability and the first pass effect. (A) Drugs given by the oral route are absorbed through the gastrointestinal wall and immediately enter the portal vein. This takes the drug to the liver before it can access the central compartment. (B) In vitro assays relevant to this process are permeation (passive diffusion in parallel artificial membrane permeation assay (PAMPA) or biological permeation in CaCo-2 cells; ordinate axis) or metabolic stability (microsomes, S9, hepatocytes) through readings such as percentage of parent compound remaining after 60 min incubation (abscissae). Compounds with corresponding values in the upper right corner would be expected to have favorable oral bioavailability. Those in the lower right or upper left would be expected to have poor oral bioavailability.

where it immediately gets shunted to the portal vein and into the liver. Thus, the drug encounters two pharmacokinetically challenging processes; absorption and metabolism; this challenge is given the name "first pass effect" (Fig. 7.23A). The total fraction of drug entering the central compartment via the oral route (denoted "F") is a product of the fraction absorbed (f_a) and the fraction that escapes the passage through the liver (f_h). Thus, $F = f_a \times f_h$, meaning that if 50% of the drug is absorbed and 50% emerges from the liver then the total oral bioavailability will be 25%. Data from two in vitro pharmacokinetic assays can be of use in predicting oral bioavailability; specifically, permeation assays and measures of stability in liver microsomes, S9, and/or hepatocytes. Clearly, a molecule that permeates cell layers quickly ($P_{app} > 10^{-5}$ cm/s) and is stable in hepatic in vitro cell preparations (> 50% parent compound remaining at 120 min) will have the highest probability of being an orally bioavailable drug. Fig. 7.23B shows how plotting these values yields a grid where the top right quadrant isolates potentially bioavailable drugs during the compound sorting process in drug development.

It can be seen from the dual nature of the first pass effect (absorption plus metabolic stability) that oral bioavailability may be limited by one of the factors or both. The maximum of the oral availability

curve (C_{max}) and the time when this peak occurs (T_{max}) are both sensitive indicators for the limiting factors in oral bioavailability. If absorption is decreased, C_{max} is decreased and T_{max} increased (peak occurs
later); when absorption is increased the reverse is true. Similarly,
when clearance is decreased, C_{max} is increased and T_{max} decreased; the
converse occurs when clearance is decreased- see Fig. 7.24. There are
ways to experimentally determine whether absorption or metabolism
is the limiting factor for a given candidate drug. Fig. 7.25 shows how
cannulation of the duodenum, hepatic vein, and arterial system can
experimentally delineate where the major limitation for oral bioavailability can be.

Since, the drug is passing through the GI tract, there are other
effects that enter into the calculation of in vivo bioavailability; these
will be discussed further in Chapter 8, Pharmacokinetics II:
Distribution and Multiple Dosing. For instance, solubility in water is
critical (see discussion of MAD and Eq. 7.1). Experimentally, a value
for F of 0.2 is adequate, while 0.5 is very good. However, there are
exceptions to this rule. For example, the F value for Etidronate, a
bisphosphonate for stabilization of bone matrix in osteoporosis, is 0.03;
in spite of this very low oral bioavailability, this is a viable drug treatment. In general, if values of $F > 0.2$ are not attained there are strategies to improve permeation, solubility, or stability; these are outlined
in Table 7.3.

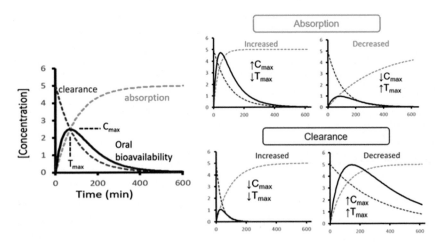

FIGURE 7.24   Oral bioavailability is described by a biphasic curve that is an amalgam
of the curves for clearance and absorption. The peak height and where along the time axis
the peak occurs depend on the relative rates of clearance and absorption.

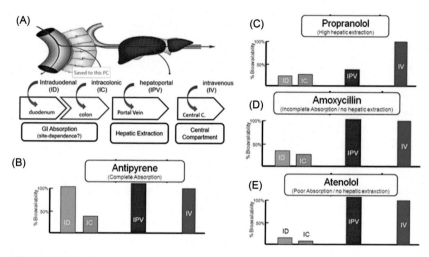

FIGURE 7.25 Drugs can be introduced at various points along the first pass continuum and compared to central compartment concentrations when introduced iv. Thus, bioavailability can be reduced by poor absorption, high metabolism or both. Panel A shows good availability both IC and IPV for antipyrine, panel C poor bioavailability for propranolol (the fact that IPV is low indicates high metabolism), panel D a problem with absorption for amoxicillin (entry IPV shows little metabolism) and panel E low absorption for atenolol (no reduction IPV). Source: *Data from L. Letendre, M. Scott, G. Dobson, I. Hidalgo, B. Aungst, Evaluating barriers to bioavailability in vivo: Validation of a technique for separately assessing gastrointestinal absorption and hepatic extraction. Pharmaceut. Res. 21 (2004) 457–1462.*

TABLE 7.3 Strategies for improving oral bioavailability.

Problem	Assay	Solution?
• Low solubility or slow dissolution	• Kinetic solubility assay	Reduce lipophilicity/make salts
• Low GI tract stability	• Stability in acidic buffer	Replace unstable groups
• Low metabolic stability	• Microsomes • Hepatocytes	Reduce lipophilicity/block metabolic sites
• Poor absorption due to low passive diffusion	• PAMPA • CaCo-2	Remove charges/hydrogen bond donors and acceptors/increase lipophilicity
• Poor absorption due to active efflux (P-gp)	• CaCo-2 • $(B \rightarrow A)/(A \rightarrow B)$	Overwhelm by improving passive diffusion/remove or alter hydrogen bond acceptors/lower molecular weight
• Extensive biliary excretion	• In vivo assays	Reduce molecular weight/remove anionic charge/block conjugation

Summary

- The structure–activity relationships for drug primary activity, pharmacokinetic properties (ADME) and safety profile can be different from each other.
- Modern drug discovery begins considering ADME at the very beginning of the discovery process.
- A discovery program likely will have limits set as to route of delivery and frequency of dosing; this defines required clearance and other ADME properties.
- The first step is to utilize chemical scaffolds with "drug-like" activity; defined limits of Log$P$, H_2O solubility, pK_a and molecular weight.
- Drug absorption (passive diffusion, transport) can be estimated in vitro as can stability to hepatic enzymes; these assays can be used to optimize ADME profiles.
- In addition, there are in vitro assays available to determine whether a molecule inhibits hepatic enzyme function (this can be predictive of DDIs) or produces induction of liver enzymes.
- Oral bioavailability results from a dual process of absorption followed by metabolism (first pass effect).
- Unmatched rates of absorption and clearance (i.e., as found in some sustained-release preparations) can be detected through "flip flop" pharmacokinetics.
- The above ADME effects are different for biologicals as these have particular issues with absorption, distribution, metabolism and excretion

References

[1] R.S. Al-awar, J.E. Ray, R.M. Schultz, S.L. Andis, J.H. Kennedy, R.E. Moore, A convergent approach to cryptophycin 52 analogues: synthesis and biological evaluation of a novel series of fragment a epoxides and chlorohydrins, J. Med. Chem. 46 (2003) 2985–3007.

[2] I. Kola, J. Landis, Can the pharmaceutical industry reduce attrition rates? Nat. Rev. Drug. Disc 3 (2004) 711–716.

[3] U. Velaparthi, P. Liu, B. Balasubramanian, J. Carboni, R. Attar, M. Gottardis, Imidazole moiety replacements in the 3-(1H-benzo[d]imidazol-2-yl)pyridin-2 (1H)-one inhibitors of insulin-like growth factor receptor- 1 (IGF-1R) to improve cytochrome P450 profile, Bioorg. Med. Chem. Lett. 17 (2007) 3072–3076.

[4] J.R. Proudfoot, Drugs, leads, and drug-likeness: an analysis of some recently launched drugs, Bioorg. Med. Chem. Lett. 12 (2002) 1647–1650.

[5] W. Curatolol, Physical chemical properties of oral drug candidates in the discovery and exploratory development settings, Pharm. Sci. Technol. Today. 1 (1998) 387–393.

[6] R.W. Clark, R.B. Ruggeri, D. Cunningham, M.J. Bamberger, Description of the torcetrapib series of cholesteryl ester transfer protein inhibitors, including mechanism of action, J. Lipid Res. 47 (2006) 537–552.

[7] C.A. Lipinski, Drug-like properties and the causes of poor solubility and poor permeability, J. Pharmacol. Toxicol. Methods 44 (2000) 235–249.

[8] C.A. Lipinski, F. Lombardo, B.W. Dominy, P.J. Feenery, Experimental and computational approaches to estimate solubility and permeability in drug discovery and development settings, Adv. Drug. Deliv. Rev. 23 (1997) 3–25.

[9] N.A. Kasim, M. Whitehouse, C. Ramachandran, M. Bermejo, H. Lennernäs, A.S. Hussain, Molecular properties of WHO essential drugs and provisional biopharmaceutical classification, Mol. Pharm. 1 (2004) 85–96.

[10] T. Otulana, J. Thipphawong, Systemic delivery of small molecules: product development issues focused on pain therapeutics, Respir. Drug. Deliv. VIII (2002) 97–104.

[11] J. Anderson, Degarelix: a novel gonadotropin-releasing hormone blocker for the treatment of prostate cancer, Future Oncol. 5 (2009). Available from: https://doi.org/10.2217/fon.09.24.

[12] R. Weinshilboun Genomic, Medicine: inheritance and drug response, N. Eng. J. Med. 348 (2003) 529–537.

[13] J.A. Galloway, R.E. McMahon, H.W. Culp, F.J. Marshall, E.C. Young, Metabolism, blood levels and rate of excretion of acetohexamide in human subjects, Diabetes. 16 (1967) 118–127.

[14] J.A. Carrillo, J. Benitez, Clinically significant pharmacokinetic interactions between dietary caffeine and medications, Clin. Pharmacokinet. 39 (2000) 127–153.

[15] Y.H. Choi, U. Lee, B.K. Lee, M.G. Lee, Pharmacokinetic interaction between itraconazole and metformin in rats: competitive inhibition of metabolism of each drug by each other via hepatic and intestinal CYP3A1/2, Br. J. Pharmacol. 161 (2010) 815–829.

Pharmacokinetics II: distribution and multiple dosing

By the end of this chapter the student will be able to put in vitro pharmacokinetic data on absorption and metabolism into the context of the in vivo environment. The student will also understand in vivo clearance and volume of distribution, and how these factors control all of pharmacokinetics. Finally, the student will be able to see how data from a limited number of in vivo experiments can be used to generally

Pharmacology in Drug Discovery and Development
DOI: https://doi.org/10.1016/B978-0-443-14124-9.00017-3

describe the pharmacokinetics of any drug. These data can also be used to predict pharmacokinetics in other species to further predict dosing in humans for clinical study.

Drugs in motion: in vivo pharmacokinetics

As shown in the previous chapter (see Fig. 7.4), a drug is nearly in constant motion from the instant it is introduced into the body until the time it leaves. Thus, the therapeutic target essentially responds to a running stream of drugs of varying concentrations. Chapter 9, In Vivo Pharmacology, discusses how this is relevant to the therapeutic response in vivo; this present chapter relates to the factors controlling the characteristics of that motion, what drug properties affect it, and how they can be measured and quantified.

New terminology

The following new terms will be introduced in this chapter:

- *Allometric scaling*: The process of using body weight to predict physiological parameters in different animal species.
- C_{max}: The maximal peak concentration of drug observed in the central compartment as a result of a given dosing regimen.
- C_{min}: The minimal concentration of drug observed in the central compartment during repeat dosing.
- *Enterohepatic circulation*: The secretion of substances from the liver into the bile duct; these substances then can be reabsorbed from the gastrointestinal tract back into the body.
- *Extraction ratio*: The amount of substance removed from a flow of drug into a removal organ (i.e., liver) expressed as a ratio of the quantity entering the organ.
- *MRSD*: Maximal recommended starting dose for a human clinical trial.
- *NOAEL*: No observed adverse effect level for a drug.
- *NOEL*: No observed effect level for a drug.
- *Nonlinear pharmacokinetics*: The pharmacokinetics seen in vivo when the clearance capacity of the body begins to be exceeded by the drug levels in the central compartment.
- τ: The dosage interval, that is, the period between dosing in repeat dosing studies.
- *Volume of distribution*: The virtual volume of water in which drug appears to be dissolved when concentrations are measured in the central compartment; it can be used to detect sequestration of drug in various parts of the body.

The central compartment and in vivo clearance

The process of permeation and absorption controls the rate of entry of a drug into the central compartment; once there, immediate factors begin the process of drug clearance from the body and/or other processes that make the drug inaccessible to the therapeutic target. One of those, namely plasma protein binding, has been discussed briefly in Chapter 7, Pharmacokinetics I: Permeation and Metabolism. This process sequesters drug away from metabolic and renal processes of removal; it will be seen later in this chapter that plasma protein binding keeps the drug in the central compartment and does not allow it to be sequestered into other tissues. This has the effect of reducing the volume of distribution of the drug (*vide infra*). While plasma protein binding reduces free drug concentration, generally, it is not a problem that needs to be addressed through medicinal chemical alteration of the molecule (see Box 8.1). This is because dosing is usually adjusted to accommodate it and limitations in free drug concentration are somewhat offset by a reduction in clearance afforded by plasma protein binding. For example, the antimuscarinic antagonists Zamifenacin and Darifenacin are of comparable potency (between twofold and fourfold differences in IC_{50}) but differ by a factor of 300 in their plasma protein binding (Darifenacin is 94% protein bound while Zamifenacin is 98.98% protein bound). In spite of this radical difference in plasma protein binding, the equieffective clinical doses of Zamifenacin and Darifenacin differ by only a factor of two. In addition, the physicochemical changes needed to change plasma protein binding are usually extensive and would probably interfere with primary activity or other ADME properties. The one realm where plasma protein is important is when clinical dose is compared to observed response and the true potency (and safety margin) of drugs needs to be calculated. This will be considered further in the next chapter (Chapter 9, In Vivo Pharmacology) on the measurement of pharmacologic effects in vivo.

Another way in which the central compartment drug concentration can change is through metabolic destruction; this is particularly true of esters as there are plasma esterases present to degrade esters to carboxylic acids. For example, the anticholinergic mydriatic drug eucatropine is destroyed in human plasma within 35 minutes. Similarly, the local anesthetic procaine is destroyed in only a few minutes.

In addition to these factors, there are three forces moving drugs out of the central compartment (see Fig. 7.4), these are: (1) distribution to other compartments in the body; (2) renal excretion and (3) hepatic metabolism. Of these, hepatic metabolism is usually the most important and this will be considered first.

BOX 8.1

Is drug plasma protein binding really a problem?

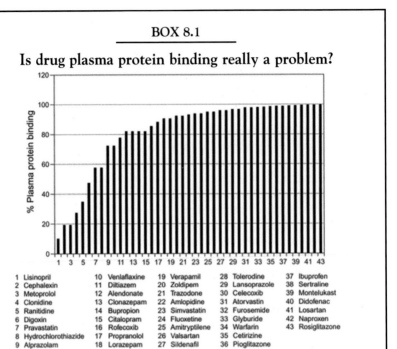

1 Lisinopril	10 Venlaflaxine	19 Verapamil	28 Tolerodine	37 Ibuprofen
2 Cephalexin	11 Diltiazem	20 Zoldipem	29 Lansoprazole	38 Sertraline
3 Metoprolol	12 Alendonate	21 Trazodone	30 Celecoxib	39 Montelukast
4 Clonidine	13 Clonazepam	22 Amlopidine	31 Atorvastin	40 Didofenac
5 Ranitidine	14 Bupropion	23 Simvastatin	32 Furosemide	41 Losartan
6 Digoxin	15 Citalopram	24 Fluoxetine	33 Glyburide	42 Naproxen
7 Pravastatin	16 Rofecoxib	25 Amitryptilene	34 Warfarin	43 Rosiglitazone
8 Hydrochlorothiazide	17 Propranolol	26 Valsartan	35 Cetirizine	
9 Alprazolam	18 Lorazepam	27 Sildenafil	36 Pioglitazone	

While plasma protein binding can cause dissimulations between the observed dosage of effective drugs and the concentration in the biophase actually producing the effect, it is not considered a roadblock to the development of drug therapies. Below are shown 43 of the 100 most prescribed drugs in the United States; it can be seen that over half are >90% plasma protein bound and some are >99.99% protein bound. In spite of this, the dosage administered accounts for this effect and these are useful therapies.

The body is a nonequilibrium system where drugs enter at a certain rate and are removed at a certain rate; the removal of a drug from the body is referred to as drug clearance. Drugs can be cleared through numerous organs in the body (i.e., liver, kidney, brain, lungs, sweat glands, etc.) and these are all treated as processes connected in parallel, except for the lungs, which are considered a series process. Drugs introduced via the oral route undergo first-pass metabolism (absorption from the gastrointestinal tract and then immediate shunting via the portal vein into the liver), while drugs introduced into the central compartment by other routes of administration are mainly cleared by the

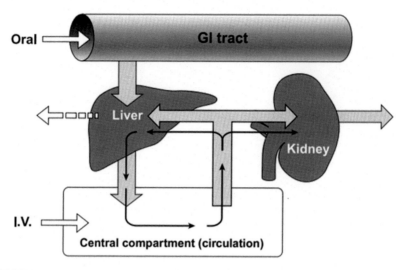

FIGURE 8.1 Clearance. Scheme depicting routes of elimination of drugs entering the body orally or directly from the central compartment. Oral drugs must pass through the liver before they enter the central compartment. The central compartment is then cleansed of the drug through repeated circulation(s) through the liver and kidneys until the drug is cleared from the body.

hepatic or renal system. The central compartment is cleansed of drug by cyclic filtering through either the liver or kidney (or both) until the drug is eliminated (see Fig. 8.1). In practical terms, for nonpolar drugs, the main organ of clearance is the liver. The efficiency of the liver as a removal organ can be quantified by an extraction ratio (E_H) given by:

$$\text{Extraction ratio} = E_H = 1 - \frac{[\text{concentration out}]}{[\text{concentration in}]} \tag{8.1}$$

Thus if a concentration of 1 mg/L enters the liver and 0.3 mg/L emerges, this would be an extraction ratio of $1 - (0.3/1) = 0.7$, that is, 70% of all drug that enters the liver is metabolized. Clearance is the rate of complete cleansing of a given volume of body water per unit time. Thus, if the liver receives 20 mL/min kg of blood (this is the Q_H of the liver blood flow for a healthy adult) and a removal process extracts 70% of this, then the hepatic clearance (CL_H) is given by $Q_H \times E_H = 20$ mL/min kg $\times 0.7 = 14$ mL/min kg. For a 70 kg male, this equals 980 mL/min. It is useful to denote levels of clearance in general terms as a fraction of liver blood flow. For a healthy male, liver blood flow is 1450 mL/min. Thus, a clearance value of 0%–40% of liver blood flow is considered low (<580 mL/min), 40%–70% medium (580–1015 mL/min) and >70% (>1015 mL/min) high clearance.

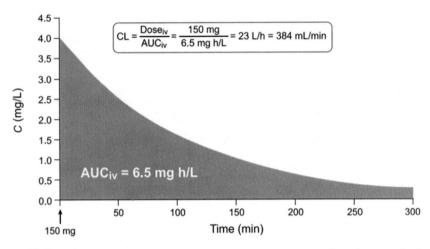

FIGURE 8.2   In vivo clearance. A single dose of drug given iv is allowed to completely clear from the body ($AUC_{iv} \rightarrow 0$ as $t \rightarrow \infty$). The calculated area under the curve (AUC) for this drug is 6.5 mg h/L. The dosage (150 mg) divided by this value yields the clearance which, in this case, is 384 mL/min (low).

Clearance is extremely important in pharmacokinetics as it determines the dose rate for clinical infusions to achieve therapeutic steady-state concentrations and the dosing schedule for repeat administration in chronic treatment. It is the single most important determinant of whether a drug is a once-a-day, twice-a-day, etc., treatment. It can be measured in vivo by comparing the exposure to the drug (expressed as the area under the concentration-time curve) and the dosage. It should be noted that when in vivo clearance is measured in this way, there is no restriction as to mechanism, that is, it may be a mixture of removal mechanisms including hepatic and renal. Thus, clearance in vivo is given by $CL = dosage_{iv}/AUC_{iv}$ (see Fig. 8.2).

One additional mechanism of drug clearance related to hepatic function is secretion into the enterohepatic circulation. The liver secretes from 0.25 to 1 L of bile each day containing anions, cations and low-molecular weight (<300) nonionized molecules. The lower molecular weight compounds are reabsorbed before being excreted into the bile duct, but molecules of high-molecular weight (approximately 500 or greater) can be secreted into the bile duct and continue on to be deposited into the gastrointestinal tract. The glucuronide conjugates of small polar structures can attain these sizes and glucuronides are known to take part in enterohepatic excretion. A practical aspect of this for clinical trials (and therapy) is the observation that some drugs that take part in this process (i.e., chloramphenicol; see Box 8.2) can demonstrate large secondary oral absorption curves after a meal as the bile is secreted into the GI tract in response to food.

BOX 8.2

The enterohepatic circulation

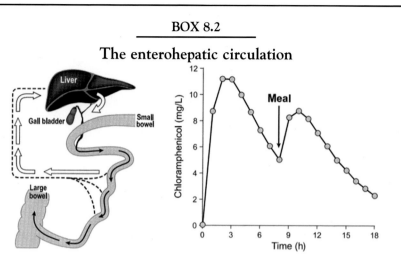

The enterohepatic circulation forms a cycle whereby drugs are secreted into the bile duct (through transport processes, such as P-gp, MDR2, MDR3, BSEP, and MRP2) from the hepatic cells. They are shunted to the gastrointestinal tract when the gall bladder secretes bile (after a stimulus such as a meal) and from there they can be reabsorbed. This is known to occur with chloramphenicol and chloramphenicol-glucuronide. These effects must be considered in clinical trials where fasting conditions can affect absorption.

Renal excretion

A main pathway for drug excretion from the body is through the kidney; this is the primary method of clearance for polar water-soluble chemicals. The kidney receives about 173 L of water a day and returns approximately 171 L back to the body. It filters water at a rate of 110–130 mL/min through a system of approximately one million nephrons (tubules) that have distinct properties (Fig. 8.3A shows one such tubule). Filtration begins at the glomerulus, an area of vasculature that has uniquely large pores that allow all but protein bound drug ($>$ m.w. 30,000) to pass. The blood passes through the glomerulus at a rate of 1200 mL/min and 10% is filtered through as plasma water. The clearance by glomerular filtration is $CL_{GF} = f_u \times GFR$ where f_u refers to the free fraction of drug (nonprotein bound) and GFR is the filtration rate (approximated at 120 mL/min). The filtrate then progresses to the proximal tubule, which has secretory pumps capable of actively transporting drugs from the circulation into the tubule. There are two main

(A)   (B)

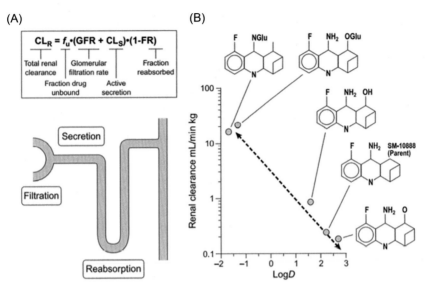

FIGURE 8.3 Renal clearance. Diagram on the left (A) shows a single renal tubule beginning at the glomerulus (where the process of plasma filtration occurs), to the collecting duct, (which deposits urine into the bladder). Free drug is filtered at the glomerulus and it can also be actively secreted into the proximal tubule. As water passes down into the loop of Henle and distal tubule, it is reabsorbed. The graph on the right (B) shows the renal clearance of a parent drug (SM-10888), an acetylcholinesterase inhibitor, and its increasingly polar hepatic metabolites. It can be seen that as the LogD value for the metabolites decreases, the renal clearance correspondingly increases. Source: *Data from D.A. Smith, B.C. Jones, D.K. Walker, Design of drugs involving the concepts and theories of drug metabolism and pharmacokinetics, Med. Res. Rev. 16 (1996) 243–266 [1].*

secretory processes; one for negatively charged molecules (weak acids) and one for positively charged molecules (weak bases). This process is saturable and designated CL_S (see Fig. 8.3).

Finally, in the loop of Henle, all but 1 or 2 mL of the 120 mL, filtered at the glomerulus, is reabsorbed. It is here that nonionized membrane-soluble drugs are also reabsorbed according to a concentration gradient. This process is controlled by urine volume (high volume = low gradient = low reabsorption). Since only nonionized drug is reabsorbed, pH and pK_a may become factors in how much drug is reabsorbed. In cases where urine pH is subject to change (i.e., pH is lowered in conditions of chronic obstructive pulmonary disease, diabetic ketoacidosis, etc.), renal clearance may change for some drugs with disease states.

Considering all of the processes in the renal tubule, the total renal clearance is given by:

$$CLR = f_u(GFR + CL_S) \times (1 - FR) \qquad (8.2)$$

where f_u is the fraction of nonprotein bound drug, GFR is the glomerular filtration rate, CL_S is the amount of drug secreted into the tubule, and FR is the fraction reabsorbed in the distal tubule and loop of Henle. Thus, if renal clearance is greater than GFR, the drug is secreted into tubules; if it is less than GFR, the drug is reabsorbed or highly protein bound. If renal clearance is equal to GFR, then it is either freely filtered or the amounts secreted and reabsorbed approach equality. In general, highly ionized drugs are filtered or secreted without being reabsorbed, causing them to appear rapidly in the urine. For example, p-amino hippuric acid is cleared in one passage through the kidneys (i.e., clearance is equal to the entire renal blood flow). Nonpolar drugs are not as highly cleared by the renal system as they are reabsorbed. However, due to the fact that this process can be dependent on urine pH, this can be variable.

Renal clearance can be measured by:

$$CLR(mL/min) = \frac{Conc_U(mg/mL) \times U(mL/min)}{Conc_{plasma}(mg/mL)} \quad (8.3)$$

where $Conc_U$ and $Conc_{plasma}$ refer to the concentration of drug in the urine and plasma, respectively, and U refers to the rate of urine flow. The importance of renal clearance can be estimated by measuring clearance in normal and renal-impaired animals. For example, Fig. 8.4 shows

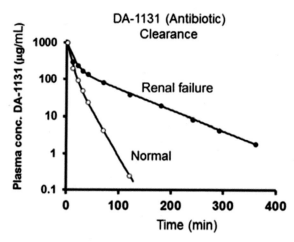

FIGURE 8.4 Clearance of the antibiotic DA-1131 in normal rats and rats with compromised renal function through treatment with uranyl nitrate. It can be seen that the clearance in normal rats is 4.2-fold faster than in renal-impaired rats renal-impaired rats indicating a dependence on renal clearance for this molecule. Source: *Data redrawn from: S. H. Kim, H.J. Shim, W.B. Kim, M.G. Lee, Pharmacokinetics of a new carbapenem, DA-1131, after intravenous administration to rats with uranyl nitrate-induced acute renal failure antimicrob. Agents Chemother. 42 (1998) 1217–1221 [2].*

the clearance of the antibiotic DA-1131 in normal rats and rats with ura-nyl nitrate-induced renal failure. It can be seen that clearance is severely reduced in renal failure animals indicating an important role of renal clearance for this molecule.

Drug distribution

Referring to Fig. 7.4, it can be seen that another major process that a molecule undergoes, when introduced into the body, is redistribution. The body is comprised of numerous compartments, and drugs, owing to their particular physicochemical properties, may sequester in some of these but not others. Knowledge of where drugs go in the body can be useful to determine the therapeutic potential of drugs; a tool to make these estimates is the volume of distribution (V_d). The volume of distribution of a drug is a virtual quantity of water into which a given drug would appear to be dissolved when the concentration is measured from the central compartment. Because the body is like a container with a hole in it, drug concentration changes with time. Therefore, to gage the volume of distribution, the concentration at the instant the drug enters the body is required. This can be measured by estimating the clearance of a single intravenous dose of molecule. Fig. 8.5A shows the decay in concentration with time of an intravenous dose of 20 mg of an experimental drug. This exponential decay curve can be linearized by plotting the natural logarithm of the concentration with time, as shown in Fig. 8.5B, allowing the extrapolation of the decay curve to time zero. This is the theoretical concentration of drug in the central compartment at the instant the drug is injected. From this concentration value and knowledge of the amount of drug injected, the apparent volume of distribution of the drug can be calcu-lated. In this case it is 20 mg $\div$ 0.5 mg/mL = 40 L. This is approximately the amount of water in a 70 kg male, suggesting that the drug is evenly distributed in the body water. This procedure can be used to detect drug sequestration. For example, when 300 mg of the antimalar-ial drug chloroquine is given in a single intravenous dose, the concen-tration at time zero by extrapolation is 40 ng/mL (0.04 mg/L) [3]. This leads to an estimation of V_d of 300 mg $\div$ 0.04 mg/L = 7500 L, a volume approximately 180 times the volume of water in a human. This inordi-nately large V_d value indicates that chloroquine distributes to other tis-sues and is not present in the central compartment (see Fig. 8.5C). When drugs leave the central compartment and concentrate in other tissues (i.e., adipose tissue, muscle), the central compartment concen-tration will be exceedingly low and this, in turn, leads to an extremely high apparent volume of distribution. Therefore, high values for V_d

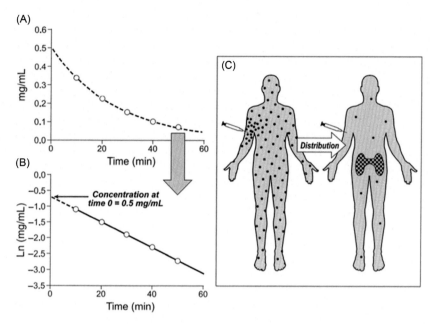

FIGURE 8.5 Volume of distribution. (A) A single dose of drug is given intravenously and the concentration with time is followed; an exponential decay is observed. (B) The ordinate drug levels are converted to natural log values to yield a straight line for the fall in concentration with time. This allows extrapolation to the theoretical concentration at time zero. This can be used to calculate the volume of distribution. (C) If a compound sequesters in a restricted compartment, then the concentrations of drug will be low in the central compartment. This will yield a high volume of distribution.

are indicative of drug sequestration out of the central compartment. The factors that can cause drugs to be sequestered in special areas of the body (away from the central compartment) are entry into separated compartments, such as the blood−brain barrier, mammary circulation, placenta, intracellular tissue binding, high lipid solubility, and trapping due to pK_a/pH combinations. Binding of drugs to plasma proteins actually decreases the volume of distribution since it prevents free drug from diffusing elsewhere into the body.

There is a temporal aspect of the distribution of drugs within the body that leads to multicompartment pharmacokinetics. The body is made up of many compartments of varying size, accessibility, and blood flow, and access to these compartments varies with time. Upon injection, drugs rapidly distribute to highly perfused organs, such as the liver, brain, kidney, and lungs, over a timescale of minutes. Over a period of hours thereafter, drugs then equilibrate according to their physicochemical properties throughout the body viscera (muscle, skin, fat).

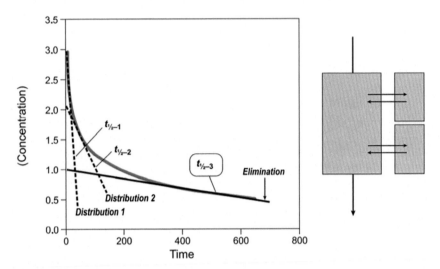

FIGURE 8.6 Drug clearance from a multicompartment system. Shown is the central compartment drug concentration (ordinates) changing with time (abscissa) as the drug clears from the body. The drug redistributes from two low capacity but rapidly equilibrating compartments and then more slowly from a larger compartment. The rate of exit from each compartment can be approximated with a $t_{1/2}$ value; $t_{1.2-1}$; and $t_{1/2-2}$ quantify redistribution while true exit from the body is quantified by $t_{1/2-3}$.

This leads to clearance curves that are more complex than those describing a single compartment. Fig. 8.6 shows clearance from a three compartment system where the first two compartments are rapidly cleared to give a steep initial component to the curve; this profile represents redistribution of the drug within the body. The final phase of the curve represents true clearance where the drug leaves the body.

At this point it is useful to discuss the concept of half-time ($t_{1/2}$) with respect to whole body pharmacokinetics. The concentration of drug leaving a single compartment, as a function of time (denoted $[C]_t$), is given by:

$$[C]_t = [C]_0 \times e^{-k_{out}t} \tag{8.4}$$

where $[C]_0$ is the initial dosage given, t is time and k_{out} is a rate constant. This can be converted to a straight line through expressing the ratio $[C]_t/[C]_0$ as a natural logarithm $(Ln([C]_t/[C]_0) = -k_{out}t)$. The time required for the concentration to fall to half its initial values $([C]_t/[C]_0 = 0.5; \quad Ln(0.5) = -0.693)$ is denoted as the half-time $(t_{1/2} = -0.693/k_{out})$. Thus, since the $t_{1/2}$ directly relates to the rate constant for decay, it is a parameter that also characterizes the rate of decay. For a drug interacting with multiple compartments, a summation of processes according to Eq. (8.4), each with their own k_{out}, can model the curve. Fig. 8.6 shows a three compartment system where the first two $t_{1/2}$ values represent redistribution, while the third $(t_{1/2-3})$ represents true clearance from the body. While redistribution is important therapeutically and can pose clinical problems (e.g., retention of drug in rapidly distributed organs, such as the brain for diazepam in *status epilepticus*), the main concern for drug development is whole body clearance. This is because the $t_{1/2}$ for removal of drug from the body dictates the duration of effect and frequency of administration.

A drug is considered cleared from the body after $5 \times t_{1/2}$ periods ($>97\%$ of the drug has left the body at that point). Similarly, if a drug is given repeatedly at intervals of every $t_{1/2}$, then it requires a period of $5 \times t_{1/2}$ to achieve steady-state concentration for therapy. For drugs, which have an inordinately long $t_{1/2}$ (i.e., chloroquine), this dictates a long-treatment period to achieve steady state (see Box 8.3). The half-time of a drug in the body is an extremely useful characteristic number

---

BOX 8.3

Long $t_{1/2}$ means long pretreatment to steady-state

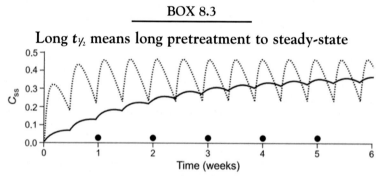

Just as five half-times represents the time it takes to nearly completely clear a drug (97%), it takes approximately five half-times to achieve a steady-state concentration of drug with repeated dosing if given every $t_{1/2}$. For drugs with very long half-times, this means that treatment may need to be prolonged to achieve a constant level of drug. Below is shown repeated dosing with a drug with an approximate $t_{1/2}$ of 40 hours (e.g., digoxin; gray tracing) and one with a $t_{1/2}$ of 200 hours (e.g., chloroquine; black tracing). Although these dosage intervals are not at $t_{1/2}$, the effect is similar, that is, it takes considerably longer to achieve a steady-state with chloroquine than it does with digoxin. Chloroquine is an antimalarial and the long pretreatment requirement compels beginning of treatment 5 weeks before travel into a malaria-risk zone.

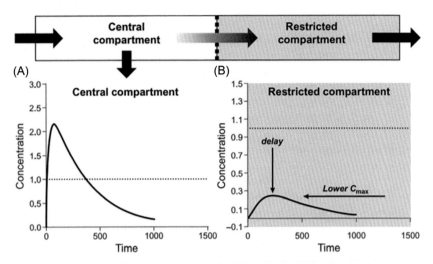

FIGURE 8.7   Drug diffusion into a restricted compartment. Top panel shows diffusion into the central compartment and subsequent diffusion from that into a restricted compartment. Panel (A) shows a hypothetical pattern of drug absorption and clearance in the central compartment. Panel (B) shows the resulting concentration of drug in the restricted compartment. Note: how the peak is observed at a later time and is of lower magnitude than that in the central compartment.

for a given drug and in vivo system; the application of this parameter to determine dosing regimens will be discussed in the next section.

If the therapeutic target resides in a compartment which has limited access (e.g., digoxin for cardiac cells) then the concentrations in the treatment compartment may be lower than those in the central compartment. They may also reach peak levels after peak levels in the central compartment have waned; this is shown in Fig. 8.7.

Concentration is usually the driving force for flow into the restricted compartment, but in vivo drug levels are temporally transient, that is, for intravenously (iv) dosing, concentrations begin high and diminish, while for oral dosing concentrations reach a peak within a given time and then also diminish. Therefore, the kinetics of central compartment concentration can be important to the restricted compartment, that is, not only is the peak level important, but also how long the concentration remains high; Fig. 8.8 illustrates this effect. Fig. 8.8A and B shows a defined central compartment peak concentration with a resulting 10% peak concentration in a restricted compartment. Fig. 8.8C shows the same drug in a system with a reduced rate of clearance; the dose has been reduced to mimic the peak concentration in Fig. 8.8A. Note how this reduced clearance leads to a greater drug concentration in the restricted compartment (29%; see Fig. 8.8D) in spite of the fact that the

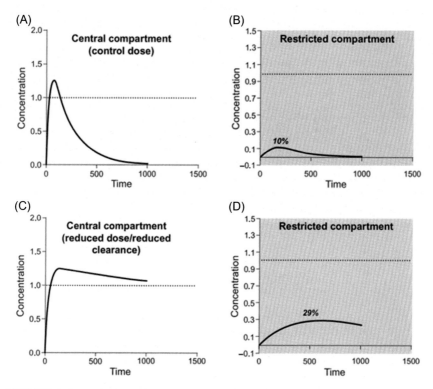

FIGURE 8.8 Diffusion into a restricted compartment is described in Fig. 8.6. Panels (A) and (B) describe a system resulting in a given set of values for absorption and clearance. Panels (C) and (D) show the same system with a reduction in clearance. The dose of the drug has been reduced to match the peak level in Panel (A). More of the central compartment concentration is able to enter the restricted compartment due to the fact that the reduced clearance allows the concentration to remain high for a longer period of time.

dosage has been reduced. This is because the concentration in the central compartment remains elevated for a longer time, allowing the slower diffusion into the restricted compartment to transfer more drug. This suggests that low clearance values for investigational drugs are optimal for transfer of drug into restricted compartments.

Drug distribution can be quantified with imaging. Using this technique, low-energy molecules directly labeled with ^{11}C, ^{12}C, ^{18}F, or ^{19}F are injected in vivo and imaged with positron emission tomography (PET). The radionuclide emits positrons, which are captured by a scanner; they are subsequently annihilated by electrons to yield gamma rays, which are captured by a multiplier and used to construct an image. An example of how PET can be used for whole-body pharmacokinetic studies is given in Box 8.4. An alternative method that does not require a radionuclide analog of the drug uses test molecules to displace

---

BOX 8.4

Visualizing pharmacokinetic compartments with imaging

Images of low-energy analogs of molecules can directly indicate where molecules go in the body and the concentrations they attain in these compartments. Below are shown levels of the triazole antifungal Fluconazole (as a radioactive analog ^{18}F-Fluconazole) measured by quantitative PET imaging. This technique allows quantitation of drug levels in different organs in the body and also shows real-time drug level as it is cleared from the body.

Source: *Redrawn from A.J. Fischman, et al., The role of positron emission tomography in pharmacokinetic analysis, Drug Metab. Rev. 29 (1997) 923—956 [4].*

---

a prelabeled PET tracer already equilibrated in the organ of choice. This technique is not applicable to whole-body pharmacokinetics but can be used to determine drug access to particular organs.

At this point, it is worth putting the concepts of clearance and volume of distribution together to consider the in vivo pharmacokinetics of drugs. The aim of this endeavor is to characterize the pharmacokinetic parameters of a new drug entity to assess how it will behave therapeutically. Thus, "how much drug should be given" and "how often" are the critical questions with regard to how pharmacokinetics will control C_{ss}, the steady-state concentration of drug in the biophase available for therapeutic application.

In vivo pharmacokinetics

Up to this point, the processes of absorption, metabolism, and excretion have been treated somewhat as if they operate in isolation but, of course, in the body, they are concurrent and, sometimes, interdependent processes. As pointed out in Chapter 7, Pharmacokinetics I: Permeation and Metabolism, the steady-state drug level in vivo is due to a delicate

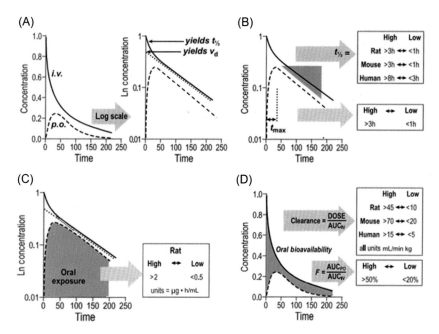

FIGURE 8.9 Pharmacokinetic parameters measured in vivo. (A) From a single intravenous dose, the clearance, $t_{1/2}$, for elimination and volume of distribution can be calculated. With a single oral dosage, the time to peak maximum can also be measured. Panel (B) shows some characteristic values for rat, mouse and human $t_{1/2}$. (C) A single oral dose also allows estimation of oral exposure. (D) A comparison of AUC_{oral} versus AUC_{iv} allows a calculation of F. Shown are values for high and low F and clearance in mouse, rat and human.

balance of drug entering and leaving the system; anything that changes that balance could also change the steady-state. A great deal of knowledge about how these processes come together for a given drug can be obtained from a minimal in vivo study (see Fig. 8.9). For example, the time course of plasma concentration of a single intravenous dose of compound can yield:

- clearance;
- volume of distribution;
- $t_{1/2}$.

Similarly, from a single oral dose, the following data can be obtained:

- F;
- t_{max};

where t_{max} is the time to peak concentration (a possible indicator of restricted absorption). It will be seen how these parameters can be used to form an idea about the in vivo stability of a compound and what dosing characteristics it will need to have in the therapeutic setting. In general, in vivo pharmacokinetic experiments can permit the study of metabolites, the measurement of excretion (notably renal excretion), and can provide estimates of species-dependent plasma protein binding. In addition, the in vivo setting presents opportunities for observing drug-drug interactions not easily detected and studied in vitro. Finally, in vivo conditions may yield estimates of clearance and other pharmacokinetic parameters that are unique to a given species or study condition; these must be identified and noted as exceptions when scaling is used to estimate pharmacokinetic parameters for humans.

In vivo pharmacokinetics brings into play the dynamics of drug movement in the body and this can affect how drugs behave to produce therapeutic effect. For instance, Rowland's hepatic clearance equation illustrates the interplay between drug presentation to the liver and removal by the liver:

$$\text{Hepatic clearance} = (\text{blood flow})(CL_{INT}/(\text{blood flow} + CL_{INT})) \quad (8.5)$$

where blood flow refers to the blood flow through the hepatic vein (90 L/h) into the liver and CL_{INT} the intrinsic rate of drug removal through metabolism. This equation illustrates how drug pharmacokinetics can differ in disease. For example, consider an investigational drug for congestive heart failure with high intrinsic clearance in healthy volunteers (1500 L/h); this yields an extraction ratio (E_H) of $1500/(1500 + 90) = 94\%$ for a clearance of $CL = \text{blood flow} \times E_H = 90 \times 0.94 = 84.6$ L/h. When tested in patients with chronic Hepatitis B, with a 50% reduced liver function, the clearance is very similar to that found in healthy volunteers: $E_H = 750/(750 + 90) = 0.89$ for a clearance value of $0.89 \times 90 = 80.1$ L/h; only a 5% reduction. However, when tested in a patient with congestive heart failure resulting in a 50% reduction in liver blood flow (to 45 L/h), the $E_H = 1500/(1500 + 45) = 0.97$ for a clearance value of 45×0.97 of 43.7 L/h (a 48% decrease in clearance); a very different result.

A different effect is seen with a drug with low intrinsic clearance (4.2 L/h) having an extraction ratio of ($E_H = 4.2/(4.2 + 90)$) of only 4.4%. This yields a hepatic clearance of $CL = \text{blood flow} \times E_H = 90 \times 0.044 = 4$ L/h. When tested in a patient with reduced liver function (alcoholic cirrhosis) with a 50% reduced liver function, the clearance is drastically reduced. Specifically, the extraction ratio is reduced to $E_H = 2.1/(2.1 + 90) = 2.2\%$ for a clearance value of $0.022 \times 90 = 2.05$ L/h, a 50% reduction. However, when tested in a patient with compromised cardiac output producing a 50% reduction in liver blood flow, the $E_H = 4.2/(4.2 + 45) = 0.085$ for a clearance value of 45×0.085 of 3.83 L/h (only a 4% decrease in clearance); again a very different result.

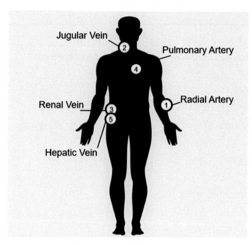

* 1 – 2 = Brain Clearance

* 1 – 4 = Lung Clearance

* 1 – 3 = Renal Clearance

* 1 – 5 = Hepatic Clearance

Total Body Clearance (CL_{tot})
CL_{tot} = Infusion Rate/ C_{ss}
(C_{ss}= concentration @ steady-state)

Extraction Ratio (E)
E= (C_{in}-C_{out})/C_{in}

Clearance = E x Q
Q= Blood Flow

FIGURE 8.10 Schematic diagram of five anatomical points on the human body from which blood samples can be drawn to measure drug levels for estimation of organ clearances.

Another element of whole body, in vivo pharmacokinetics is the estimation of drug clearance for various organ systems; these can be obtained by comparing the differential concentrations of drugs measured at various entry points in the body. Fig. 8.10 shows five entry points where drug level measurement can be taken and the calculations that yield various organ clearances.

Oral bioavailability

Oral bioavailability (F) is directly measured as the ratio of area under the curve (AUC) obtained by the oral route divided by the AUC produced by the same dosage given intravenously or, if the doses are different, then $F = (\text{dose}_{iv} \times \text{AUC}_{po})/(\text{dose}_{po} \times \text{AUC}_{iv})$. Thus, F values are the fraction of a dosage given via the oral route that makes its way into the central compartment (i.e., it is bioavailable). Experimentally, a value of F of 0.2 is adequate while 0.5 is very good. However, there are exceptions to this rule. As noted in Chapter 7, Pharmacokinetics I: Permeation and Metabolism, some bisphosphonates have extremely low F values yet, since they integrate nearly irreversibly into the bone matrix, eventually therapeutic levels accumulate. The AUC_{po} is proportional to the rate of drug absorption and the rate of clearance (usually hepatic); therefore, any factor that alters these rates will alter the value of F for a drug. Table 8.1 shows some gastrointestinal tract effects that

TABLE 8.1   GI effects on oral bioavailability.

	Increased	Decreased
Stomach emptying	Hunger, exercise, metoclopramide	Narcotics, antidepressants
Increased absorption	Decreased absorption	
Intestinal motility	Gastroenteritis/decreased transit time	Narcotics, anticholinergics, tricyclics
Decreased absorption	Increased absorption	
Chemical interaction	Chelation of tetracyclines with metal ions	
Decreased absorption		

can subsequently affect oral bioavailability; in general, these stem from changes in the rate of absorption. These are uniquely in vivo effects that cannot be adequately predicted in vitro.

Drug–drug interactions

Drug-drug interactions are commonly encountered in the liver (see Chapter 7, Pharmacokinetics I: Permeation and Metabolism), but can also occur in vivo wherever drugs compete for saturable processes. Some of these interactions occur at the level of drug transport. For example, digoxin is a substrate for the efflux transporter P-gp, but dosage is adjusted to account for this. However, if a P-gp inhibitor is given in vivo (i.e., verapamil, quinidine, cyclosporine-A), then digoxin toxicity can result as levels rise. Neurotoxicity to the antidiarrheal loperamide is also observed when coadministered with quinidine. In general, when dealing with the complex physiology of the body, there are numerous ways in which one drug can interfere with the therapeutic action of another; some of these are given in Table 8.2.

Nonlinear pharmacokinetics

The aim of pharmacokinetic studies is to derive predictions about central compartment concentrations with a given dosage. A possible

TABLE 8.2 Some drug–drug interactions detected under in vivo conditions.

Victim		Perpetrator	Mechanism	Outcome
Ketoconazole	+	Cimetidine	Altered gastric pH. Altered GI transit	Reduced dissolution of ketoconazole; reduced absorption
Warfarin	+	Phenobarbitol	Induction of metabolism	Increased metabolism of warfarin→reduced anticoagulation
Theophylline	+	Cimetidine	Inhibition of metabolism	Cimetidine reduces clearance of theophylline leading to adverse effects
Digoxin	+	Hydralazine	Increased renal blood flow	Increased renal clearance of digoxin
Penicillin	+	Probenicid	Increased renal blood flow. Increased tubular secretion	Prolonged half-life of penicillin allowing single dose therapy
Aspirin	+	Antacids	Increased renal blood flow. Increased tubular secretion	Reduced tubular absorption of salicylate due to increased urine pH

complication in this endeavor is the observation of "nonlinear pharma-cokinetics." While this may not lead to overt drug-drug interactions, this phenomenon can lead to capricious relationships between dose and drug blood levels. To discuss this further, it is useful to describe "linear" pharmacokinetics. This occurs when drug levels are well below the clearance capacity of the body. If clearance is approximated by a saturable process following Michaelis–Menten kinetics (i.e., hepatic clearance, renal transport) where the maximal velocity of the clearance is V_{max} and the sensitivity of the system to drug is K_m (this is the concentration of drug that half saturates the process), then the velocity of this process divided by the concentration of drug gives intrinsic clearance (CL_i):

$$CL_i = \frac{1}{[A]} \times \frac{[A]V_{max}}{([A] + K_m)} = \frac{V_{max}}{[A] + K_m} \tag{8.6}$$

It can be seen that when $[A] << K_m$ (when the concentration of drug is well below the saturation point of the process), the $CL_i \approx V_{max}/K_m$. Since, these are constant parameters of the system, the clearance is a constant, that is, there is a constant rate of removal of drug (in volume/time units, e.g., mL/min) from the system. If the drug is given intravenously at a given dosage rate (e.g., Dr infusion is μg/min), then the plasma steady-state concentration is linearly related to the dosage rate

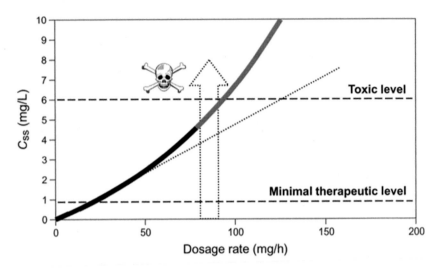

FIGURE 8.11   Nonlinear pharmacokinetics. The linear dotted line shows linear pharmacokinetics whereby the capacity of the system to clear the drug is not saturated.
Changes in dosage rate (abscissa) produce a correspondingly linear change in steady-state
concentration of drug in the central compartment (C_{ss}). Under conditions of nonlinear
pharmacokinetics (where the capacity of the system to clear the drug is diminished with
concentration), increased dosage rates cause an abnormally large increase in C_{ss}, as
denoted by the curvature in the line.

(C_{ss} (μg/mL) = Dr (μg/min) $\div$ CL$_i$ (μL/min)). This linear relationship
can be used clinically to control therapeutic C_{ss} levels by adjusting the
dosage rate (see Fig. 8.11). However, if the drug level rises to concentrations, which begin to approach or exceed the capacity of the clearance system ([A] $\rightarrow$ K_m), the relationship between Dr and CL$_i$ becomes
nonlinear and follows Eq. (8.6) (Fig. 8.11). As this region of concentration is approached within the dosage rate, the normally linear curve
becomes curvilinear and C_{ss} levels can become alarmingly high. This
can become a problem in drug therapy and it also poses a problem for
predictive pharmacokinetics.

Under conditions of linear pharmacokinetics, the exposure to a drug
(as measured by the area under the plasma concentration-time curve)
increases with drug dosage (see Fig. 8.12). However, the characteristic
feature of AUC versus dosage with linear kinetics is that a plot of
AUC/dosage versus dosage is a horizontal straight line (Fig. 8.12).

Fig. 8.13 shows conditions of nonlinear pharmacokinetics. It can be
seen that AUC may still increase with dosage, and the line relating
AUC versus dosage may even be straight, but this does not necessarily
constitute linear pharmacokinetics. The important feature is to note that

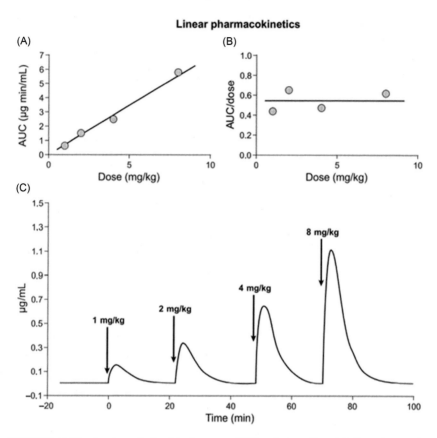

FIGURE 8.12 In vivo relationship between AUC and dose (Panel (A)) under conditions of linear pharmacokinetics. Panel (B) shows the horizontal relationship between AUC/dose ratios and dose. Panel (C) shows the actual AUC increases with dosage.

for this experiment, the plot of AUC/dosage versus dosage is not horizontal indicating that, as dosage increases, clearance is diminishing (nonlinear pharmacokinetics). It is essential to identify nonlinear pharmacokinetics in the clinic as it can control how a drug is used therapeutically (e.g., control of plasma steady-state concentration with dosage rate, determination of time to steady-state, unresponsive recovery after cessation of dosing). In terms of drug development and the use of in vivo animal systems to predict pharmacokinetics in humans, it is also important to detect such conditions, since nonlinear kinetics can cause slow drug elimination (e.g., the $t_{1/2}$ for Phenytoin changes from 12 hours to 1 week) and an increased time to steady-state conditions. This can greatly decrease the predictive value of data from an in vivo system demonstrating nonlinear pharmacokinetics.

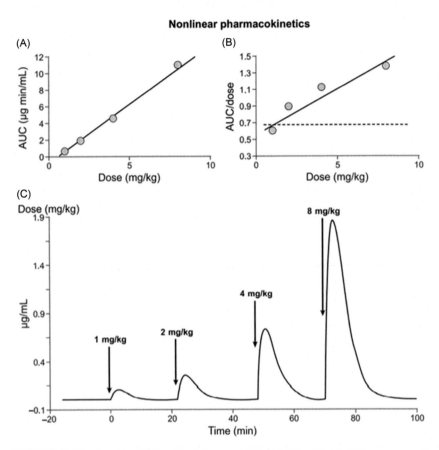

FIGURE 8.13 In vivo relationship between AUC and dose (Panel (A)) under conditions of nonlinear pharmacokinetics. Note that the relationship between AUC and dose may still appear linear. Panel (B) shows that the relationship between AUC/dose ratios and dose is not horizontal. Panel (C) shows the actual AUC increases with dosage.

There are a number of mechanisms in vivo that can lead to nonlinear pharmacokinetics:

- *Decreased absorption*: Saturated gut wall transport (Riboflavin), saturated gut wall metabolism (Salicylamide).
- *Renal effects*: Active tubular secretion (Penicillin G), active tubular reabsorption (Ascorbic acid), alteration in urine pH (Salicylic acid), alteration in urine flow (Theophylline), nephrotoxicity (Gentamycin).
- *Effects on metabolism*: Capacity-limited metabolism (saturate the enzyme capability of metabolic system—Phenytoin), autoinduction (the compound induces its own metabolism by increasing CYP450

BOX 8.5

Nonlinear pharmacokinetics: where more is not necessarily better

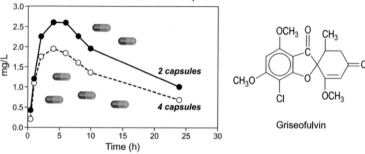

There are a number of situations where in vivo pharmacokinetics are nonlinear; many of these are encountered in the complicated process of oral dosing. Griseofulvin is an oral microcrystalline antifungal antibiotic used to treat fungal infections. It is nearly insoluble in water (12 mg/mL) and is dosed orally as a microsized or ultramicrosized powder. The limited solubility of griseofulvin in the gastrointestinal tract produces a unique profile with respect to dosing. Specifically, plasma levels with two capsules are actually higher than if four capsules are given.

Source: *Data drawn from: M. Rowland, T. Tozer, Clinical Pharmacokinetics: Concepts and Applications, Lippincott, Williams & Wilkins, Baltimore, MD, 1995 (pp. 450−451) [5].*

levels—Carbamazepine), cosubstrate depletion (when cosubstrate for conjugation is depleted leading to reduced elimination—Theophylline), product (metabolite) inhibition (Phenylbutazone).
- *Saturation of efflux transport*: for example, P-gp saturation.

In addition to decreased absorption effects, nonlinear pharmacokinetics can produce a decrease in bioavailable drug caused by problems with solubility (i.e., Griseofulvin; see Box 8.5). This can be seen as an abrupt maximum in AUC with increasing dosage. For example, 100 mg/kg of the hepatoprotective agent YH439 produces an AUC of 32 mg/min mL in rats; increasing the dosage to 500 mg/kg produces an AUC of only 37 mg/min mL, indicating a limit to the solubility of this compound [6].

The principal aim of pharmacokinetic studies is to estimate and model the ability of a new chemical entity to be adequately absorbed

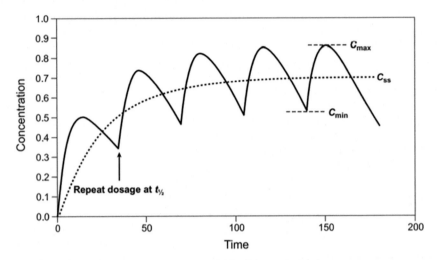

FIGURE 8.14   Repeat dosing at $t_{1/2}$ intervals leads to a steady-state concentration (C_{ss}) after approximately 5 $t_{1/2}$ periods. The actual temporal relationship between C_{ss} and time is characterized by a peak value (C_{max}) and a minimum value (C_{min}), also referred to as the trough.

in vivo and to have the properties to allow it to remain in the bloodstream for a length of time suitable for therapeutic effect. This estimation can be made using observations of the effects of multiple dosing. Fig. 8.14 shows the effect of repeated oral dosing to achieve a level of C_{ss} (steady-state plasma concentration) adequate for therapy. It can be seen from this figure that if the drug is given at intervals of every $t_{1/2}$, then as discussed previously, a steady-state will be reached within five $t_{1/2}$ periods. This steady state will still have variation in drug levels with time characterized by a C_{max} and a C_{min}. Clearly, the C_{max} must remain below predicted toxic levels while C_{min} (also called a "trough" concentration) must remain above minimally therapeutic levels. It is at this point that the importance of $t_{1/2}$ as a characteristic of a given in vivo system can be seen, as this parameter characterizes the ability of a drug to remain in the body for therapeutic effect. In vivo the $t_{1/2}$ is given by:

$$t_{1/2} = \frac{V_d}{\text{clearance}} \qquad (8.7)$$

Thus, high clearance produces a low $t_{1/2}$ (rapid excretion from the body) while a low clearance yields a high $t_{1/2}$. Similarly, a high volume of distribution yields a high $t_{1/2}$ (large V_d values indicate sequestration of the drug in compartments with subsequently retarded efflux) and a low V_d a correspondingly low $t_{1/2}$.

The $t_{1/2}$, the parameter that indicates how long the drug remains in the body, is a major parameter of whole-body *in vivo* pharmacokinetics. This value makes it an important determinant of how the drug will be used and what its value will be therapeutically. However, the presence of drugs in the body is not necessarily synonymous with their therapeutic availability. As shown by Eq. (8.6), a large $t_{1/2}$ can be obtained through a low clearance or a high volume of distribution. This latter mechanism may not be a therapeutically advantageous way to get a large $t_{1/2}$ since all this means is that the drug distributes into parts of the body through restricted diffusion and these may not be the same regions where the drug is required therapeutically. For instance, if the drug distributes into adipose tissue, the $t_{1/2}$ will be large due to a large volume of distribution but the drug may not be where it needs to be therapeutically. Thus, in general, choosing a drug candidate with a large volume of distribution to obtain a large $t_{1/2}$ is not a good therapeutic strategy. However, this effect can be used effectively to fine tune $t_{1/2}$ for therapeutic candidates.

In general, the volume of distribution of molecules is correlated with $LogP$ and pK_a values in that high $LogP$ and basic pK_a lead to molecules with larger volumes of distribution and vice versa. Therefore, medicinal chemical manipulation of $LogP$ and pK_a can be used to adjust the volume of distribution and thus, the $t_{1/2}$. Fig. 8.15 shows the adjustment of $LogP$ for the calcium antagonist nifedipine ($LogP = 2.9$) to $LogP = 3.3$ for amlodipine changes the respective volumes of distributions from 0.79 to 17 L/kg; this changes the $t_{1/2}$ values to be 1.9 hours (dosage

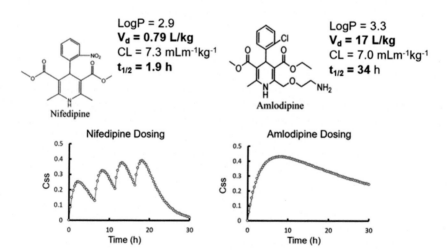

LogP = 2.9
V_d = 0.79 L/kg
CL = 7.3 mLm^{-1}kg^{-1}
$t_{1/2}$ = 1.9 h

Nifedipine

LogP = 3.3
V_d = 17 L/kg
CL = 7.0 mLm^{-1}kg^{-1}
$t_{1/2}$ = 34 h

Amlodipine

FIGURE 8.15 Adjustment of $t_{1/2}$ through modification of volume of distribution with $LogP$ values. Nifedipine has a low volume of distribution (0.79 L/kg) and a low $t_{1/2}$ (1.9 h); modification of $LogP$ from 2.9 to 3.3 with amlodipine increases the volume of distribution to 17 L/kg and correspondingly the $t_{1/2}$ to 34 h.

$4 \times$ day) for nifedipine to 34 hours (once a day) for amlodipine. A similar effect is seen with a change in the pK_a for erythromycin ($V_d = 0.95$ L, $t_{1/2} = 2$ h) through introduction of a second basic center to azithromycin ($V_d = 33$ L, $t_{1/2} = 69$ h).

The $t_{1/2}$ is a very important parameter as it links the original remit of a new drug discovery group to what will need to be dealt with in the evaluation of experimental candidate molecules. Usually, the characteristics of a desired drug profile are known at the outset of a discovery program. For example, the chemical target may be an oral, once-a-day treatment. The $t_{1/2}$ can be linked to dosage frequency and thus be used to assess candidate suitability. Defining a desired C_{min} for target coverage and also a C_{max} for safety, a ratio of C_{max}/C_{min} can be determined. This is related to the dosage rate (denoted as τ for the period between doses) by the $t_{1/2}$ with the following equation:

$$\frac{C_{max}}{C_{min}} = \frac{1}{e^{-\frac{0.693\tau}{t_{1/2}}}} \tag{8.8}$$

This equation can be used to set useful guidelines for what the $t_{1/2}$ of an investigational compound needs to be for a given dosing regimen. Fig. 8.16A gives a graphical representation of the parameters used for Eq. (8.8). Fig. 8.16B shows the C_{max}/C_{min} ratios for three molecules of varying $t_{1/2}$. In this example, it can be seen that if a dosing period of 12 hours is required, then a compound with a short half-life ($t_{1/2} = 2.3$ hours) would be completely inadequate.

Eq. (8.8) can be useful for predicting dosage interval. For example, assume that an experimental HIV-1 entry inhibitor with a $t_{1/2}$ of 6 hours has a K_i for blocking HIV-1 entry of 100 nM. For protection against HIV-1 entry, it is proposed that a $10 \times K_i$ concentration would be needed in the target compartment at all times; for a molecule of molecular weight of 389, this would be a minimum concentration required for therapy (C_{min}) of 0.4 µg/mL. It is also known that a 10 mg dose gives a C_{max} value of 2.5 µg/mL, well below the toxic level of 10 µg/mL. Using 2.5 µg/mL as C_{max}, this sets C_{min}/C_{max} at $0.4/2.5 = 0.17$ µg/mL. Rearranging Eq. (8.9):

$$\tau = \frac{- \text{Ln}\left[\frac{C_{min}}{C_{max}}\right] \times t_{1/2}}{0.693} \tag{8.9}$$

which predicts a τ value of 15.3 hours. Thus a 10 mg dose given every 12 hours should produce adequate target coverage for this investigational drug.

It is important to note that clearance is the major determinant of the dosing interval and that simply increasing the dosage of a highly cleared drug will not increase $t_{1/2}$ or the dosage interval τ. Fig. 8.17A

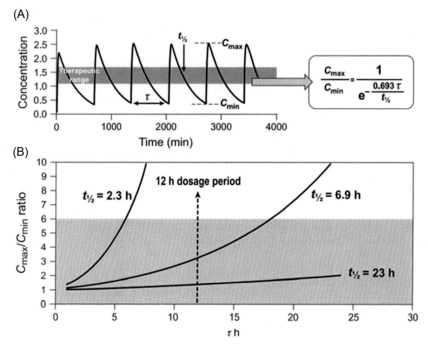

FIGURE 8.16 Repeat dosing showing C_{max}, C_{min} values and τ as the period between doses. Panel (A): Equation to the right shows the relationship between the ratio of C_{max}/C_{min}, $t_{1/2}$ and τ. Panel (B) shows C_{max}/C_{min} ratios as a function of τ for drugs of differing $t_{1/2}$. If the shaded area represents a maximum desired C_{max}/C_{min} ratio (higher ratios may indicate toxic concentrations or escape from minimal therapeutic concentrations), then it can be seen how a required dosage period of 12 h limits the choice of molecule (based on $t_{1/2}$ values).

shows how increasing the dosage will increase C_{max} (up to possible toxic levels) but will only minimally increase the duration of effect.

In contrast, Fig. 8.17A shows how a decrease in clearance will subsequently enable increased τ and give better target coverage. There are cases where an increased dosage may be adequate, if the periods of exposure are sufficient for target coverage and the drug is very safe (see Box 8.6).

Another strategy to achieve a suitable τ value to meet compliance is to use a formulation, such as coated tablets to retard absorption to avoid high (and possibly toxic) C_{max} levels (see Box 8.7).

Scaling data to predict human pharmacokinetic behavior

In vitro and in vivo pharmacokinetic studies are usually done in a variety of animal species in an effort to characterize the ADME

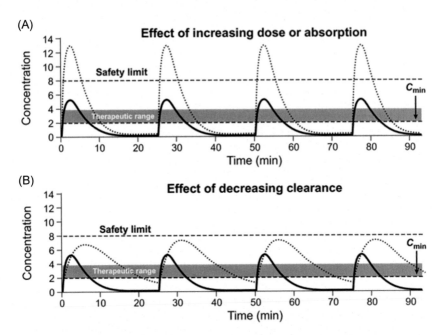

FIGURE 8.17 The effect of increasing dosage when the $t_{1/2}$ will not allow a convenient dosage period. Panel (A): It can be seen that little therapeutic coverage is gained from simply increasing the dosage under conditions of linear pharmacokinetics. Also, peak values may well extend beyond safety limits. Panel (B): In contrast, a reduction in clearance can increase target coverage to a point where a substantially longer τ value can be attained.

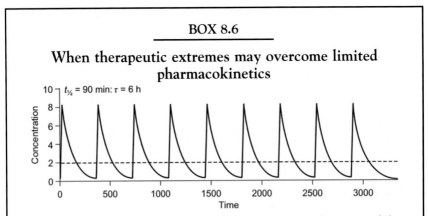

BOX 8.6

When therapeutic extremes may overcome limited pharmacokinetics

Usually, the half-time of a drug dictates the dosage frequency if the C_{max}/C_{min} ratio needs to be kept within a certain limit. A high dosage may be used to increase C_{min}, but with this comes a correspondingly high C_{max}, which could pose problems with safety. However, if the drug is inordinately safe, then it may be possible to give fairly large doses at intervals ($\gg t_{1/2}$) that are more amenable to better patient compliance. This approach may give drug exposure periods of sufficient magnitude to be therapeutic. One such drug is Augmentin (amoxycillin/clavulanate combination) used for the treatment of pediatric otitis.

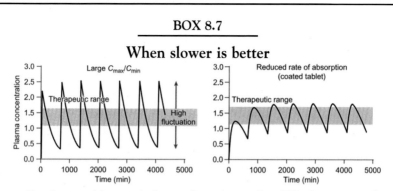

BOX 8.7

When slower is better

For drugs with marginal $t_{1/2}$ values, it may be difficult to reconcile adequate therapeutic coverage and a dosage regimen compatible with reasonable patient compliance. The left panel shows multiple dosing with a drug that is rapidly absorbed and cleared. A high dosage may provide target coverage but the fluctuation in concentration (C_{max}/C_{min} ratio) is unacceptably high. However, by reducing the rate of absorption (through coated tablets) and increasing the dosage, a better and less fluctuating steady-state concentration may be achieved.

properties of a given molecule and also to predict the pharmacokinetics that will be observed in humans. An important tool in this endeavor is the process of allometric scaling. This is a method of predicting parameters in various species based on body weight. The basic equation for this is:

$$Y = a \times W^b \tag{8.10}$$

where Y is the physiological parameter in question, a and b are fitting parameters and W is body weight. It is used in pharmacokinetics in the logarithmic form:

$$\log(Y) = \log(a) + b\log(W) \tag{8.11}$$

The basis for this equation is the relationship between observed and calculated values of physiological parameters and body weight; some of these are shown in Table 8.3.

The liver blood flow of various species, as a function of body weight, is shown in Fig. 8.18; the straight line results from fitting the data to Eq. (8.11).

TABLE 8.3   Physiological parameters of various animal species.

	Body weight (kg)	Blood flow liver (mL/min)	Kidneys (mL/min)	Urine (mL/day)	GFR (mL/min)
Mouse	0.02	1.8	1.3	1	0.28
Rat	0.25	13.8	9.2	50	1.31
Rabbit	2.5	177	80	150	7.8
Monkey	5	218	138	375	10.4
Dog	10	309	216	300	61.3
Human	70	1450	1240	1400	125

	Total body water (mL)	Compartment intracellular fluid (mL)	Volumes extracellular fluid (mL)	Plasma volume (mL)
Mouse	14.5	–	–	1
Rat	167	92.8	74.2	7.8
Rabbit	1790	1165	625	110
Monkey	3465	2425	1040	224
Dog	6036	3276	2760	515
Human	42,000	23,800	18,200	3000

GFR, renal glomerular filtration rate.

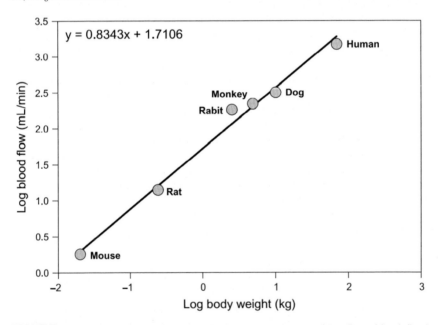

FIGURE 8.18   Allometric scaling. Graph shows a regression of Log(liver blood flow) on Log(body weight) according to the allometric scaling equation (Eq. 8.10). If hepatic metabolism is the primary method of clearance and is a constant percentage of liver blood flow in the range of species shown, then a graph of clearance in the animal species will be linear with the same slope, allowing prediction of clearance in humans.

The same can be done for most physiological parameters, such as volume of distribution and renal clearance. From these relationships, measurements taken in a range of species can be used to extrapolate the value for humans. If the molecule in question is cleared by the same mechanisms in all species, then scaling works well (although a larger body weight species is recommended for accurate scaling to humans; see Box 8.8).

Allometric scaling can also be used to identify species that demonstrate idiosyncratic pharmacokinetics for a given compound. Fig. 8.19 shows the scaling data for the antibiotic CS-023; it can be seen that the data for the monkey lies off the linear regression scaling line. Subsequent data showed that CS-023 is abnormally well reabsorbed in the kidney tubules of monkeys, thereby identifying the reason for the aberrant pharmacokinetics [7].

Once sufficient studies have been undertaken to predict suitable pharmacokinetics in humans, the data is applied to estimate the

BOX 8.8

The statistical geometry of allometric scaling

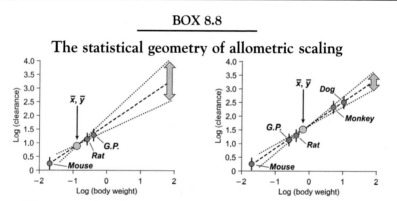

The main tool in allometric scaling is a linear regression of the equation (specific example for clearance):

$$\log(\text{clearance}) = \log(A) + b\log(\text{body weight})$$

Theoretically, any three animal species could define a straight line for scaling to values for humans. However, the error for the slope of a regression line is the rotation about the mean x and y values, and the further away the extrapolated value is from the mean x and y, the greater the error in estimation. Therefore, it is usually imperative to have an animal species of larger body weight to define the regression line for an accurate estimate for humans (70 kg)

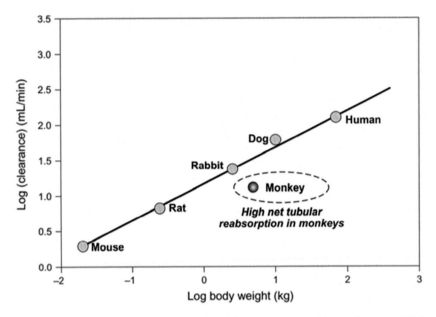

FIGURE 8.19 Allometric scaling regression for the antibiotic CS-023 clearance. While values for mouse, rat, rabbit, dog, and human reside on the linear regression, values for monkey diverge. Subsequent study showed this species had an abnormally high net renal tubular reabsorption, causing an aberrant reduction of clearance in this species [7].

starting dosage for human studies. There are numerous factors involved in this procedure affecting safety and predictability of effect; these include the NOEL (no observed effect level) and NOAEL (no observed adverse effect level) in animals. The NOAEL can be used to predict the MRSD (Maximum Recommended Starting Dose) in humans by:

$$MRSD = NOAEL_{animal} \times \left[\frac{SA_{human}}{SA_{animal}}\right] \times \left[\frac{1}{10} \text{safety factor}\right] \qquad (8.12)$$

where SA refers to body surface area given by:

$$\text{Body surface area}\,(\text{m}^2) = 1.85 \times \left(\frac{W}{70}\right)^{2/3} \qquad (8.13)$$

In general, Chapter 7, Pharmacokinetics I: Permeation and Metabolism, and this chapter have described the types of in vitro and in vivo experiments that can be done to characterize the ADME properties of new chemical entities. Fig. 8.20 summarizes the steps that can be taken in vivo, first with single and then with multiple dose studies to determine in vivo pharmacokinetics. These data can then be used in

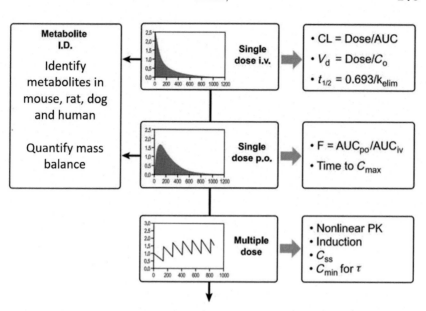

FIGURE 8.20 Summary of in vivo pharmacokinetics studies. Intravenous and oral doses can provide estimates of clearance, volume of distribution, $t_{1/2}$, t_{max}, and F. Analysis of plasma samples in different species also allows identification of metabolites. Multiple dose studies allow detection of nonlinear pharmacokinetics, possible induction effects, C_{ss} and estimation of τ values.

allometric scaling experiments both to choose the appropriate species for toxicology and efficacy studies, and also to project how best to progress to testing in humans.

Summary

- The kidney filters and excretes polar water-soluble compounds. Nonpolar compounds are filtered but may be reabsorbed.
- The extent of distribution of a drug can be determined by measuring the volume of distribution.
- Reduction in whole body clearance can be useful to increase drug distribution into restricted body compartments.
- Observing the decay, with time, of drug levels from a single iv dose can yield estimates of clearance, volume of distribution, and $t_{1/2}$. A single oral dose can yield values for oral absorption (F).
- The $t_{1/2}$ can be altered by changing the volume of distribution of drugs through altered pK_a or $LogP$ values.

- While there are in vitro experiments that can yield data to characterize specific processes relevant to in vivo pharmacokinetics (i.e., absorption, metabolism), there are factors encountered in vivo that can modify in vitro predictions.
- For example, solubility and other absorption effects in the gastrointestinal tract can modify the impact of first pass metabolism. Similarly, renal effects are not accounted for in vitro.
- In vivo experiments can detect complex mechanisms of drug-drug interactions and nonlinear pharmacokinetics.
- Nonlinear pharmacokinetics should be identified both as a therapeutic challenge and also as a factor in evaluating animal data to predict pharmacokinetics in humans and other species.
- Multiple dosing is used in vivo to achieve a therapeutic steady-state level of drug adequate for therapy (C_{ss}). The $t_{1/2}$ for elimination is an important determinant of the frequency of dosing possible to achieve adequate C_{ss}.
- In general, the rate of drug clearance is the dominant factor in determining frequency of dosing needed to attain adequate C_{ss}.
- Allometric scaling is a procedure whereby the pharmacokinetic data obtained in a range of animal species can be used to predict the pharmacokinetics in humans.
- Allometric scaling can also be used to detect aberrant pharmacokinetics in any single species.

References

[1] D.A. Smith, B.C. Jones, D.K. Walker, Design of drugs involving the concepts and theories of drug metabolism and pharmacokinetics, Med. Res. Rev. 16 (1996) 243–266.
[2] S.H. Kim, H.J. Shim, W.B. Kim, M.G. Lee, Pharmacokinetics of a new carbapenem, DA-1131, after intravenous administration to rats with uranyl nitrate-induced acute renal failure antimicrob, Agents Chemother. 42 (1998) 1217–1221.
[3] L.L. Gustafsson, O. Walker, G. Alvain, B. Beermann, F. Estevez, L. Gleisner, Disposition of chloroquine in man after single intravenous and oral doses, Br. Clin. Pharmacol. 15 (1983) 471–479.
[4] A.J. Fischman, The role of positron emission tomography in pharmacokinetic analysis, Drug. Metab. Rev. 29 (1997) 923–956.
[5] M. Rowland, T. Tozer, Clinical Pharmacokinetics: Concepts and Applications, Lippincott, Williams & Wilkins, Baltimore, MD, 1995, pp. 450–451.
[6] W.H. Yoon, J.K. Yoo, J.W. Lee, C.-K. Shim, M.G. Lee, Species differences in pharmacokinetics of a hepatoprotective agent, YH439 and its metabolites M4, M5, and M7 after intravenous and oral administration to rats, rabbits and dogs, Drug. Metab. Dispos. 26 (1998) 152–163.
[7] T. Shibayama, Y. Matsushita, A. Kurihara, T. Hirota, T. Ikeda, Prediction of pharmacokinetics of CS-023 (RO4908463), a novel parenteral carbapenemantibiotic, in humans using animal data, Xenobiotica. 37 (2007) 91–102.

In vivo pharmacology

By the end of this chapter, the reader will understand the various pharmacokinetic and pharmacodynamic factors involved in the production of in vivo drug responses, as well as some of the ways in which these can be quantified and predicted in simple in vitro experiments. Also, readers will see that since the body is an open system (not in equilibrium) the kinetics of the interaction of drugs with targets become paramount and a major determinant of overall in vivo activity.

Whole body drug response

The tremendous technological advances over the past 200 years in medicine and pharmacology overshadow the equally tremendous history of empirical drug discovery done in vivo over the past 5000 years. Considering ideas set forth in the Ebers papyrus (a very early source of ancient "prescriptions"; see Box 9.1), the modern period of in vitro testing comprises only 4%−5% of the time empirical medicine has been

Pharmacology in Drug Discovery and Development
DOI: https://doi.org/10.1016/B978-0-443-14124-9.00016-1

BOX 9.1

The Ebers Papyrus: prescriptions from antiquity

Another	for	controlling	fast-flowing	urine:

seeds	grass,	one;	cyperus grass,	one;	beer,

one quarter liter;   cook   strain; to be taken for day one

The Ebers papyrus (so called because it was purchased in Luxor by Georg Ebers in 1873) is one of the oldest surviving medical records known. Thought to be written in approximately 1500 BC, it contains nearly 700 "prescriptions" (some dating from 3000 BC) for the treatment of maladies. Although many of these prescriptions are magical formulas and remedies, some hold kernels of pharmacological logic. For example, for night blindness, the "liver of ox" was suggested. Since night blindness can be caused by a deficiency in Vitamin A, and since the liver is an excellent source of Vitamin A, this prescription should produce a useful effect. A partial translation of the Ebers papyrus by Carpenter and colleagues [1] gives an intriguing example of ancient in vivo pharmacology.

practiced; the other 95%–96% of the effort has been drug discovery done in vivo.

Within this period the trial and error testing of herbal remedies forms a rich history of early drug discovery (e.g., see Withering and the Discovery of Digitalis; Box 9.2).

In addition to observing desired therapeutic activity, the clinical testing of new drugs has led to the observation of "side-effects" some of which have provided insights into therapies for different diseases (see Box 9.3).

BOX 9.2

Withering, Dropsy and the Foxglove Plant

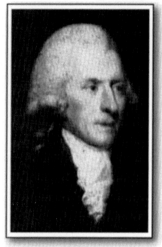

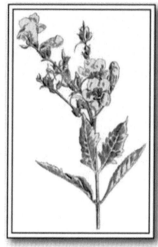

William Withering
(1741–99)

Foxglove
(Gerardia Quercifolia)

While working at Birmingham General Hospital in 1779, the British physician William Withering noticed a woman with "cardiac dropsy" (fluid swelling from congestive heart failure) improve remarkably after ingesting a local herbal remedy. He learned about the remedy from an old woman herbalist and went on to determine that the active ingredient was digitalis. In the years following, he systematically explored different preparations (gathered at various times of the year) to document 156 cases of the use of digitalis. In 1785, he published his famous paper, "An Account of the Foxglove and Some of its Medical Uses." This treatise describes clinical trials and notes on the therapeutic effect of digitalis and its toxicity; it is a classic chronicle of in vivo drug discovery and development. This subject became a topic of dissention when a physician colleague of Withering, Erasmus Darwin, was called for a second opinion and published the paper "An Account of the Successful Use of Foxglove in Some Dropsies and in Pulmonary Consumption." This led them to become estranged and led to a bitter argument over what Withering considered academic plagiarism.

With this history as a backdrop, modern pharmacology and drug discovery combine the rigor of in vitro testing (where drug concentration is known) and pharmacokinetic modeling of drug response in vivo. All the

---

BOX 9.3

New drugs from side-effects

Ethanolamines

CH_2—$CH_2N(CH_3)_2$

Ethylenediamines

$NCH_2CH_2N(CH_3)_2$
CH_3CH_2

Phenothiazines
(Promethazine)

$NCH_2CH_2N(CH_3)_2$
CH_3

In vivo

Chlorpromazine
(Antipsychotic)

Cl

$NCH_2CH_2CH_2N(CH_3)_2$

One of the main problems in drug discovery is the need for drug-like properties and adequate safety in molecules to allow testing in humans for proof of concept. When a drug meets these criteria, it can be an extremely useful tool for the exploration of other possible useful activities through the observation of secondary effects (so-called "side-effects"). Thus, the observed diuresis with the antibacterial sulfanilamide led to the development of the diuretic furosemide. Similarly, the development of the antidiabetic tolbutamide arose from observations with the antibacterial carbutamide. One of the most difficult areas of drug development is in diseases of the central nervous system. This is because of the subjectivity and complexity involved in the interpretation of CNS effects for diseases, such as depression and psychosis. In the 1950s, efforts to develop antihistamines led to compounds that caused patients to be "disinterested in their surroundings." This CNS side effect was recognized as possibly of value to patients who have constant unwanted sensory input in schizophrenia. This led to the development of chlorpromazine, the first drug for that disorder.

---

previous chapters are aimed at methods and strategies to obtain a molecule that will be therapeutically useful in vivo. This chapter considers the two topics of pharmacodynamics (primary activity at the therapeutic target) and pharmacokinetics (delivery of a therapeutic dose in vivo to the target organ) and combines them to discuss the final in vivo activity of a drug. The third main element of discovery, namely safety pharmacology, will be discussed in the next chapter.

When a drug enters the body, it encounters a complex and dynamic system that has its own basal activity combined with reflex mechanisms designed to counter any perturbation. As seen in Fig. 9.1, a drug introduced

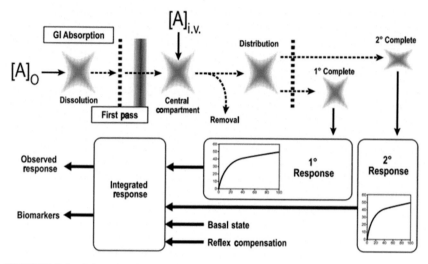

FIGURE 9.1 Schematic diagram of the route of travel of a drug given either intravenously (i.v.) or orally in an in vivo system. The production of observed effect is seen as a function of the primary therapeutic (desired) drug action modified by secondary effects, interaction with the basal physiological tone of the system, and in vivo reflexes.

orally must dissolve in the gastrointestinal tract, be absorbed through the lumen, and pass through the liver before it can enter the central compartment. Drugs introduced intravenously already gain access to the central compartment. From there, drugs can be destroyed by enzymatic degradation, bound by plasma proteins, distributed to other compartments of the body, further destroyed by hepatic metabolism, or directly excreted by the renal (or other) system. During this process, quantities of drugs in body compartments can interact with tissues to produce pharmacologic responses. Some of these may be beneficial (therapeutic response) and others may counter the therapeutic effect or produce other effects that may compromise normal cellular activity. These latter interactions can raise safety issues. In general, the observed response to a drug takes into consideration the pharmacokinetic factors that can affect the magnitude of the dose given, the integration of all the responses produced by the drug, the effect of body reflexes, and finally, the interaction of the drug with the ongoing basal physiological activity of the system.

New terminology

- *Biomarkers*: An observed finding that can be associated with a drug effect, disease, or physiological state. These can be physiological readings, chemical or biochemical substances, or images.

- *Pharmacodynamic-pharmacokinetic dissociation:* This occurs when a target coverage exceeds the period that the drug is actually in the receptor compartment (persistent binding allows drug effect even though free drug has been cleared).
- *ROC curves:* Receiver operated characteristic curves are used to evaluate procedures; in this case, the effectiveness of biomarkers as predictors of disease or drug effect.
- *Target coverage:* A term that encompasses the degree to which and the length of time a biological target is associated with (bound to) a drug molecule.

The "Dose" in dose—response

Chapter 7, Pharmacokinetics I: Permeation and Metabolism and Chapter 8, Pharmacokinetics II: Distribution and Multiple Dosing, extensively consider the properties required of a molecule to reach the target organ in the body and be present there for a sufficient length of time to be therapeutically useful. There are examples of where pharmacokinetics can completely dominate how a drug works in vivo (see Box 9.4).

This chapter will now relate the pharmacokinetically available dose with observed in vivo responses. It should be recognized that drug levels are measured in the body from samples taken from the central compartment and these may be quite different from the drug levels in the compartment actually containing the biological target for therapy (see Fig. 9.2).

There are factors in the central and therapeutic compartment, which can alter the concentration of drug producing an observed effect; two of these are plasma protein binding (PPB) and restricted diffusion.

PPB was discussed in Chapter 7, Pharmacokinetics I: Permeation and Metabolism, as a factor causing divergent values for dosages given in vivo and those that are actually free to produce a response. While not an extremely important factor in candidate selection of molecules, it can obscure whole body pharmacokinetics (see Box 9.5).

It is also important when the clinical dose is compared to the observed response, and the true potency (and safety margin) of drugs needs to be calculated. PPB is a saturable process; therefore, its importance may change with dosage level. Fig. 9.3A shows the aberration of central compartment drug levels by PPB. It can be seen that as the drug level saturates the amount of protein available, the central compartment concentration approaches the dosage given. Depending on the amount of protein and concentration of drug, the dosage level at which this occurs varies. As seen in Fig. 9.3B, the observed response to a drug that is 97% protein bound occurs at concentrations considerably greater than

BOX 9.4

The route of drug administration can mean the same drug can become a different drug

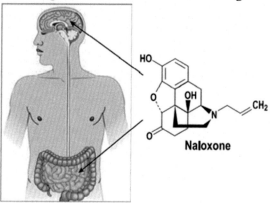

Naloxone

The route of administration of a drug in vivo can be a means of increasing the delivery of the drug to a given organ to optimize the active concentration at the therapeutic target. It can also effectively reduce the side effects of a drug in vivo. For example, β-adrenoceptor bronchodilators in asthma reach the constricted bronchioles at a maximal concentration through aerosol and then dissipate through the body to arrive at the heart (a major organ for side-effects) at a much lower concentration. The opioid receptor antagonist naloxone can actually yield completely different clinical profiles when given by different routes in vivo. When administered intravenously for an opiate overdose, the drug gains access to the brain where it is needed. If given via the oral route it acts exclusively on bowels to treat constipation during pain therapy without affecting the central pain-reducing effects of opiates.

the true free drug concentration, since only 3% of the added drug is free to produce a physiological response.

PPB can be species-dependent; therefore, it is important to quantify it from actual in vivo samples to normalize dosing data. Fig. 9.4 shows a convenient apparatus for this; plasma samples are placed into a centrifuge tube separated into compartments by a semipermeable membrane. This allows aqueous media and dissolved-free drug to pass to the bottom layer and protein (and protein-bound drug) to be retained on the membrane after centrifugation. Thus, plasma samples from in vivo

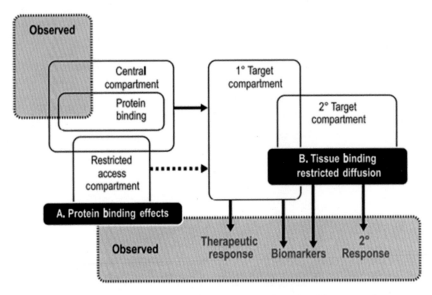

FIGURE 9.2 Shaded areas represent the experimentally accessible points of an in vivo experiment. Plasma samples from the central compartment can be assessed for levels of free and protein-bound drugs and linked to observed effects either directly or through biomarkers.

experiments can be rapidly assessed for free drug for evaluation of true dose-response sensitivity. Shown in this figure is the 350% variation in PPB of the antibiotic CS-023 with species [3].

If the therapeutic compartment (containing the target of interest for primary activity) has restricted diffusion for entry, then differences between drug levels in the central compartment and the therapeutic compartment (beyond those caused by PPB) can be further exacerbated. In such a compartment, the rate at which the drug achieves steady-state concentration at the biological target is given by:

$$[A_t] = (1 - e^{-(Q/V)t}) \tag{9.1}$$

where $[A_t]$ is the concentration in the compartment at time t, the rate of diffusion is Q and the volume of the compartment is V. As in all in vivo systems, there is a rate of dissolution from the compartment through either degradation within the compartment or bulk diffusion out as clearance reduces the central compartment drug level. In restricted access compartments Q may be inordinately low, causing a fall in steady-state concentration into the therapeutic compartment beyond that seen in the central compartment. These are local effects and the means to measure them may not be available except through a technology amenable to detailed analysis, such as imaging (see Box 8.4).

BOX 9.5

Plasma protein binding (PPB) can obscure pharmacokinetics

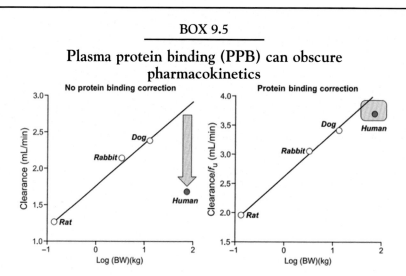

Source: Data drawn from: E. Van Hoogdalem, Y. Soeishi, H. Matsushima, S. Higuchi, Disposition of the selective α1A-adrenoceptor antagonist tamsulosin in humans: comparison with data from interspecies scaling, J. Pharm. Sci. 86 (1997) 1156–1161 [2].

While PPB may not seriously alter drug development strategy (see Box 8.1), it should not be ignored when pharmacokinetic profiles of compounds and/or quantitative relationships between dose and response in vivo are required. The figure below shows the difference in the veracity of predictions for human clearance made through allometric scaling. When PPB is not measured and corrected for, the regression for the α_{1A}-adrenoceptor antagonist tamsulosin shows how the observed value falls considerably short of the allometric projection. This difference is greatly reduced when corrections are made for free drug concentration.

Another factor made evident from Eq. (9.1) is the relative volume of the therapeutic compartment; if this is large then differences in the concentration gradient (between the central (measurable) compartment and therapeutic (restricted) compartment) may be further compromised. Since the body is comprised of numerous diffusion-limited compartments, these effects constitute some of the main reasons for difficulty in equating the in vitro drug response with the dose administered in vivo.

As discussed briefly in Chapter 7, Pharmacokinetics I: Permeation and Metabolism, another factor in evaluating in vivo responses is the production of pharmacologically active metabolites. These must be

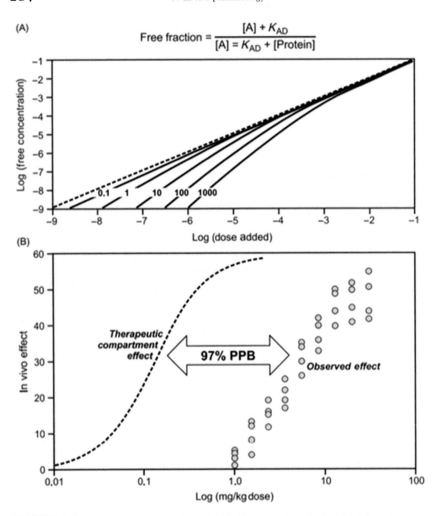

FIGURE 9.3 Plasma protein binding. (A) Ordinates reflect the level of free drug as a function of drug added to an in vivo system containing protein that can bind the drug. As the level of added drug increases, the binding becomes saturated and the level of free drug then equals the level of added drug. This effect is inversely proportional to the amount of protein in the system. (B) Dose–response curve of observed effect (ordinates) as a function of added drug (open circles) for a drug that is 97% protein bound. Thus, a level of 3 mg added results of only approximately 0.09 mg free drug available for response. The dotted line represents the true sensitivity of the response system to the drug.

identified so that an in vivo response can be correctly ascribed to the parent compound or an active metabolite. For example, Fig. 9.5 shows the production of hydroxyhexamide from the parent acetohexamide [4]; the $t_{1/2}$ of the parent is 58 minutes while that of the metabolite is much

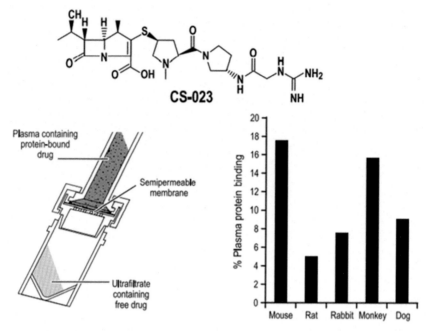

FIGURE 9.4 Apparatus in left panel allows separation of protein-bound drug (deposited on membrane) and free drug (captured in lower vessel) by centrifugation. Bar graph on right shows plasma protein binding for the antibiotic CS-023 in different animal species. Source: *Data from T. Shibayama, Y. Matsushita, A. Kurihara, T. Hirota, T. Ikeda, Prediction of pharmacokinetics of CS-023 (RO4908463), a novel parenteral carbapenemantibiotic, in humans using animal data, Xenobiotica 37 (2007) 91−102.*

longer ($t_{1/2} = 141$ minutes). Response is produced by both of these molecules; therefore, depending on the extent of metabolism in various species, the $t_{1/2}$ for the response could vary considerably. Table 9.1 gives a partial list of drugs that produce active metabolites in vivo.

What constitutes drug response?

Assuming that a suitable estimation can be made of the levels of active drug in the target compartment, the other variable to be considered is response. Usually, response is defined by the therapeutic endpoint of the drug. For example, a bronchodilator for asthma is aimed at relaxation of hypersensitive and constricted bronchioles to alleviate constricted breathing. Ideally, the effect of a drug in vivo can be visualized in real time within a timescale that can be associated with dosage of drug. For example, aspirin given for a fever produces a fairly rapid reduction in body temperature. There are many drug responses,

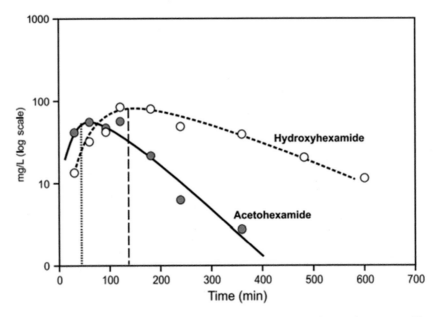

FIGURE 9.5 Production of an active metabolite from acetohexamide in vivo. The effects of the active metabolite are considerably more prolonged than those of the parent. *Source: Data from J.A. Galloway, R.E. McMahon, H.W. Culp, F.J. Marshall, E.C. Young, Metabolism, blood levels and rate of excretion of acetohexamide in human subjects, Diabetes 16 (1967) 118–127.*

however, which occur only on chronic dosing (reduction in viral load in AIDS) or do not produce immediately observable effects. To monitor these types of responses, biomarkers are often used. Biomarkers in medicine furnish an indicator of the physiological or pathophysiological state of an organ that can be monitored as a surrogate for drug effectiveness. They can be direct observations (such as insulin levels, heart rate, etc.) or biochemical products of a reaction associated with a drug or pathological process (see Box 9.6).

Biomarkers can be cells, molecules, genes, gene products, enzymes, or hormones. Several biomarkers are associated specifically with disease, such as serum low-density cholesterol for cardiovascular disease, blood pressure for hypertension, and P53 gene or matrix metalloproteinases for cancer. Fig. 9.6 shows plasma drug levels of the anticancer drug dasatinib in immunodeficient mice implanted with K562 human chronic myeloid leukemia xenograft tumors. In this case, the tumor produces a unique biomarker in the form of BCR-ABL, a constitutively active tyrosine kinase [5]. It can be seen that the biomarker levels track drug levels, thereby linking the drug to the response. One of the most useful types of biomarkers is imaging, as in the use of rubidium

TABLE 9.1 Drugs that form active metabolites through hepatic metabolism.

Drug	Metabolite
Acetylsalicylic acid	Salicylic acid
Amitriptyline	Nortriptyline
Carbamazepine	Carbamazepine 10,11-epoxide
Chlordiazepoxide	Desmethyl chlordiazepoxide
Codeine	Morphine
Diazepam	Desmethyldiazepam
Enalapril	Enalaprilat
Encainide	O-Desmethylencainide
Fluoxetine	Norfluoxetine
Imipramine	Desipramine
Isosorbide dinitrate	Isosorbide 5-monobitrate
Meperidine	Normeperidine
Morphine	Morphine 6-glucuronide
Prazepam	Desmethyldiazepam
Prednisone	Prednisolone
Primidone	Phenobarbital
Procainamide	N-Acetylprocainamide
Sulindac	Sulindac sulfide
Verapamil	Norverapamil
Zidovudine	Zidovudine triphosphate

chloride to evaluate the perfusion of heart muscle. Imaging biomarkers tend to be more closely associated with expressed phenotype of diseases and can furnish a better association between dose and therapeutic effect. In addition, imaging is versatile, offers continuous assessments of therapy over time, can be done in animals and humans (thereby yielding translational data), and is noninvasive. Now well established, imaging is relatively simple as a method of measuring drug response (as well as pharmacokinetics; see Box 8.4). One of the most important areas for imaging as a measure of drug response is cancer, where tumor size can be immediately measured after drug treatment [6].

Table 9.2 gives a partial list of common biomarkers used in medicine to assess drug effectiveness and disease state.

BOX 9.6

Biomarkers: nature's messengers for physiological state

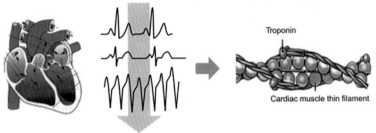

Troponin

Cardiac muscle thin filament

Reduction in blood flow to the heart (through blockage of one or more blood vessels) in conditions, such as unstable angina or heart attack can cause chest pain, shortness of breath, nausea, sweating, and dizziness. If prolonged, this condition can lead to damage to the heart muscle in the form of an infarction and thus can be life-threatening. There are cases where myocardial infarctions may be "silent" or clinically unrecognized and in these cases, a biomarker can be a valuable indication of possible cardiac damage. The most reliable biomarker used by physicians for detection of cardiac damage from such episodes is the detection of troponins in the blood. Although troponins exist in other cell types, cardiac troponin I is unique, and thus can be specifically identified. This makes troponin I the only specific biomarker for cardiac muscle. Levels rise 4–6 hours after infarction and may remain elevated for up to 7 days, thereby leaving a lasting record of the event.

Considering biomarkers as indicators of effect can be speculative, that is, there may be a number of possible biomarkers available for the disease state and the effectiveness of drug treatment. To evaluate these, receiver operated characteristic (ROC) curve analysis can be useful. This procedure was introduced during World War II to characterize the ability of radar operators to discern friendly versus hostile aircraft. In this procedure, a regression of the fraction of truly positive events that are correctly identified as positive (CPF) are made upon the fraction of truly negative events that are correctly identified (CNF). This is then used as a ROC curve to assess biomarkers; an example of this is shown in Fig. 9.7.

Another aspect of measuring drug response in vivo is the variation in the magnitude of drug response with the existing normal physiological basal tone of the system. For example, the physiological heart rate is

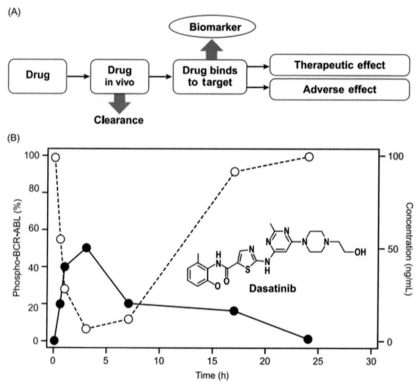

FIGURE 9.6 Biomarkers. (A) Schematic diagram of the production of a biomarker produced by a system in direct response to the action of a drug. (B) Biomarker for cancer (BCR-ABL, a constitutively active tyrosine kinase produced by the tumor) shown as open circles (dotted line) as a function of time. Filled circles show central compartment concentrations of an antitumor drug dasatinib. Source: *Drawn from F.R. Luo, Z. Yang, A. Camuso, R. Smykla, K. McGlinchey, K. Fager, et al., Dasatinib (BMS-354825) pharmacokinetics and pharmacodynamic biomarkers in animal models predict optimal clinical exposure, Clin. Cancer Res. 12 (2006) 7180–7186.*

somewhat elevated as a result of the basal endogenous activity of the sympathetic nervous system. There are situations where in vitro testing of drugs in systems devoid of basal activation may yield data different from that observed in vivo because of this factor. The most obvious cases occur for weak partial β-adrenoceptor agonists. Fig. 9.8 shows how a partial agonist may increase physiological activity in conditions of low physiological tone and decrease activity under conditions of high physiological tone.

Finally, the body has mechanisms to counter imbalance and attain stability; some of these are neuronal reflexes and it is difficult to predict drug effects on these processes from in vitro experiments. Reflexes can

TABLE 9.2   Some common biomarkers.

Biomarker	Denotes
• Prostate specific antigen (PSA)	Prostate cancer
• Human papilloma virus	Environmental exposure to toxic substances
• ↑Dimethylarginine	Cardiovascular disease
• ↑Insulin levels	Diabetes
• C-reactive protein (CRP)	Inflammation; can be indicator of effectiveness of anti-inflammatory therapy
• ↑Cholesterol	Cardiovascular disease
• ↑Creatinine kinase	Biomarker of muscle damage
• ↑Fibrinogen in venous blood	Cardiovascular disease; also, an acute phase protein in inflammation

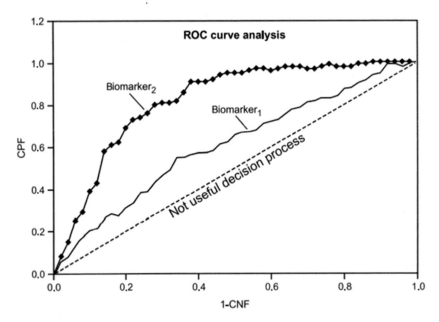

FIGURE 9.7   Receiver operating characteristic (ROC) curve analysis. Ordinate values (fraction of events that are correctly correlated with biomarker; CPF) plotted as a regression on 1—the fraction of negative events that are correctly identified with the biomarker (1-CNF). The dotted straight line indicates random chance (50%–50% chance of prediction with biomarker). Skewed lines in the top left quadrant reflect increasing ability of the test to correctly predict outcomes. This particular curve shows that biomarker$_2$ is a better predictor of the event than biomarker$_1$.

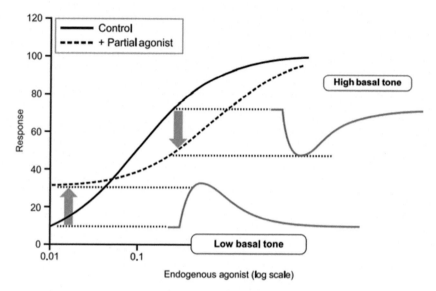

FIGURE 9.8 Dose-response curves to an endogenous full agonist in vivo in the presence and absence of a single concentration of partial agonist. Solid line represents system response to the full agonist in the absence of partial agonist. Dotted line shows the response to the full agonist in the presence of a concentration of partial agonist. In conditions of low basal tone (low concentrations of endogenous full agonist), the partial agonist will produce stimulation. Under conditions of high endogenous basal tone (higher ambient concentration of endogenous full agonist), the partial agonist will produce antagonism.

be important determinants of drug utility; for example, unabated hypotension through blockade of pressor α-adrenoceptor activation robs the patient of reflexes to counter postural hypotension; this can lead to fainting when patients stand. Box 9.7 shows a reflex mechanism that produces a favorable drug effect.

As discussed in Chapter 3, Predicting Agonist Effect (see Figs. 3.1 and 3.2) tissue-related factors can control sensitivity to hormones, transmitters, and synthetic agonists. Specifically, the amount of target in the cell (e.g., densities of cell surface receptors) and how efficiently the target is coupled to cellular response mechanisms can produce a wide range of sensitivities. The Black—Leff operational model (see Chapter 3, Predicting Agonist Effect) can be used to relate the power of agonists to activate a given organ system; this can be done in vitro in a test system. Fig. 9.9A shows the in vitro dose-response curves to two agonists, a standard and a test compound. From this type of analysis, the relative efficacy (relative τ values) and relative affinities for the target can be measured. If a dose-response curve to the standard agonist is available in vivo, then the change in sensitivity of the in vitro test system versus the in vivo therapeutic system can be made through quantification of

BOX 9.7

Reflexes become important to drug activity

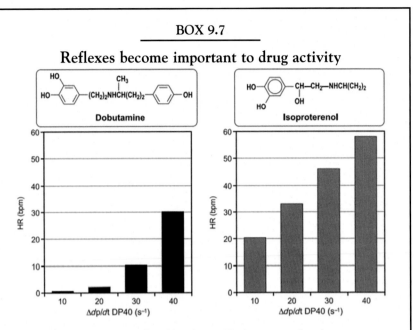

Source: *Data from: T.P. Kenakin, S.F. Johnson, The importance of α-adrenoceptor ago-nist activity of dobutamine to inotropic selectivity in the anaesthetized cat, Eur. J. Pharmacol. 111 (1985) 347–354 [7].*

β-Adrenoceptor agonists produce increased force of contraction (measured as the rate of rise of left ventricular pressure, $\Delta dp/dt$); theoretically, this effect could be of benefit in congestive heart failure as, in this disease, cardiac contractility is reduced and considerable congestion occurs due to inefficient left ventricular emptying. A major limitation to the use of β-agonists is the fact that they also promote debilitating increases in heart rate; this is shown for isoproterenol where increases in contractility ($\Delta dp/dt40$) are accompanied by increased heart rate. The same problematic heart rate effect is not seen with the β-agonist Dobutamine (panel on right). This is because Dobutamine possesses a low level of α-adrenoceptor activation, which slightly elevates vascular tone. This, in turn, activates the baroreceptor reflex to repress increases in heart rate. The slight activation of the baroreceptor reflex allows Dobutamine to be of limited use as an inotropic drug in humans; this effect is only seen in vivo.

the change in τ for the standard agonist. Under these circumstances, the relative power of the test agonist can then be assessed. This is shown in Fig. 9.9B where it can be seen that the in vivo system is considerably

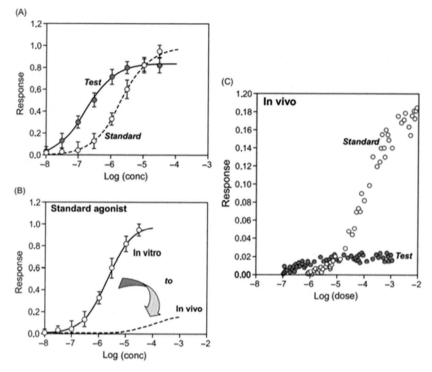

FIGURE 9.9 Application of the Black–Leff operational model of agonism (Chapter 3, Predicting Agonist Effect) for the prediction of agonist response in vivo. (A) Effects of a standard and test agonist in an in vitro test system. These data furnish estimates of the relative efficacy (τ values) and affinities of the agonists. (B) Measure of the change in sensitivity from the in vitro system to the in vivo system for the standard agonist. This gives an estimate of the change in τ value for the standard agonist in going from the in vitro to the in vivo system. (C) The change in τ value for the standard agonist is applied to the test agonist (applied to the relative τ value determined in vitro) to predict the dose–response curve to the test agonist in vivo. It can be seen from this case that the relative τ values determined in Panel (A) predict that essentially no agonism to the test agonist will be seen in vivo.

less sensitive than the in vitro system. The change in sensitivity from the in vitro to the in vivo system is then applied to the test agonist (see Fig. 3.6) for prediction of the sensitivity of the in vivo system to the test agonist. As shown in Fig. 9.9C, the relative efficacy of the test to standard agonist coupled with the reduction in sensitivity of the in vivo system (compared to the in vitro system) predicts that little, if any, response will be observed in the in vivo system to the test agonist. These types of predictions can be very useful in assessing in vivo responses (or lack of responses) to agonists.

The importance of kinetics in vivo

In vitro experimentation to optimize drug activity emphasizes intensity of effect (i.e., potency, efficacy, etc.). However, for open (in vivo) systems, the kinetics of effects are equally, and sometimes more, important. Therefore, the duration of effect becomes a critical variable in the assessment of drug activity. If the duration is linked to elimination pharmacokinetics, then assuming that final elimination can be described by a single compartment after drug distribution throughout the body, concentration with time is given by:

$$[C]_t = (Dose/V_d)e^{-kt} \tag{9.2}$$

where V_d is the volume of distribution, k is an elimination rate constant, and t is time. Defining $t_{duration}$ as the time the concentration is above an arbitrary therapeutically defined minimal level (C_{min}), and setting $k = 0.693(t_{1/2})^{-1}$, Eq. (9.2) defines the duration of action as:

$$t_{duration} = 1.44t_{1/2}(\ln[Dose] - (V_dC_{min})) \tag{9.3}$$

Under these circumstances, the duration of action is proportional to the $t_{1/2}$ for drug elimination if effect is linked to pharmacokinetics. The various procedures described in Chapter 7, Pharmacokinetics I: Permeation and Metabolism and Chapter 8, Pharmacokinetics II: Distribution and Multiple Dosing, can be used to estimate $t_{1/2}$ and a measure of duration of the drug action can be made.

Since drug response is linked to kinetics in open systems, observed potencies can be affected by the time following dosage that the measurements are taken. Fig. 9.10 shows a dose-response curve to an agonist as a function of time; it can be seen from this figure that the time at which response is measured can have important effects on the reported potency of the agonist in vivo.

There also can actually be large discrepancies between clinically effective responses to drugs and the initial biochemical events that trigger them. Fig. 9.11 shows the time course for alleviation of the symptoms of depression as a function of treatment with a monoamine uptake inhibitor. While the fairly rapidly observed biochemical event (increased neurotransmitter present in the synaptic cleft) coincides with the biochemical mechanism of the drug, it takes a considerable length of time for the system to remodel itself as a result of this biochemical effect to finally produce the therapeutic effect. These are extreme discontinuities between the initiation of the pharmacologic effect and the eventual return to normal physiology. Similar effects are seen in cancer chemotherapy where complete elimination of tumors may require prolonged biochemical treatment.

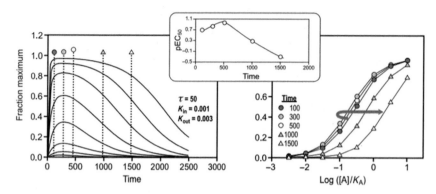

FIGURE 9.10 Influence of the analysis of agonism, at different time-points, on the observed potency of the agonist. It can be seen that the time-point at which the agonism is measured controls the location of the dose-response curve to the agonist along the drug concentration axis, that is, potency is a function of time in an open system. Inset shows pEC_{50} of the agonist with time.

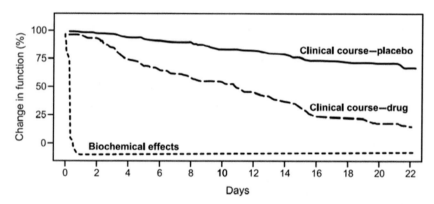

FIGURE 9.11 Effect of an antidepressant on clinical depression with time. For antidepressant drugs that are inhibitors of monoamine transport (dopamine, serotonin, norepinephrine), a rapid increase in the synaptic cleft concentration of neurotransmitter is observed within 1–2 days. The measurable improvement in subjective indices of depression, however, requires a much longer time to become evident. Thus, there is a discontinuity between the biochemical effect and the therapeutic effect.

There are a number of common circumstances where central compartment pharmacokinetics is not the only consideration in defining duration of drug effect in vivo. For instance, if the therapeutic target resides in a diffusion-restricted compartment, then efflux to and from this compartment may be slower than it is from the central compartment, and duration may be longer than that predicted from central compartment pharmacokinetics. In a restricted compartment, drug that has

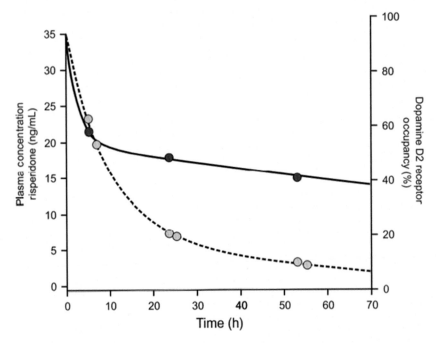

FIGURE 9.12   Separation of kinetics of drug level and drug target occupancy of dopamine D2 receptors by risperidone. Filled circles show the time course of dopamine receptor occupancy measured in human brain in vivo through imaging; this process has a $t_{1/2}$ of
80.2 h. Open gray circles show the plasma concentrations of risperidone; $t_{1/2} = 17.8$ h.
*Source: Drawn from A. Takano, T. Suhara, Y. Ikoma, F. Tasuno, J. Maeda, T. Ichimiya, et al.,
Estimation of the time-course of dopamine D2 receptor occupancy in living human brain from
plasma pharmacokinetics of antipsychotics, Int. J. Neuropsychopharmacol. 7 (2004) 19–26.*

diffused from the target may rebind due to confined volume effects or
binding to high affinity "exosites" within the compartment [8]. These
effects are difficult to predict reliably although imaging of distinct
regions may be an option. Fig. 9.12 shows how reversal of the brain
dopamine D2 receptor occupancy of the antipsychotic drug risperidone
with time (as observed through imaging) is considerably slower than
the clearance of the drug from the central compartment. Specifically,
the $t_{1/2}$ for clearance from the central compartment is 17.8 hours while
the $t_{1/2}$ for offset from receptors in the brain is 80.2 hours [9].

   One mechanism to predict the duration of the effect that can be evaluated in vitro is the kinetics of binding of the molecule to the biological
target. The kinetics of the receptor dissociation can be extremely important to in vivo target coverage (a term encompassing dissociation of the
drug from the target with time in vivo). If the offset of the antagonist
from the receptor is slow, then the antagonism can far outlast the

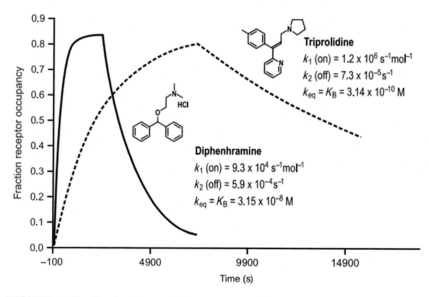

FIGURE 9.13 Graph of theoretical association and dissociation patterns for two antihistamines of known potency. Addition of the antagonist leads to an increasing receptor occupancy until a plateau is reached, while washing causes reversal of occupancy with antagonist dissociation. Diphenhydramine is a rapidly acting antagonist while triprolidine is slow.

presence of the antagonist in the receptor compartment. The kinetics of offset from the receptor once the antagonist is bound is given by:

$$\rho_{t-off} = \rho_e e^{-k_2 t} \tag{9.4}$$

The potency of the antagonist is given by the equilibrium dissociation constant of the antagonist-receptor complex defined as the ratio $K_B = k_2/k_1$. For example, Fig. 9.13 shows association and dissociation curves for two antihistamines; diphenhydramine has a potency of 31.5 nM and triprolidine has a potency of 3.14 nM. While these antagonists differ in potency, they also differ widely in kinetics. The rate of dissociation (from the receptor) of diphenhydramine is 8.1 times the rate of dissociation of triprolidine, causing the antagonism by diphenhydramine to be much more transient than an equiactive dose of triprolidine in an open system. Differences in dissociation kinetics need not necessarily be obvious from antagonist potency. Since a near infinite range of k_2 and k_1 values can yield the same K_B, it can be seen that antagonists of identical potencies can have a wide range of onset and offset kinetics. For example, a nanomolar potency antagonist (i.e., $K_B = 10^{-9}$ M) can have a rate of onset of 5×10^5/s mol and a rate of offset of 5×10^{-4}/s (consider this a "rapid" offset antagonist) or a rate of onset of 10^5/s mol and offset of 10^{-4}/s ("slow" offset). While these molecules are equipotent in a closed system at equilibrium (i.e., in an in vitro assay), they will give widely different temporal target coverage in vivo.

Specifically, the "slow" antagonist will give a much longer coverage of the receptor than the "fast" antagonist. Box 9.8 shows how the serotonin antagonists altanserin and ritanserin, which are similar in potency, have vastly different target coverage capabilities.

Dissociation kinetics of the antagonists can become very important in light of the fact that the exposure of the target to the antagonist in vivo is transient. If dissociation kinetics are slow then a transient exposure of target to antagonist may "load" the system and antagonism may persist long after the receptor compartment is free of antagonist.

Fig. 9.14 shows the receptor occupancy for antagonists of varying offset kinetics after a transient exposure of antagonist in vivo. It can be seen that slow rates of offset can cause persistent receptor occupancy by the antagonist that do not follow the pharmacokinetics of antagonist concentration in the receptor compartment.

Very slow antagonist dissociation can be useful in producing long periods of target coverage, even after the molecule has been cleared from the body. Fig. 9.15A shows dissociation curves for the chemokine CCL3 and three allosteric HIV-1 entry inhibitors from the therapeutic target, namely the CCR5 chemokine receptor. It can be seen that the $t_{1/2}$ values for aplaviroc, maraviroc, and Sch-C are considerably longer than 24 hours [11]. Fig. 9.15B shows a simulated target coverage for aplaviroc in contrast to plasma concentration. It can be seen that the association with the target continues long after aplaviroc has been cleared. For aplaviroc, the slow dissociation kinetics allows it to be a once-per-day treatment even though the pharmacokinetics of concentration in the plasma does not support that regimen of dosing. In this case, the target coverage was assessed by noting that lymphocytes derived from patients 24 hours after treatment still failed to be infected by HIV-1, indicating that aplaviroc is still bound to CCR5 at that time. Dissociation between the pharmacokinetic concentration of drugs in the central compartment and their target coverage in vivo offers a tool to pharmacologists for the improvement of in vivo therapy. Due to this fact, the in vitro measurement of drug-target dissociation rate becomes an important part of the characterization of the activity of drugs, as much as the measurement of steady-state equilibrium measures of potency and efficacy.

Summary

- The ultimate therapeutic value of a molecule is determined by its effect in vivo; factors, such as PPB, endogenous physiological tone,

BOX 9.8

Target residency may be more important than potency

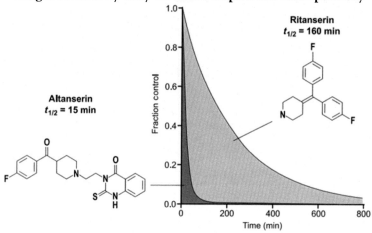

Source: *Data from: J.E. Leysen, W. Gommeren, Drug-receptor dissociation time, new tool for drug research: receptor binding affinity and drug-receptor dissociation profiles of serotonin-S2, dopamine D2 and histamine H1 antagonists and opiates, Drug Dev. Res. 8 (1986) 119–131 [10].*

The absolute potency of receptor antagonists is an important parameter since it is directly linked to the amount of drug that must be present in the target compartment to produce an antagonist effect. However, since the body is an open system, the concentration of drug varies with time; therefore, the target is exposed to a "wave" of drug for a certain period and then the pool is removed from the target compartment. Therefore, the amount of time it takes for the antagonist to dissociate from the receptor becomes an integral factor in the amount of time the antagonist can produce target coverage (i.e., be associated with the target to cause a therapeutic effect). This dissociation time can be somewhat different from the potency; thus, it becomes another factor in the antagonist profile. The serotonin antagonists altanserin and ritanserin have relatively similar potencies (altanserin $pK_B = 9.37$ and ritanserin $pK_B = 9.05$) but the $t_{1/2}$ for dissociation of ritanserin is more than 10 times greater. This would produce considerably better target coverage in vivo.

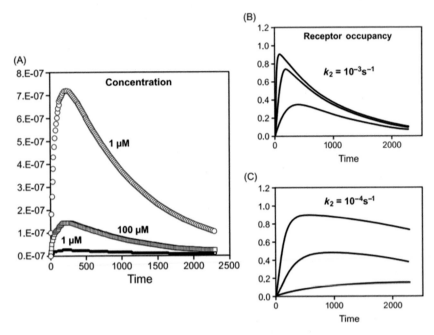

FIGURE 9.14 Correspondence between antagonist target coverage and antagonist absorption concentration in the central compartment. Panel (A) shows the absorption and pharmacokinetics for an antagonist. Panel (B) shows the corresponding receptor occupancy with time for the antagonist if it has a rapid dissociation ($k_2 = 10^{-3}$ s^{-1}). Panel (C): Receptor coverage with time if the same antagonist had a much slower rate of dissociation ($1/10 \times$ to yield $k_2 = 10^{-4}$ s^{-1}).

and reflexes can obscure the relationship between free drug concentration and observed effect.
- The response to a drug may be observed directly or through a surrogate, such as a biochemical biomarker. In addition, there may be temporal dissociation between the actual biochemical events initiated by the drug and the eventual lasting therapeutic response.
- The Black–Leff operational model (Chapter 3, Predicting Agonist Effect) can be very useful in translating in vitro agonist effect into predicted effects in vivo.
- Since in vivo systems are open systems, response must be linked with time of exposure to drug.
- The kinetics of drug movement within the body is immensely important to the in vivo activity of drugs either through restricted diffusion to and from the compartments containing the therapeutic

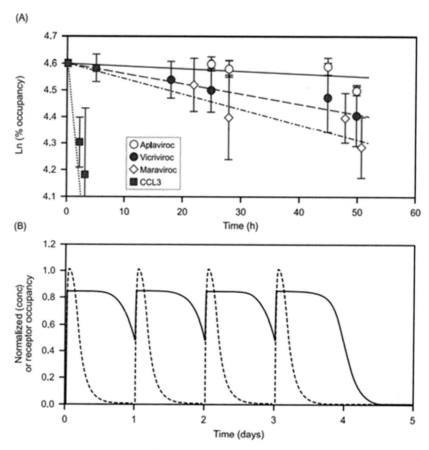

FIGURE 9.15 Real-time kinetics of target coverage. (A) Rate CCR5 receptor occupancy (log scale) by allosteric HIV-1 entry inhibitors (Aplaviroc, Vicriviroc, and Maraviroc) and chemokine CCL3 as a function of time. (B) Simulated target coverage (solid lines) for aplaviroc in once-a-day dosage regimen with pharmacokinetic levels of drug shown as dotted lines. *Source: Panel (A): Data from C. Watson, S. Jenkinson, W. Kazmierski, T.P. Kenakin, The CCR5 receptor-based mechanism of action of 87340, a potent allosteric non-competitive HIV entry inhibitor, Mol. Pharmacol. 67 (2005) 1268–1282 [11].*

target or through the actual rate of dissociation of the drug from the target itself.

- A slow rate of drug-target dissociation can greatly augment otherwise rapid and inadequate pharmacokinetics for therapy (Pharmacodynamic-Pharmacokinetic dissociation).
- It is important to quantify the rate of drug–target dissociation as an integral part of the profile of a given drug candidate (in addition to potency and efficacy).

References

[1] S. Carpenter, M. Rigaud, M. Barile, T.J. Priest, L. Perez, J.B. Ferguson, An Interlinear Transliteration and English Translation of Portions of The Ebers Papyrus Possibly Having to do With Diabetes Mellitus, Bard College, Annandale-on-Hudson, NY, 1998.

[2] E. Van Hoogdalem, Y. Soeishi, H. Matsushima, S. Higuchi, Disposition of the selective α1A-adrenoceptor antagonist tamsulosin in humans: comparison with data from interspecies scaling, J. Pharm. Sci. 86 (1997) 1156–1161.

[3] T. Shibayama, Y. Matsushita, A. Kurihara, T. Hirota, T. Ikeda, Prediction of pharmacokinetics of CS-023 (RO4908463), a novel parenteral carbapenemantibiotic, in humans using animal data, Xenobiotica. 37 (2007) 91–102.

[4] J.A. Galloway, R.E. McMahon, H.W. Culp, F.J. Marshall, E.C. Young, Metabolism, blood levels and rate of excretion of acetohexamide in human subjects, Diabetes. 16 (1967) 118–127.

[5] F.R. Luo, Z. Yang, A. Camuso, R. Smykla, K. McGlinchey, K. Fager, Dasatinib (BMS-354825) pharmacokinetics and pharmacodynamic biomarkers in animal models predict optimal clinical exposure, Clin. Cancer Res. 12 (2006) 7180–7186.

[6] M. Rudin, R. Weissleder, Molecular imaging in drug discovery and development, Nat. Rev. Drug. Discov. 2 (2003) 123–131.

[7] T.P. Kenakin, S.F. Johnson, The importance of α-adrenoceptor agonist activity of dobutamine to inotropic selectivity in the anaesthetized cat, Eur. J. Pharmacol. 111 (1985) 347–354.

[8] G. Vauquelin, S.J. Charlton, Long-lasting target binding and rebinding as mechanisms to prolong in vivo drug action, Br. J. Pharmacol. 161 (2010) 488–508.

[9] A. Takano, T. Suhara, Y. Ikoma, F. Tasuno, J. Maeda, T. Ichimiya, Estimation of the time-course of dopamine D2 receptor occupancy in living human brain from plasma pharmacokinetics of antipsychotics, Int. J. Neuropsychopharmacol. 7 (2004) 19–26.

[10] J.E. Leysen, W. Gommeren, Drug-receptor dissociation time, new tool for drug research: receptor binding affinity and drug-receptor dissociation profiles of serotonin-S2, dopamine D2 and histamine H1 antagonists and opiates, Drug. Dev. Res. 8 (1986) 119–131.

[11] C. Watson, S. Jenkinson, W. Kazmierski, T.P. Kenakin, The CCR5 receptor-based mechanism of action of 873140, a potent allosteric non-competitive HIV entry inhibitor, Mol. Pharmacol. 67 (2005) 1268–1282.

10

Safety pharmacology

By the end of this chapter, the reader will be aware of the breadth of assays and testing procedures available to assess the safety of a new drug entity. In addition, readers will be able to identify rapid in vitro tests that can detect serious toxicity in molecules at a very early stage. Finally, this chapter should yield an understanding of toxicity due to elevated drug exposure (intrinsic toxicity) versus that due to stochastic opportunity (idiosyncratic toxicity) showing how the latter is difficult to predict in drug testing and thus poses a serious risk in the drug development process.

Introduction

In addition to having primary activity and being able to enter the body, access the appropriate tissue, and have sufficient target presence to achieve

Pharmacology in Drug Discovery and Development
DOI: https://doi.org/10.1016/B978-0-443-14124-9.00012-4

therapeutic utility, a drug must cause no harm to the host. Therefore, the third important structure-activity relationship that must be explored for a drug is safety pharmacology. The human body is a finely tuned symphony of biochemical reactions and physiological functions, and miscues can cause the system to go awry. It is unrealistic to suppose that extreme amounts of almost any substance will not eventually cause harm; as put by Paracelsus (1493−1541):

> ... all things are poison and nothing is without poison. Solely the dose determines that a thing is not poison ...

The concept of "safety" can also be relative. As pointed out in the discussion of target validation in Chapter 1, Pharmacology: The Chemical Control of Physiology, one of the criteria in the choice of a favorable target for an antagonist is that the knockout mouse (genetically altered such that the target is not expressed in tissues) is healthy, that is, the organism can do without the target. Thus, it was observed that CCR5 knockout mice (lacking the CCR5 receptor) were healthy, thereby indicating that the CCR5 receptor is redundant and not required for life. While this spurred on pursuit of CCR5 as a target for HIV-1-mediated AIDS infection, the idea that CCR5 is redundant and not required for health was later shown to be simplistic. In this case, there is a human counterpart to the CCR5 knockout mouse, namely a population of people possessing a Δ32 CCR5 deletion in the receptor that causes it not to be expressed on the cell surface; in essence, human equivalent "knockouts." These people appeared to have normal health; however, as data accumulated this concept of "healthy" began to be questioned. Specifically, it had been shown that Δ32 subjects have a higher than average incidence of health abnormalities (i.e., greater incidence of liver disease and sclerosing cholangitis [1], risk of death in Nile Virus disease [2], greater mortality after liver transplantation [3], and mild immunodeficiency [4]). The point of these data for this chapter is to suggest that chemical intervention in *any* physiological function almost necessarily brings with it a risk of imbalance and consequent harm. Therefore, it is a defensible statement to suggest that all drugs, if given in sufficient dosage, may have harmful side-effects and pharmacological safety is simply a matter of relative benefit to risk of harm. This chapter will consider this benefit-to-risk ratio for drugs.

New terminology

The following new terms will be introduced in this chapter:

- *Carcinogenesis*: The creation of cancer where normal cells are transformed into cancer cells.

- *Cytotoxicity*: The quality of being toxic to cells to detrimentally affect cell metabolism, function, growth, and to subsequently induce damage.
- *Idiosyncratic toxicity*: Toxic effects due to stochastic probability occurring when a combination of favorable conditions coalesces.
- *Intrinsic toxicity*: Toxicity due to an elevation of dosage above a threshold for toxicity, that is, it is observed whenever this dosage is exceeded.
- *MTD*: Maximum tolerated dose—applies to long-term studies and refers to the largest dose that causes no obvious signs of ill health.
- *Mutagenesis*: Induction of genetic change in a cell through alteration of cell genetic material (usually DNA).
- *NOAEL*: No observed adverse effect level—the largest dose causing no observed toxicity or undesirable physiological effect.
- *NOEL*: No observed effect level—the threshold for producing a pharmacologic or toxic effect.
- *NTEL*: No toxic effect level—the largest dose in most sensitive species that produces no toxic effect.

Safety versus toxicity

Drug safety is often discussed in terms of "toxicology" when it is really more appropriate to focus on the term safety, defined as "the condition of being safe from undergoing... hurt, injury." Presupposing that a drug will cause harm if used inappropriately or in too high a dose, the aim is to define the conditions whereby a drug can be used effectively to heal with minimal risk of toxicity (defined as "containing or being a poisonous material... capable of causing death or serious debilitation"). The notion of "do no harm" for drug therapy does not lead to uniform safety standards for all drugs for all diseases. The notion of a "safety margin" depends upon the therapeutic indication of the drug, the intended patient population, the competitive environment, and the present standard of care. While a safe drug is an extremely important prerequisite to drug therapy, no drug at all for a devastating disease is also negative. In addition, kinetics can be extremely important (as discussed for hepatic enzyme inhibition—see Chapter 7, Pharmacokinetics I: Permeation and Metabolism); reversible toxicity should not be assessed with the same criteria as irreversible toxicity. As shown in Box 10.1, lead, a well-known toxic agent, has levels of toxicity associated with different kinetics with a half-time for release of years in bone this is known as a "body burden." A "body burden" of toxicity, such as that for doxorubicin, exists mainly because of the irreversible nature of the adverse effect. Irreversible toxicity usually is unacceptable in human clinical trials. It also is important if there is a biomarker for the toxicity. If the toxicity can be monitored then it may be detected and the treatment stopped before development into an irreversible toxicity.

BOX 10.1

Sinks, pools, and body burden for toxic drugs.

Toxicity can be related to real-time kinetics as well as dosage. For example, lead is a well-known toxic element. Upon absorption, it is nearly completely taken up by red blood cells where it has a long $t_{1/2}$ of 36 days. However, while in this pool it can diffuse into soft tissue, such as brain, muscle, spleen and heart and it is in these organs that it does the damage. Moreover, lead can also diffuse into bone where it has a remarkably long $t_{1/2}$ of 10–27 years [5]. This type of toxic pool is referred to as the "body burden" of lead since it essentially is with the patient for most of his or her life. Such long-term burdens can be important as in the case of doxorubicin treatment for cancer. Doxorubicin produces irreversible cardiac damage; therefore, patients are limited to a lifetime dosage level of $<550 \, mg/m^2$ of body surface area. Once this level has been achieved, clinicians are no longer allowed to prescribe doxorubicin for cancer treatment.

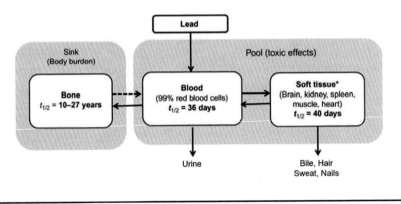

The hazard of toxicity can also depend on how the drug is used. For example, the drug theophylline is used intravenously in emergency rooms for acute bronchoconstriction in children. While a serum concentration of $15 \, \mu g/mL$ produces life-saving bronchodilation, $25 \, \mu g/mL$ causes mild side-effects, which become potentially serious at $35 \, \mu g/mL$ and severe at $42 \, \mu g/mL$. Thus, less than a threefold increase in serum plasma levels can lead to toxicity. The key to theophylline's value is the fact that it is used in a strictly controlled setting (intravenous administration under a physician's supervision with constant surveillance). In this case, the "safety" of theophylline is an extremely qualified parameter. It is also important to determine the mechanism of action of the toxic event as some toxicities may be species-dependent and not relevant to human health.

There is an obvious interplay between the severity of the disease being treated and the severity of the toxicity. Thus, the toxicity standards for a drug designed for the casual treatment of weight loss to be used in a huge population of subjects would be greater than for a life-saving drug in a limited population of AIDS patients for which there was no alternative. When the toxicity is catastrophic, such as the fatal cardiac effects of Torsades des Pointes, then it is extremely important to detect the risk for any new drug; specific applications of toxicity tests can be used. A number of assays can be used to predict this toxicity, among them inhibition of the hERG potassium channel, prolongation of the QTc interval in the electrocardiogram, and arrhythmia in the isolated perfused heart (Langendorff heart preparation). Fig. 10.1 shows an analysis of three assays used to study hERG channel inhibition leading to Torsades des Pointes. There are a number of types of predictions that can be made. If the number of toxic events for any compound is quantified and compared to the relative number of clinically toxic events observed in humans, a 4×4 grid can be constructed by comparing truly positive, truly negative, false positive, and false negative events. From these, predictions of the sensitivity and specificity of toxicity and also the predictive value of the model can be made. The objective of determining sensitivity is hazard identification and elimination of toxicity with a goal to minimize the risk of progressing compounds with known safety pharmacology issues. The objective of specificity is risk assessment while the predictive value of the test relates to risk management and mitigation. This will, in turn, help us understand the inherent mechanisms of compound liabilities. As can be seen from the data shown, all three tests yielded fairly uniform values for all indices although slight differences can be seen (i.e., the optimally sensitive assay is QTc prolongation, while specificity and predictive value are best with the hERG assay [6]). There are categories of toxicity based on mechanism:

- *Undesired but expected effects*: These result from the primary pharmacology of the drug occurring by the therapeutic mechanism but in tissues other than the primary therapeutic organ. These usually cannot be avoided. Examples of this type of toxicity are digital tremor with β_2-adrenoceptor bronchodilators. Since β_2-adrenoceptors mediate bronchodilation and unwanted response (digital tremor), any such agonist will produce both effects. Restricted route of administration (aerosol) is used to minimize these side-effects.
- *Desired excessive effects*: These result from the primary pharmacology of the drug acting on the therapeutic organ. An example of this is insulin-induced hypoglycemic reaction. These also cannot be avoided and come with excessive dose.

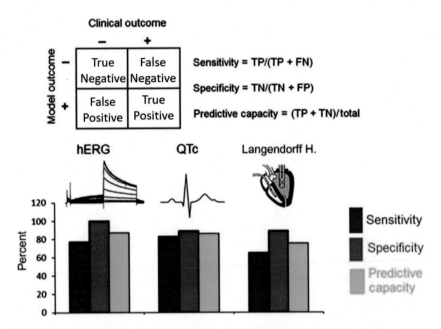

FIGURE 10.1   Predicting catastrophic toxic effects; *Torsades de Pointes*. Three assays, hERG channel inhibition, QTc prolongation in vivo, and Langendorff perfused hearts, predict dissociation of atrial-ventricular electrical communication and arrhythmia. Comparison of events in the model and events in patients lead to indices of sensitivity, specific and predictive capacity of the assays. These data indicate that all three assays are relatively uniform for the prediction of *Torsades de Pointes*. *Source: Data from J.-P. Valentin, R. Bialecki, L. Ewart, T. Hammond, D. Leishmann, S. Lindgren, et al., A framework to assess the translation of safety pharmacology data to humans, J. Pharmacol. Toxicol. Methods 60 (2009) 152–158.*

- *Undesired unexpected effects*: These occur by mechanisms different from the primary therapeutic mechanism of action of the drug. An example of this is the dry mouth coming from antimuscarinic effects of antihistamines, such as diphenhydramine.
- *Poorly predictable effects*: These are the most problematic in that they are difficult to detect. They consist of drug allergies, idiosyncratic effects, mutagenesis, carcinogenesis, and drug dependency.
- There are other classifications of toxicity used, such as the Type A to E listing of adverse drug reactions (see Box 10.2).

Safety pharmacology

There is a basic difference between safety assessment and determining primary drug efficacy. In the latter, researchers know what to look for; in safety assessment they do not. A hazard cannot be characterized until it is identified. Therefore, safety pharmacology involves the dual

---

BOX 10.2

A classification system for adverse reactions.

An adverse drug reaction (ADR) can be defined as any undesired, noxious, or unintended event occurring from a normal dosage (used for prophylaxis, diagnosis, or treatment) of the drug. The Federal Drug Administration regards any outcome leading to death, risk of death, hospitalization, disability, or required intervention to prevent permanent impairment or damage as adverse; these account for approximately 5% of all hospital admissions per year. Treatment failure, intentional, or accidental overdose are not considered ADRs. Below is one classification of ADRs based on drug mechanism of action.

Mechanistic Classifications of Adverse Drug Reactions

Classification	Characteristics	Example
Type A	• Result of Pharmacology of the Drug Target type	• High levels of anticoagulants lead to hemmorhage
Type B	• Idiosynchratic reaction and/or activation of secondary target	• fenfluramine activation of cardiac 5-HT_{2B} receptors
Type C	• chemically mediated , oxidative stress, phospholipidosis, haemolysis	• acetaminophen (paracetamol) hepatotoxicity
Type D	• delayed after chronic treatment / cancers	• fetal hydantoin syndrome with phenytoin
Type E	• end of treatment (withdrawal)	• seizures after sudden withdrawal of phenytoin

Source: Data from B.K. Park, M. Pirmohamed, N.R. Kitteringham, Idiosyncratic drug reactions: a mechanistic evaluation of risk, Br. J. Clin. Pharmacol. 34 (1992) 377–395 [7].

---

tasks of hazard identification and risk assessment. Hazard identification basically examines the profile of a drug and analyzes the potential harmful effects that can, and do, occur. Risk assessment then quantifies the probability that they will occur during clinical or accidental exposure. From this point other analyses are done to yield possible dose-response relationships for these effects. This involves issues, such as reversibility and determination of NOAEL (no observed adverse effect level; see Chapter 8, Pharmacokinetics II: Distribution and Multiple Dosing) and parameters for clinical monitoring. Other features of these analyses include examination of physical risk factors (age, gender, and susceptible patient populations), environmental risk factors (conditions present that may enhance toxicity/pharmacological

interactions), and genetic risk factors (genetic determinant for susceptibility to toxicity, known gene polymorphisms).

Safety assessment of drugs is an extremely important endeavor in
that if a hazard is not identified, patients may be harmed. Moreover, in
the drug development process, resources increase exponentially as candidate molecules reach the end of the development process; to reduce
the expenditure of large resources, candidates that will not be successful
due to toxicity must be identified as soon as possible (see Box 10.3).

As safety testing begins, a number of lines of investigation are initiated (see Table 10.1):

- *Safety pharmacology*: Detection of undesirable pharmacodynamic
  effects on specific organ systems. Some of these tests are simple

---

BOX 10.3

Costly discoveries.

A prospective drug has incurred nearly 90% of its cost of discovery
and development by the time it is in Phase III testing. Therefore, it is of
paramount importance that an unsuitable molecule be eliminated from
development before costs rise to this level. However, even more devastating is the discovery of serious toxicity after a drug has been
approved and is on the market. Below are four examples of drugs that
demonstrated rare but extremely serious toxicity after marketing, causing them to be withdrawn from the market.

Oculolucocutaneous Reactions — Practolol

Liver Damage — Troglitazone

Cardiovascular Damage — Vioxx

Torsades des Pointes — Terfenadine

TABLE 10.1 Safety pharmacology testing during different stages of drug development.

Development phase	Safety activity
Lead to candidate	• Acute toxicology • hERG • Ames test/cytotoxicity • Early safety prediction • 2° receptors
Candidate selection to first human dose	• Genotoxicity • Safety pharmacology dose ranging • 14–28 days toxicology studies
Patient phase 2a/2b studies	• 3/6/9/12 months toxicology studies • Reproductive toxicology studies • Immunotoxicology studies
Phase 3 clinical studies	• Carcinogenesis • Reproductive toxicology

in vitro experiments that can be done very early on in the development process, much like in vitro ADME studies (CaCo-2, hepatic enzymes; *vide infra*).

• *Genetic toxicity*: Examination of possible gene mutations and chromosomal damage.
• *Single/repeat dosing studies*: Detailed examination of target toxicity and local tolerance.
• *Reproductive toxicity*: Effects on embryo-fetal development, fertility, parturition, postnatal development.
• *Carcinogenicity*: Risk of development of tumors.
• *Special studies*: Immunotoxicology, phototoxicology, environmental health, and safety.

A major tool in these endeavors is the repeat dosing study. In this procedure, the goal is to develop an understanding the relationship between the exposure to drug and observed untoward effects, and also to assess the potential for reversibility. Responses can be directly observed or the study may seek to find biomarkers for effects. The overall aim is to assess organ toxicity and safety associated with repeat dosing to predict risk in humans; the object is to specifically define the no observed effect level (NOEL), maximal tolerated dose (MTD), and NOAEL. The first step in this process is to achieve high exposures of systems to the drug in vivo. For this, pharmacokinetic effects may need to be observed at doses extended far beyond what is required therapeutically, that is, dosing must continue (and exposure be increased) until adverse effects are detected [8]. Therefore, cases of limited exposure due to solubility (see Chapter 8, Pharmacokinetics II: Distribution and Multiple Dosing, for discussion of solubility limitation for exposure to the hepatoprotective agent YH439) can be problematic. In these cases, extended exposure protocols may be required, which may not be applicable to therapeutic dosing. Fig. 10.2 shows the effects of some solvents used for administration of experimental candidate molecules to optimize solubility and, ultimately, exposure.

An element of perspective should also be used in assessing the risk of high exposures. The sweetener saccharin has been used since the 1800s but was only subjected to rigorous safety testing in the 1970s. In these tests, it was linked to bladder cancer in rats and subsequently recalled from the market. It was later recognized that the doses at which this occurred would have required a human to ingest grams of saccharin every day from birth until 80 years of age. Moreover, the effect was *unique to rats* since there was a characteristic combination of high urine pH, level of calcium phosphate, and a special protein in rat urine causing microcrystallization of these doses of saccharin. These eventually caused damage to the lining of the bladder where, over time, active production of cells to repair the damage led to tumor formation. The salient points for the assessment

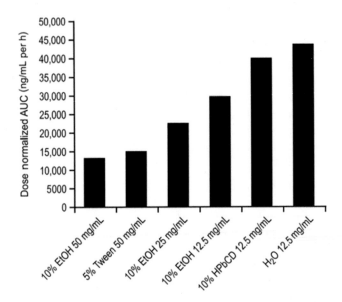

FIGURE 10.2 Effect of using various solvents for a new drug entity with limited solubility for intravenous administration to *Cynomolgus* monkeys. It can be seen that a 300% increase in exposure can be achieved through judicious use of solvent. A list of solvents used to increase drug exposure in vivo is shown in the right panel. *Source: Data from M.N. Cayen, Prediction of pharmacokinetics and drug safety in humans, in: P.L. Bullock (Ed.), Early Drug Development, John Wiley and Sons, New York, NY, 2010, pp. 89–129 [9].*

of the safety of saccharin; however, are that the doses were enormously high and the effect was specific to the rat.

Safety studies are done with a control group (vehicle only) and exposure to low doses (one- to fourfold multiples of efficacious dose), mid-doses (to determine dose-responsiveness), and high doses (to identify organ toxicity). Hopefully, these types of studies will give an understanding of the range between efficacy and toxicity, the maximum achievable dose, the kinetics of achieving those doses and an idea of the anticipated toxicity. Endpoints for such studies are body weight and food consumption, ophthalmological effects, electrocardiography, clinical observations, mortality, organ weights, and hepatic cytochrome P450 analyses. Also, macroscopic and microscopic examination of tissue is done; this can be extensive as thousands of tissue samples are analyzed (in addition to thousands of samples for clinical pathology, hematology, blood coagulation, clinical chemistry, and urinalysis). There are several schemes for conducting such repeat dosing experiments; two common ones are shown in Fig. 10.3.

As safety testing progresses, there is increasing rigor with respect to how data is collected, how much data is collected, and how it is analyzed. Fig. 10.4 shows a progression to good laboratory practice (GLP) studies where particular attention is paid to accurate documentation of effects, calibration, and maintenance of instruments used in the studies (with attention to application of internal and external audit of procedures), and validation of relevant technology with the aim of reporting data in a regulated environment. Some studies conducted at this stage are given in Table 10.2.

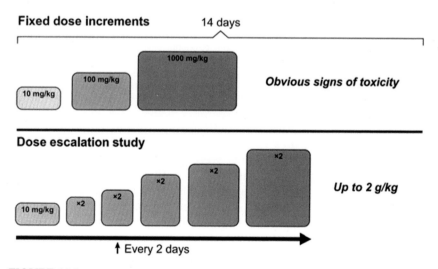

FIGURE 10.3   Dosing schemes for conducting repeat dose safety studies.

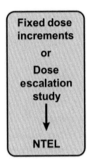

Non-GLP

Fixed dose increments

or

Dose escalation study

↓

NTEL

Detailed single dose tox study in 2 species

From expected therapeutic dose to well above NTEL

Multiple dose-ranging study

Drug given daily or twice daily for 2 weeks

GLP

Long-term studies of variable makeup depending on regulatory body and predicted drug usage

FIGURE 10.4   Repeat dose testing for observance of no observed effect level (NOEL), no observed adverse effect level (NOAEL) (also referred to as NTEL for no toxic effect levels). Once this has been done and progress is indicated, then good laboratory practice (GLP) studies can be initiated.

TABLE 10.2   Types of toxicity tested for in GLP and non-GLP studies.

Exploratory (non-GLP) studies

• In vitro screens • In silico screens • Cytotoxicity • Immunotoxicity	• Hepatotoxicity • Embryotoxicity • Single and repeat dose range finding studies in two species

Regulatory (GLP) studies

• Safety pharmacology • Genotoxicity • 28-day repeat dose toxicity and recovery in two species • 3–12 months' chronic toxicity in two species	• 24 months carcinogenicity in two species • Reproductive toxicity in one species covering: • Fertility implantation • Fetal development • Pre/postnatal effects

Overall, traditional pharmacology predicts only 10%–70% of all human adverse effects. In a study of 150 drugs, when only rodents were used, 40% of human toxic events were observed, in contrast to 60% when a nonrodent species was used; when both a rodent and nonrodent species were included, the maximal detection of toxic effects were observed (up to 70%) [10]. In spite of best efforts to detect adverse effects, if late-stage toxicity is observed that has been missed in early safety testing, the question arises "why did this occur?" and "how can we be assured that it will not occur with the next candidate?" The basis of the answers to these questions lies in some of the basic assumptions made in safety testing. First, it is assumed that animal toxicity will translate to human toxicity and this encompasses assumptions about similar metabolites being formed and similar pharmacokinetics and sensitivity of organs to hazards. One prevalent problem is that animals are bred for health while drugs are usually targeted toward unhealthy individuals. This has led to proposals that more safety testing should be done in animal models of disease (i.e., rat models of type II diabetes, heterozygous p53 knockout mice for chemically induced carcinogenicity, lipopolysaccharide (LPS)-induced inflammation (vide infra), and heterozygous superoxide dismutase-knockout mice to unveil mitochondrial toxicity). Another problem is that animals are bred for homogeneity to yield consistent experimental results, while the human population is much more diverse (60% of human genes may be alternatively spliced). In addition to the previously discussed case of bladder cancer with saccharin occurring only in rats, many other differences between animals and humans have been noted, such as increased liver weight to ketotifen only in dogs but not humans and renal necrosis to efavirenz in rats but not humans. For these reasons there are proposals to utilize human tissue to a greater extent in safety testing in an effort to obviate differences due to species. Thus, human blood vessel endothelial cells [11], hepatocytes [12], and human kidney proximal cells [13] have been used in safety studies for drug testing.

Another important difference is the relative exposure to populations of varying sizes. Specifically, even in the most rigorous safety testing studies, the number of animals exposed to a drug is very much smaller than the number of humans that will be exposed to the drug as it becomes widely available to the greater human population (perhaps 1000−2000 animals exposed as opposed to 1,000,000 humans). Also, the dosage regimen given to animals in safety studies is tightly controlled whereas in the human population, dosages may sometimes be capricious (missed dosage, multiple dosages at one time, etc.). For example, Fig. 10.5 shows the increasing exposures of a drug to different populations as it progresses through development. For a drug such as Vioxx, which had a toxic event of one in every 113,927 patients, no clinical trial could have been devised to detect such an event (an incidence of 0.0009%). Clearly, the number of subjects required for any given clinical trial to detect an adverse event depends upon the rarity of the event and also the baseline random occurrence for the event, that is, to assess the risk for a given drug to produce cardiac arrhythmia, the natural rate of occurrence of cardiac arrhythmia must be considered.

Fig. 10.6 shows predictions for the number of subjects required in clinical trials to statistically detect a drug-related adverse event. As shown in the figure, for an adverse event with baseline occurrence of 4/1000, it would require approximately 2500 patients to detect the adverse event

Toxicity through stochastic opportunity

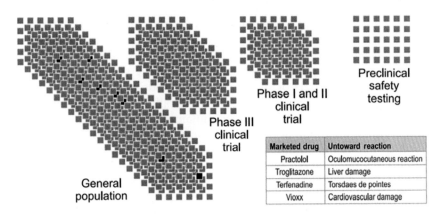

FIGURE 10.5 Schematic diagram of increasing population exposure to a drug as it moves from discovery to development, and eventually to the marketplace in the general population. Shown in the box are four drugs found to produce serious toxic effects only when released to the greater population (see also Box 10.3).

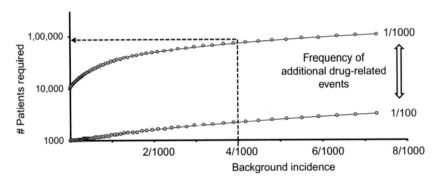

FIGURE 10.6 Relationship between number of patients required in a clinical study to detect adverse events with a frequency of 1/1000 (gray-filled circles) and 1/100 (open circles). The abscissae represent the natural frequency of the same adverse event occurring without drug. Source: Redrawn from H.-G. Eichler, F. Pignatti, B. Flamion, H. Leufkens, A. Breckenridge, Balancing early market access to new drugs with the need for benefit/risk data: a mounting dilemma, Nat. Rev. Drug Discov. 7 (2008) 818–8.27 [14].

caused by the drug if the drug produced a fairly common rate of occurrence (1/100). If the drug-related event were rare (1/1000), this would require nearly 100,000 patients to be detected. Thus, the common adverse event could have been detected in phase 3 clinical trials but the rare event only once the drug was approved and released to the general population.

This also raises the question of the type of toxic effect involved, specifically if it depends on concentration (where exceeding a therapeutic window will always lead to toxicity) versus toxicity due to stochastic opportunity. This latter classification of toxic effect (known as idiosyncratic) depends more on when a combination of rare conditions is encountered. It can be dependent on population, in that some populations may never show the effect. For these types of drugs, various probabilities must be considered including the probability of exposure to the drug, environmental risk factors, and host risk factors (i.e., genetic predisposition to effect). These topics will be discussed further with mutagenicity and cancer, and idiosyncratic liver toxicity.

Early safety tests

Just as with pharmacokinetics, there are avenues of exploration to assess safety that can be initiated very early on in the discovery and development process. For example, in silico analysis of chemical structure can give guidance to chemists in terms of the identification of known substructures (toxicophores) that are present in known toxic compounds; these can be avoided in the optimization of primary and ADME activity. Such so called "non-testing" methods have advantages in the design of libraries and medicinal chemistry efforts in lead optimization including [15]:

- higher throughput
- less expense
- less time consuming
- constant optimization possible
- higher reproducibility, if the same model is used
- low compound synthesis requirements
- potential to reduce the use of animals

There are limitations in this approach including:

- unknown quality of training set experimental data
- transparency of the program (what is being modeled?)
- descriptors sometimes confusing
- applicability domain sometimes not clear
- ADME features, especially metabolism, not taken into account
- carcinogenicity prediction does not work on nongenotoxic compound

Fig. 10.7 shows a number of common toxicophores present in known mutagenic compounds.

In addition to in silico studies, there are some simple and inexpensive in vitro tests that can be done to assess possible harmful activity in molecules. These are:

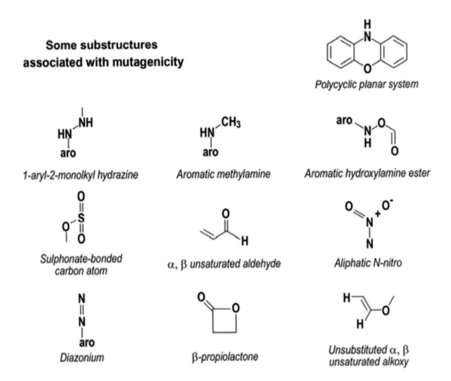

Some substructures associated with mutagenicity

Polycyclic planar system

1-aryl-2-monolkyl hydrazine   *Aromatic methylamine*   *Aromatic hydroxylamine ester*

Sulphonate-bonded carbon atom   *α, β unsaturated aldehyde*   *Aliphatic N-nitro*

Diazonium   *β-propiolactone*   *Unsubstituted α, β unsaturated alkoxy*

FIGURE 10.7 Some known toxicophores identified as being common to mutagenic compounds. *Source: Data from J. Kazius, R. McGuire, R. Bursi, Derivation and validation of toxicophores for mutagenicity prediction, J. Med. Chem. 48 (2005) 312–320 [16].*

Interaction with receptors mediating autonomic function

There are hundreds of extracellular receptors present on cell membranes that control the autonomic nervous system (sympathetic and parasympathetic control of cardiovascular, endocrine, gastrointestinal, and central nervous system functions). Inappropriate activation of some of these by a drug intended for some other use can be detrimental; therefore, candidate molecules must be screened for any autonomic receptor activity. For example, activation of α-adrenoceptors (vasoconstriction leading to hypertension), β-adrenoceptors (tachycardia), and antagonism of these (hypotension, cardiac failure) can lead to immediate and serious effects. While these effects are important, they are not difficult to detect in assays aimed at in vitro receptor function (and subsequent in vivo cardiovascular and behavioral studies). A list of common autonomic receptors that are routinely tested is given in Table 10.3.

Despite measurement of the effects of compounds on autonomic receptors, the assessment of the relative "safety" with respect to

TABLE 10.3 Some common autonomic receptors for unwanted side effects.

General toxicity	GI tract toxicity	Cardiovascular toxicity
5-HT_{2A}	5-HT_{1A}	5-HT_4
5-HT_{2B}	5-HT_{1P}	α_{1A}-Adrenoceptor
α_{1A}-Adrenoceptor	5-HT_{2A}	α_{1B}-Adrenoceptor
α_{1B}-Adrenoceptor	5-HT_{2B}	α_{2A}-Adrenoceptor
α_{2A}-Adrenoceptor	5-HT_3	α_{2B}-Adrenoceptor
Adenosine 2A	5-HT_4	α_{2C}-Adrenoceptor
Adenosine A1	α_{2A}-Adrenoceptor	Adenosine 2A
β_1-Adrenoceptor	α_{2B}-Adrenoceptor	Adenosine A1
β_2-Adrenoceptor	α_{2C}-Adrenoceptor	Adenosine A3
Bradykinin B2	CCK2	Angiotensin AT1
Cannabinoid CB1	Dopamine D2	β_1-Adrenoceptor
Dopamine D2	δ-Opioid	β_2-Adrenoceptor
Histamine H1	EP2	Bradykinin B1
μ-Opioid	EP3	Bradykinin B2
Muscarinic m1	Gastrin	Cannabinoid CB1
Purinergic P2Y1	Histamine H2	CGRP
	μ-Opioid	Dopamine D2
	Motilin	Endothelin A
	Muscarinic m2	Endothelin B
	Muscarinic m3	Histamine H3
	SST1	Muscarinic m1
	VIP	Muscarinic m2
		Muscarinic m3
		Muscarinic m4
		Nicotinic Ach
		NPY_1
		Thromboxane A2
		Vasopressin V_{1a}
		Vasopressin V_{1b}

unwanted activity can be subjective and target-dependent. For example, the anti-Parkinson disease drug pergolide is 36-fold less potent on 5-HT_{2B} receptors than therapeutic dopamine D2 receptors. In addition, the AUC for pergolide ED_{50} for Parkinsonism treatment is less than six times the ED_{50} for 5-HT_{2B} receptor activation. Notwithstanding this 216-fold safety margin, devastating 5-HT_{2B} receptor-mediated valvular heart effects were observed with pergolide causing withdrawal from the market—see Box 10.4.

BOX 10.4

The best laid plans can go Awry.

Apparently, safe guidelines for molecules can still mask untoward difficulties after drug approval. The drug pergolide for treatment of Parkinson's disease has an apparently adequate margin of selectivity for dopamine D2 receptors (the therapeutic receptor) over 5-HT_{2B} receptors (mediating devastating cardiac valvular disease effects). The figure shows the in vitro selectivity of pergolide for dopamine D2 over 5-HT_{2B} receptors (36-fold). In addition, it was known that the C_{max} value for pergolide therapeutic effects for 3 × daily dosing was considerably below the AUC required for 5-HT_{2B} activity. Specifically, the C_{max} value was only 20% of the concentration required for 5-HT_{2B} activation. In spite of these apparently favorable circumstances, pergolide was found to produce debilitating cardiac valvular disease effects in patients, requiring its removal from the market.

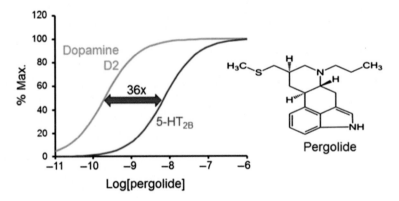

Source: *Data from P.Y. Muller, M.N. Milton, The determination and interpretation of the therapeutic index in drug development. Nat. Rev. Drug Discov. 11 (2012) 751–762 [17].*

Blockade of hERG potassium channels

This is an extremely serious effect whereby the ST segment in the human electrocardiogram is prolonged to the point where the critical communication between pacemaker cells in the atrium and the ventricle fails. This leads to a catastrophic cardiac event called *Torsades de Pointe*, which can cause syncope and sudden death. The biological target mediating this event is the human ether-à-go-go related gene coding for the $K_V11.1$ potassium channel in the heart. This protein controls a repolarizing potassium current in the myocardium essential for the conduction of electrical current across the membrane to facilitate synchronous heartbeat. So important is this potential hazard, a number of approved drugs have been taken off the market when hERG activity was discovered (Fig. 10.8). There are simple binding or in vitro electrophysiological assays available to detect hERG activity, which can be done early on in the development process. Definitive identification of QT prolongation is routinely explored through examination of EKG in vivo. There are documented cases where medicinal chemists have retained primary activity but eliminated this serious side-effect through structural changes in molecules.

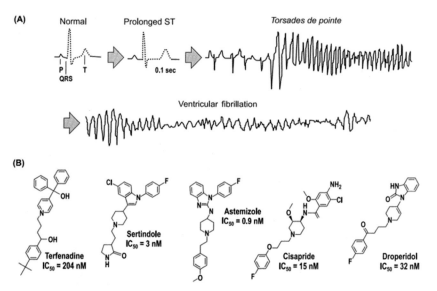

FIGURE 10.8 (A) Blockade of the hERG potassium channel in the heart leads to QT segment prolongation in the electrocardiogram and subsequent arrhythmia and ventricular fibrillation (*Torsades de pointe*). (B) Five drugs with nanomolar potency for this effect that have been withdrawn from the market.

Cytotoxicity

This refers to any effect that eventually could lead to cell death (cyto from the Greek *kytos* meaning hollow and toxic from the Greek *toxikon* meaning arrow poison). Cells are extremely complex bodies with a temporally diverse lifetime (i.e., different processes are important to life at different times); therefore, defining drug effects that will interfere with these processes can be speculative if no clear lethal effect is seen. A commonly used simple assay is the MTT cell proliferation assay (see Fig. 10.9). The basis for this assay is the fact that mitochondrial function is essential to cell health; addition of the substrate for mitochondrial reductase MTT (3-(4,5-dimethylthiazol-2-yl)-2,5-diphenyltetrazolium bromide), which is colored yellow, leads to the formation of formazan in healthy mitochondria (colored purple). This furnishes a simple colorimetric assay for cell health where comparison of the color of cell cultures (one control and one drug treated) leads to estimates of the number of living cells.

It should be noted that drugs that affect metabolic function can give conflicting signals in the MTT test. A test that can differentiate selective mitochondrial toxicity from other cytotoxicities is the circumvention of the "Crabtree Effect"—see Box 10.5. There are numerous other ways to show cellular toxicity, from cessation of growth to losing membrane integrity (and subsequent production of necrosis). Membrane integrity can be measured with trypan blue or propidium iodide substances that are normally excluded from healthy cells. Cells can also activate a genetic program of cell death (apoptosis), which produces distinctive markers. In general, cell nuclear morphology, mitochondrial function,

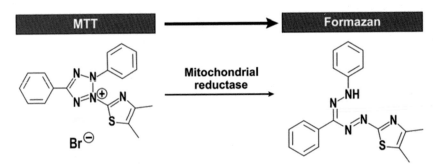

FIGURE 10.9 MTT cell proliferation assay for cytotoxicity. Mitochondrial function is assessed through the level of activity of mitochondrial reductase converting the yellow substrate MTT (3-(4,5-dimethylthiazol-2-yl)-2,5-diphenyltetrazolium bromide) to the purple product formazan. Colorimetric comparison of control cells and cells exposed to a test compound in varying concentrations can yield a dose-response curve for remaining living cells in culture.

BOX 10.5

Predicting mitochondrial toxicity with the Crabtree effect.

The Crabtree effect (named after the English biochemist Herbert Grace Crabtree) occurs in metabolically adapted cell lines that are grown in hypoxic/anaerobic conditions with high glucose. These cells have a reduced need for oxidative phosphorylation by the TCA cycle and depend on glycolysis as their major source of energy instead of mitochondria; therefore, these cells also have a reduced susceptibility to mitochondrial toxicants. The addition of galactose circumvents the Crabtree effect and increases the reliance of cells on mitochondrial oxidative phosphorylation; these cells are more sensitive to mitochondrial toxicity. Therefore, the testing of possibly toxic compounds on cells grown in hypoxic/anaerobic conditions versus those under high-galactose tone unveils selective mitochondrial toxicity. The antidepressant imipramine produces cytotoxicity but probably not through effects on mitochondria since cells primarily relying on mitochondria for energy are not more sensitive. In contrast, the insecticide rotenone produces selective toxicity in cells requiring mitochondria for energy (presence of galactose) indicating mitochondrial toxicity.

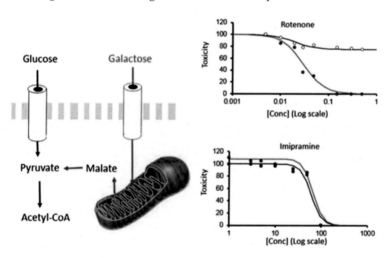

Source: Data from L.D. Marroquin, J. Hynes, J.A. Dykens, J.D. Jamieson, Y. Will, Circumventing the Crabtree effect: replacing media glucose with galactose increases susceptibility of HepG2 cells to mitochondrial toxicants. Toxicol. Sci. 97 (2007) 539−547 [18].

plasma membrane integrity, and speed of proliferation can all be used to measure cell health, and all of these effects can be readily obtained from in vitro assays in cell culture.

Mutagenicity

The ability of a drug to induce mutations in a cell can be indicative of possible carcinogenic activity. A simple and rapid test for drug mutagenicity is the Ames test. Developed by Bruce Ames and his group at the University of California, Berkeley, this tests the ability of a molecule to produce changes in the DNA of a modified *Salmonella typhimurium* (a bacteria modified to maximize the probability of mutation). Specifically, unlike native bacteria, the Ames bacterium is engineered such that it cannot synthesize histidine (and therefore requires it in the medium to live and grow). If no mutation occurs, the culture containing the Ames bacteria will die. However, if mutation occurs, it often confers the capability to synthesize histidine (and thus live in histidine-free media) upon the organism. Therefore, if cells grow in histidine-free media, it is likely that a mutation has occurred (see Fig. 10.10).

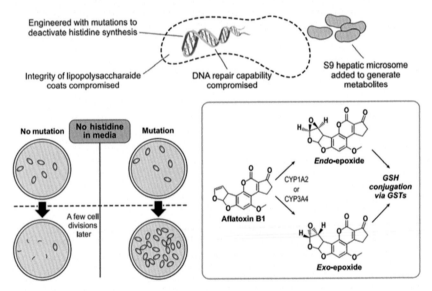

FIGURE 10.10 The Ames test. Engineered *Salmonella typhimurium* (which cannot grow in histidine-free medium unless a mutation has occurred) is cultured in histidine-free medium. If compound is added and the culture grows, it is likely that a mutation has been induced by the compound. Inset shows an example of a mutagenic product formed from aflatoxin by the hepatic enzyme CYP3A4.

The bacterium and media are altered in other ways to maximize the probability of mutation. Specifically, the LPS coat of the bacterium is compromised to allow maximal entry of compounds and the DNA repair capability of the bacterium is reduced. In addition, S9 hepatic enzyme fraction (see Chapter 7, Pharmacokinetics I: Permeation and Metabolism) is added to the medium to maximize the probability of formation of metabolites that would be seen in vivo with the compound. This is a rapid and extremely useful test but as with all tests of stochastic probability it is not always predictive (see Box 10.6).

BOX 10.6

The problem of predicting mutagenicity.

Dioxin (common name for 2,3,7,8-tetrachlorodibenzo-*p*-dioxin) is an extremely toxic substance that, when ingested, can lead to enzyme induction, immunotoxicity, reproductive and endocrine effects, developmental toxicity, chloracne, and tumor promotion. In spite of its clearly documented mutagenic activity, dioxin is not positive in the Ames test [19]. Nitroglycerin (commonly used for the treatment of angina), on the other hand, is mutagenic in the Ames test. These data highlight the stochastic nature of mutagenicity and the difficulty of predicting it.

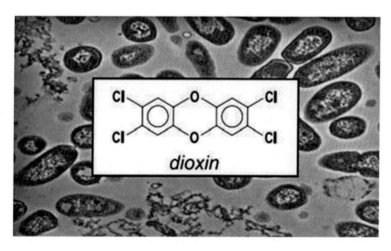

Hepatic toxicity

As discussed in Chapter 7, Pharmacokinetics I: Permeation and Metabolism and Chapter 8, Pharmacokinetics II: Distribution and Multiple Dosing, the liver is the primary organ of detoxification for the body. Moreover, the liver receives the highest initial dose of all drugs given orally due to the first-pass effect. Therefore, it perhaps should not be surprising that drug-induced liver injury (DILI) is the most frequent cause of withdrawal of approved drugs; this organ is on the front line for the detection of toxic effects. DILI is one of the primary causes of idiosyncratic adverse drug reactions. This effect results from formation of reactive metabolites (electrophilic molecules species, which can bind covalently proteins and DNA). Fig. 10.11 shows how blockade of the bile salt export pump (BSEP) exacerbates formation of reactive species in hepatic cells to cause cell stress, which, in turn, activates the immune system. Chemical trapping agents, such as reduced glutathione (GSH),

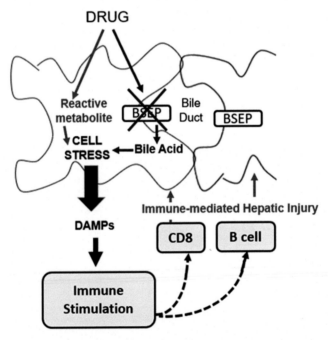

FIGURE 10.11 One exacerbation of hepatic cell stress is the inhibition of the BSEP (bile salt export pump). This leads to elevated bile salts resulting release of DAMP's (endogenous danger molecules) that are released from damaged cells to activate the immune system, i.e., T or B cells. *Source: Redrawn from J.G. Kenna, J. Uetrecht, Do in vitro assays predict drug candidate idiosyncratic drug-Induced liver injury risk? Drug Metab. Dispos. 46 (2018) 1658–1669.*

form stable adducts with reactive species and are used to identify reactive metabolites through high resolution accurate mass spectrometry.

There are two general types of DILI: intrinsic hepatotoxicity (occurs in all individuals in a dose-dependent, and thus predictable, manner) and idiosyncratic hepatotoxicity (results from a succession of unlikely events). This latter type of hepatotoxicity is much more difficult to detect since it depends on the frequency of reaction in animal studies invariably involving small numbers. In addition, interspecies variation and genetic variability play a significant role in these effects (there are 1.4 million single nucleotide polymorphisms in the human genome and 78 polymorphisms of the hepatic enzyme CYP2D6 alone). Some features of intrinsic and idiosyncratic hepatotoxicity are compared in Table 10.4.

It is difficult to deal with idiosyncratic hepatotoxicity; for example, the drug for arthritis diclofenac produces serious hepatotoxicity in 6 of every 100,000 patients (8–20% of those develop diclofenac jaundice and die of liver failure). Such an extremely low incidence (0.006%) makes it difficult to detect and difficult to predict in new drug testing. Thus, only one half of new drugs that produce hepatotoxicity in clinical stages of development show *any* animal toxicity. One hypothesis put forward to explain some of the capriciousness surrounding idiosyncratic hepatotoxicity is that, in these cases, the threshold for observing intrinsic hepatotoxicity is greater than the lethal dose (thus it is never routinely observed). However, genetic, environmental, stress (i.e., arthritis, viral hepatitis, bacterial infection, periodontal disease, asthma), and other factors may shift the threshold for this intrinsic hepatotoxicity to much lower levels periodically and when this occurs idiosyncratic hepatotoxicity appears (see Fig. 10.12).

One experimental approach to predict this is to chemically stress the liver to mimic these threshold lowering effects; this can be done with nontoxic doses of gram-negative bacterial source LPS [20]. This procedure has been shown to sensitize the liver to the toxic effects of carbon tetrachloride, monocrotaline, cocaine, aflatoxin B1, diclofenac, and sulindac. In addition, there are a number of physiologically based biochemical assays that can be used to assess liver function (and liver damage). For example, phospholipidosis (excessive accumulation of intracellular phospholipids in liver) can result

TABLE 10.4 Comparison of intrinsic and idiosyncratic hepatotoxicity.

Intrinsic	Idiosyncratic
• Affects all individuals at some dose • Clearly dose-related • Predictable latent period after exposure • Predictable with routine animal testing	• Attacks only susceptible individuals • Unclear relation to dose • Variable onset relative to exposure • Not predictable with routine animal testing • Variable liver pathology

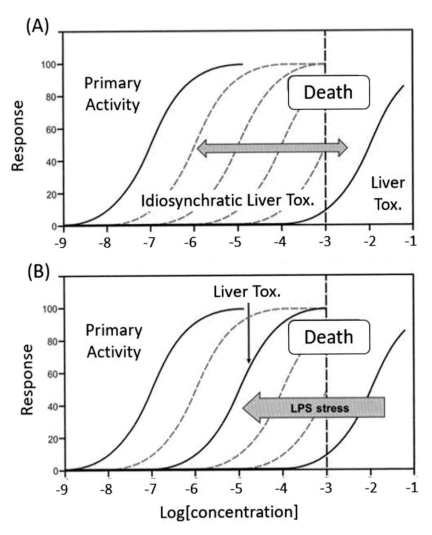

FIGURE 10.12 Idiosyncratic hepatotoxicity. (A) Extremely rare hepatotoxic events may be so because, for a given compound, the intrinsic hepatotoxicity threshold in a normal liver may lie above the lethal dose (and thus, may never be seen). However, conditions of stress may move this threshold to much lower levels to unveil hepatotoxicity which may then appear randomly. (B) Experimental procedures such as LPS stress (see text) may reduce the threshold for liver toxicity and thus, uncover what would be seen as rare idiosyncratic hepatotoxicity in a larger population. Source: *Drawn from R.A. Roth, P.E. Ganey, Intrinsic versus idiosyncratic drug-induced hepatotoxicity: two villains or one? J. Pharmacol. Exp. Ther. 332 (2010) 692–697.*

from inhibition of the enzymatic activity of phospholipases and binding of drugs to phospholipid (complexes not broken down by phospholipases). Some drugs that cause this are antibacterials, antipsychotics, antidepressants, antianginals, antimalarials, antiarrhythmics, and cholesterol-lowering agents. Another mechanism that can lead to phospholipidosis for cationic amphiphilic drugs (CAD) is the trapping of drugs in the lysosome. Intrahepatic cholestasis (impairment of bile formation leading to jaundice) is another biochemical hepatotoxic reaction seen with cyclosporin A, rifamycin, rifampicin, glyburide, and troglitazone. Finally, steatosis is another toxic biochemical hepatic reaction resulting from drug interferences with hepatic lipid processing, subsequent accumulation of triglycerides and inflammation; steatotic accumulation of fatty acids has led to the recall of marketed drugs.

Summary

- The main aim of safety pharmacology is to define the optimal way in which potentially valuable drugs can be utilized without causing harm.
- An important difference between testing for primary activity and ADME properties and safety is that, in the former, what to look for is defined; in safety testing, it is not known what should be looked for. Under these circumstances, a great many tests must be undertaken to develop confidence that harmful effects will not be seen.
- There are generally two types of toxicity: intrinsic toxicity, which is related to drug exposure (if enough drug is administered, the effect will appear) and stochastic opportunity (idiosyncratic). This latter event is rare and difficult to predict.
- Even with exhaustive testing, once a drug enters the greater population, very rare negative events (the probability of which may be infinitesimal in drug development testing) may be found.
- There are a number of chemical groups known for conferring toxicity on drugs ("toxicophores") and molecules containing these are avoided in drug libraries
- There are some common simple in vitro tests to quickly detect chemical scaffolds that interact with autonomic receptors, block the hERG channel, are cytotoxic, and may be mutagenic. These can be carried out early in the development process.
- Hepatotoxicity is a very common toxic drug effect due to the fact that high concentrations of drugs reach the liver. Moreover, the liver is designed to chemically interact with drugs. Sensitization of liver assays to toxic effects may assist in the detection of rare idiosyncratic hepatotoxicity.
- Biochemical tests associated with hepatic metabolism can be used to detect early signs of hepatotoxicity (i.e., steatosis, phospholipidosis).

References

[1] R. Eri, J.R. Jonsson, N. Pandeya, D.M. Purdie, A.D. Clouston, N. Martin, CCR5-delta32 mutation is strongly associated with primary sclerosing cholangitis, Genes Immun. 5 (2004) 444–450.

[2] W.G. Glass, D.H. McDermott, J.K. Lim, S. Lekhong, S.F. Yu, J. Pape, CCR5 deficiency increases risk of symptomatic Nile virus infection, J. Exp. Med. 203 (2006) 35–40.

[3] C. Moench, A. Uhrig, A.W. Lohse, G. Otto, CC chemokine receptor 5delta32 polymorphism-a risk factor for ischemic-type biliary lesions following orthotopic liver transplantation, Liver Transpl. 10 (2004) 434–439.

[4] E. De Silva, M.P. Stumpf, HIV and CCR5-Δ32 resistance allele, FEMS Microbiol. Lett. 241 (2004) 1–12.

[5] M.B. Rabinowitz, G.W. Wetherill, J.D. Kopple, Kinetic analysis of lead metabolism in healthy humans, J. Clin. Invest. 58 (1976) 260–270.

[6] J.-P. Valentin, R. Bialecki, L. Ewart, T. Hammond, D. Leishmann, S. Lindgren, A framework to assess the translation of safety pharmacology data to humans, J. Pharmacol. Toxicol. Methods. 60 (2009) 152–158.

[7] B.K. Park, M. Pirmohamed, N.R. Kitteringham, Idiosyncratic drug reactions: a mechanistic evaluation of risk, Br. J. Clin. Pharmacol. 34 (1992) 377–395.

[8] P. Greaves, A. Williams, M. Eve, First dose of potential new medicines to humans: how animals help, Nat. Rev. Drug. Discov. 3 (2003) 226–236.

[9] M.N. Cayen, P.L. Bullock, Prediction of pharmacokinetics and drug safety in humans, in: P.L. Bullock (Ed.), Early Drug Development, John Wiley and Sons, New York, NY, 2010, pp. 89–129.

[10] R. Dixit, U.A. Boelsteri, Healthy animals and models of human diseases in safety assessment of human pharmaceuticals, including therapeutic antibodies, Drug Discov. Today. 12 (2007) 236–342.

[11] C. Schleger, S.J. Platz, U. Deschl, Development of an in vitro model for vascular injury with human endothelial cells, Altex. 21 (Suppl. 3) (2004) 12–19.

[12] J.T. MacGregor, J.M. Collins, Y. Sugiyama, C.A. Tyson, J. Dean, L. Smith, In vitro human tissue models in risk assessment: report of a consensus-building workshop, Toxicol. Sci. 59 (2001) 17–36.

[13] W. Li, D.F. Choy, M.S. Lam, T. Morgan, M.E. Sullivan, J.M. Post, Use of cultured cells of kidney origin to assess specific cytotoxic effects of nephrotoxins, Toxicol. In Vitro. 17 (2003) 107–113.

[14] H.-G. Eichler, F. Pignatti, B. Flamion, H. Leufkens, A. Breckenridge, Balancing early market access to new drugs with the need for benefit/risk data: a mounting dilemma, Nat. Rev. Drug Discov. 7 (2008) 818–8.27.

[15] H. Raunio, In silico toxicology: non-testing methods, Front. Pharmacol. 2 (33) (2011) 1–8.

[16] J. Kazius, R. McGuire, R. Bursi, Derivation and validation of toxicophores for mutagenicity prediction, J. Med. Chem. 48 (2005) 312–320.

[17] P.Y. Muller, M.N. Milton, The determination and interpretation of the therapeutic index in drug development, Nat. Rev. Drug Discov. 11 (2012) 751–762.

[18] L.D. Marroquin, J. Hynes, J.A. Dykens, J.D. Jamieson, Y. Will, Circumventing the Crabtree effect: replacing media glucose with galactose increases susceptibility of HepG2 cells to mitochondrial toxicants, Toxicol. Sci. 97 (2007) 539–547.

[19] L.E. Geiger, R.A. Neal, Mutagenicity testing of 2,3,7,8-tetrachlorodibenzo-p-dioxin in histidine auxotrophs of Salmonella typhimurium, Toxicol. Appl. Pharmacol. 59 (1981) 125–129.

[20] R.A. Roth, P.E. Ganey, Intrinsic versus idiosyncratic drug-induced hepatotoxicity: two villains or one? J. Pharmacol. Exp. Ther. 332 (2010) 692–697.

11

The science of finding drug molecules I: applying pharmacology to discovery/target identification and validation

Pharmacology in Drug Discovery and Development
DOI: https://doi.org/10.1016/B978-0-443-14124-9.00001-X

Introduction

Pharmacology is the study of drugs and drug action; it has relevance to therapeutics (i.e., pharmacology as taught in a medical school to prospective medical practitioners) and also to the continued quest for new drugs. The previous chapters of this book are dedicated to this latter pursuit and this chapter specifically delineates where pharmacological principles impact the practical process of new drug discovery and development. By the end of this chapter, the reader will understand the logical progression of a drug discovery and development process and the various elements involved (i.e., target- vs system-based strategies, target validation, screening, lead optimization, and the incorporation of drug-like activity).

New terminology

- *Constitutive screening*: These employ receptor systems that are spontaneously active (usually through receptor overexpression). Binding of molecules to these constitutively active receptors produces a change in the constitutive activity which is used to identify the binding process.
- *DNA-encoded libraries*: In these collections of molecules for screening, the chemicals are linked to strands of DNA, which are then used to identify the molecule from mixtures.
- *"First in Class"* drugs: Projects aimed at these target diseases for which there is no current treatment.
- *Fragment-based screening*: Small chemical groups are screened to determine binding to a target site. When these are identified, they are chemically synthesized into a larger molecule that becomes the candidate scaffold.
- *"Me Too"* drugs: These emanate from programs aimed at improving existing drugs to eliminate their shortcomings.
- *Systems-based discovery*: These programs aim to identify unique phenotypic pharmacologic behaviors in human primary cell systems that can lead to new modalities for treatment.
- *Target-based discovery*: These programs are specifically aimed at finding molecules for a defined biological target thought to be associated with the disease.
- *Virtual screening*: This employs electronic docking of virtual molecules (encoded electronic structures) to identify structures that optimally bind to targets.

Unique aspects of pharmacology in the discovery process

There are important elements of pharmacology involved in therapeutics. While there are thousands of drugs available in the practitioner's armamentarium, they can be organized effectively with four basic ideas for the clinician:

- Mechanism of action
- Dosage
- Pharmacokinetic properties
- Safety issues

Once the mechanism of action of a given drug is known, it becomes a member of family and learnings from each of the members can assist in the understanding of the use of that drug. The therapeutic application of the drug naturally emerges from knowledge of the mechanism and the dosage becomes a factor that can be obtained from specific product information (and thus does not require prior knowledge for drug use). Due to the independence of structure-activity relationships governing primary activity, safety, and PK (see Fig. 7.5), the pharmacokinetics of any given agent can be unique and thus must be associated with the specific information for a given drug. Similarly, safety issues can be unique as well and these must be associated separately with each drug.

The issues are different when pharmacology is applied to new drug discovery and development. The major feature of pharmacology as a discipline in drug discovery is the ability to accommodate the differences in organ behavior between various drugs, that is, one drug can have different behaviors in different organs under different physiological or pathological conditions. This apparently capricious behavior stems from the complex interplay of drug affinity and efficacy and the intrinsic sensitivity of different organs to drug stimulation. For example, Fig. 11.1 shows dose-response curves to the a-adrenoceptor agonists norepinephrine and oxymetazoline in two different tissues. The anococcygeus muscle is very sensitive to a-adrenoceptor stimulation and the high affinity but low efficacy agonist oxymetazoline is threefold more potent than norepinephrine. In contrast, in the less sensitive vasa deferentia, the low efficacy of oxymetazoline causes it to be a less active agonist than the high efficacy of epinephrine. These types of differences will occur in vivo, but they can be predicted by pharmacologic techniques. Thus, pharmacology can convert descriptive data (what the experimenter sees in a given experimental assay) through universal scales to predictive data with the capability of determining the activity of the drug in a variety of physiological circumstances.

The heart of a new drug discovery program is the biologist-chemist interface. Biology deals with the status of systems that can vary from day

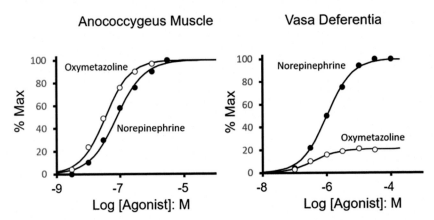

FIGURE 11.1   Responses to two a-adrenoceptor agonists, oxymetazoline (high affinity, low efficacy), and norepinephrine (low affinity, high efficacy) in two tissues. The anococcygeus muscle is very sensitive and vasa deferentia are of lower sensitivity. Note the reversal of relative agonism of the agonists just from differences in tissue sensitivity. Source: Redrawn from T.P. Kenakin, The relative contribution of affinity and efficacy to agonist activity: organ selectivity of noradrenaline and oxymetazoline with reference to the classification of drug receptor, Br. J. Pharmac. 81 (1984) 131–141.

to day (i.e., viability of the live experimental preparations, etc.), thus even descriptive data for drugs and drug activity, such as EC_{50} values for agonists, can be variable. In contrast, chemistry is a physical science with more immutable indices of activity and these vary much less. A problem can arise when chemists, who require immutable parameters to plan future syntheses, receive variable subjective biological data. Given this, it is incumbent upon biologists to describe pharmacological and physiological activity in chemical terms with invariant indices; pharmacology can provide these in the form of chemical affinity and efficacy.

There are basically four lines of predictive data that can essentially characterize a new drug molecule and enable the prediction of therapeutic activity. These are:

- Affinity
  - This will define the lower limit of the concentration of the ligand required to interact with the biological target.
- Efficacies
  - The efficacy of the ligand is in large part dependent upon the nature of the assay used to measure the activity (see Chapter 2, Drug Affinity and Efficacy). Therefore, a given drug can have many efficacies and these should be measured to determine the efficacy "fingerprint" of the ligand to assist in defining the therapeutic phenotype response it produces.

- Orthosteric versus allosteric interaction
  - It is important to know if the new ligand binds to the natural endogenous ligand-binding site (orthosteric interaction) or to a separate binding site on the target that is different from the endogenous ligand-binding site (allosteric site). This latter type of interaction opens many more options with respect to the activity of the natural system with new ligand binding than does an orthosteric interaction.
- Kinetics of target coverage
  - The rate of offset of the ligand from the target is critical to the amount of time the drug will associate with the target in vivo where concentration is never constant. Thus, the target coverage can be quite different from drug potency.

The previous chapters of this book are dedicated to the assays and techniques required to obtain these data. The following chapter will discuss the context in which these pharmacological data are utilized in the drug discovery process.

Clearly, it is important to try to design new drugs that will have predicted therapeutic activity. From that standpoint, pharmacological assays should be designed to yield data to determine what a given new drug will do under a variety of physiological circumstances. However, there are a number of unknown variables when a drug is administered in vivo (i.e., various organs may have different receptor levels and efficiencies of receptor coupling) so a useful minimal strategy is to use pharmacological assays to reveal what a given new drug can do (and perhaps will do if the conditions are appropriate). For example, determining that a given antagonist does not have negative efficacy will determine that, even under conditions of constitutive receptor activity, the ligand will not produce inverse agonism. It should be possible to determine the basic properties of a new ligand to show the possible behaviors it may and may not manifest in vivo.

Most drug discovery projects begin with a central remit whereby the objective is defined. For example, a disease in a therapeutic area is identified along with a proposed physiological outcome from drug treatment (pharmacological efficacy) and a type of molecule proposed to have that effect, that is, asthma, β_2-adrenoceptors on human bronchiole smooth muscle, and agonist. In addition, some details about the drug therapy might be identified such as "once per day oral dosage." As of 2008, it has been reported that 50% of all new drug failures are due to lack of efficacy [1]. In this case, "efficacy" is a term relating to effectiveness in treating the target disease, not necessarily drug efficacy as defined pharmacologically in Chapter 2, Drug Affinity and Efficacy.

This inordinately high failure rate suggests that a better definition of "efficacy" for target compounds is warranted. Historically, a biological target was identified (i.e., particular receptor, enzyme, ion channel, etc.) along with a behavior change for that target; as stated above a ligand to produce agonism at the human β_2-adrenoceptor for the treatment of asthma might be supposed to be a useful treatment for the disease. With increased definition of pharmacological agonism through multiple agonist assays (see Chapter 2, Drug Affinity and Efficacy), a better definition of what aspect of the biological target activity needs to be exemplified for therapy now can be obtained. Thus, the process of "target validation" has given way to "pathway validation" to better define target efficacy. As noted in Chapter 2, Drug Affinity and Efficacy, instead of simple agonism at the parathyroid receptor to treat osteoporosis new evidence suggests that selective parathyroid-receptor mediated β-arrestin-2 activation may be the key to effective treatment in osteoporosis. Another aspect of the discovery strategy involves the general approach to the disease state. Specifically, a solely "target-based" approach has been seen to be part of the reason for the 50% failure rate of new drugs; a counter-idea to this is to consider a "systems-based" approach to disease. With this approach, complex collections of physiological processes in the form of cells or whole organs may be used to yield the primary activity data for new potential drug molecules.

The projected success of a given project can also relate to the therapeutic area. For instance, central nervous system (CNS) diseases are uniquely difficult. The human brain controls all bodily functions either conscious or unconscious, and breakdown of brain function can lead to a wide variety of diseases from depression, anxiety, epilepsy, mania, degenerative disorders, pain, obsessive disorders, and schizophrenia to name a few. The current drugs available for CNS disorders form a diverse list; muscarinic receptor agonists/antagonists, serotonin uptake inhibitors, dopamine agonists, serotonin partial agonists, benzodiazepines, barbiturates, opioids, tricyclics, neuroleptics, and hydantoins. The brain is very complex and not well understood and many of these agents were discovered through empirical observation and not through logical hypothesis-based programs. In addition, there can be a distinct lack of animal models to predict human CNS behavior, lack of validated biomarkers, propensity for CNS-active drugs to produce side effects, and the presence of a substantial pharmacokinetic barrier for access (the blood brain barrier). Accordingly, while other therapeutic areas have a 15% success rate for new drug therapy, the rate for CNS drugs is less than half that value (7%). Moreover, the time to market for therapeutic areas range from 6 to 7.5 years (cardiovascular 6.3 years, gastrointestinal 7.5 years), the time for CNS drugs is 12.6 years. In addition, for optimal CNS drug therapy, often polypharmacological activity is required, that is, drugs must interact with multiple targets in the brain. For instance, the atypical antipsychotic clozapine boasts activity at histamine H4 receptors, dopamine D2, and dopamine D4 receptors, $5-HT_{2A}$, $5-HT_{2C}$, and $5-HT_6$ receptors while a major metabolite (desmethylclozapine) is an allosteric modulator at muscarinic receptors. It makes the definition of candidate molecules much more complex, if polypharmacological activity is required.

Discovery programs may vary in terms of their objectives as well. For instance, a program aimed at obtaining a molecule that improves an already existing drug or at least aims to provide a molecule for an established disease state must answer four basic questions:

- Is the molecule active at the primary target?
- Is the molecule promiscuous? (selectivity)
- Is the molecule toxic?
- Is the molecule absorbed, distributed appropriately through the body and have an adequate $t_{1/2}$?

If, on the other hand, the program breaks new ground and is aimed at a "first in class" molecule or is in a totally new therapeutic area, then there are additional questions, which may be relevant to the program:

- How is the molecule different from all other molecules and available therapy?
- How does this effort utilize the newest knowledge of disease state and pharmacology in this therapeutic area?

Under these circumstances, the program will require more assays and more complex structure activity efforts to identify candidates.

Target- versus system-based discovery strategies

A target-based approach to new drug discovery is based on the premise that the single target mediates the important aspect of the pathophysiology and the best approach to treating the disease is through very selective action at the particular target. Historically, many excellent and important drugs have resulted from target-based programs. Classic examples of success are β-blockers, such as propranolol (selective β-adrenoceptor blockade), histamine H_2 receptor blockers for antiulcer therapy (selective histamine H_2 receptor blockade), albuterol for asthma (selective $β_2$-adrenoceptor agonism), and sumatriptan for migraine (selective $5-HT_{1B}$ and $5-HT_{1D}$ receptor agonism). This latter drug is especially impressive as a selective agent because of the huge number of 5-HT receptor subtypes (15) and the vast number of physiological processes that 5-HT receptors control (i.e., central nervous system effects involved in anger, aggression, body temperature, mood, sleep, sexuality, appetite, metabolism, vomiting, GI-tract function, and vascular contraction of basilar and cranial arteries). On the other hand, many disease states are complex combinations of conditions leading to the notion that disease can be considered a systems problem. For example, many pathophysiological processes occur in asthma, which can lead to a hyper-responsive airway and subsequent bronchospasm. Historically, the initiators of response were not the target of drug therapy but rather the final response of these processes, namely bronchospasm, was reversed with bronchodilators. Specifically, powerful β_2-adrenoceptor agonists such as albuterol were given as acute treatment to reverse bronchospasm. While effective, this amounts to a system override and not a cure for the underlying disease (see Fig. 11.2).

Depending on the nature of the system, it may not be optimal to confine drug treatment to a single component of the system. For instance, in cases where a particular tumor leads to the overexpression of a particular kinase enzyme, it may be supposed that this particular kinase is essential to the survival of the tumor. Accordingly, selective blockade of the kinase might be a route to selectively damaging the tumor over healthy tissue. However, there are cases where the physiological tumor system may have alternative routes around targets making selective target-based therapy ineffective. Systems can be thought of as collections of nodes connecting signaling pathways. Not all such nodes are equal with some being considered "redundant" nodes (elimination of this type of node does not destroy the system as it has alternative routes around the node) and "fragile" nodes, which are critical to the survival of the system. Elimination of the fragile nodes can lead to optimal destruction of the system. The target-based approach to drug therapy presupposes the identity of the nodes in a system and targets those for

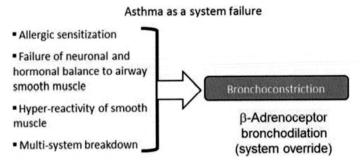

FIGURE 11.2 The pathological factors in asthma that lead to bronchoconstriction are reversed by β_2-adrenoceptor agonists in the form of a system override of the asthma disease system.

destruction. If the identification is incorrect (i.e., if the particular kinase in the tumor is a redundant node), then drug therapy will fail. Therefore, another alternative to drug discovery is to begin with the complete system and test new drugs on those and not a preidentified target; this is referred to as systems-based discovery.

Progression scheme for drug discovery

Whether the strategy for discovery is target-based or system-based, the chronological progression of the workflow is very similar. As shown in Fig. 11.3, the first steps involve the identification of the components of the program (i.e., therapeutic area, biological target, and/or signaling pathway, target pharmacological activity, such as agonism, antagonism, etc.). The next major components of discovery programs are the chemicals available for biological testing and the pharmacological assays available to search for activity.

There are various teams of scientists involved in the discovery process and these may vary with the stage of the program. The initial discovery team involved in the first phases of a program concentrates on

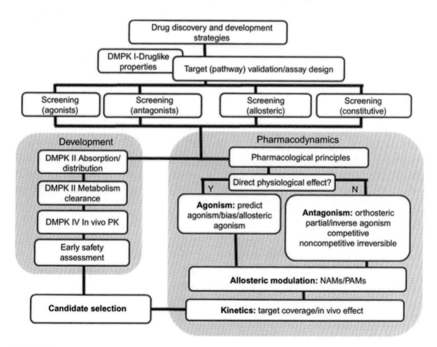

FIGURE 11.3 A logical progression path for new drug discovery encompassing pharmacodynamics, pharmacokinetics, and early measures of drug safety.

developing the assays needed for screening and lead optimization, collecting the data needed for target/pathway validation, developing the critical path for the program, and defining the criteria for success. The main aim of this team is to take the program through the screening process; the endpoint is the acquisition of hit molecules for progression. In addition, informatics becomes involved to create the tools needed to collect data from all assays and compile them to a form that can be easily accessed by biologists and chemists. The next phase involves synthetic chemistry. Once the array of hit molecules is assessed for chemical tractability, certain scaffolds are chosen for modification through synthetic chemistry. This stage may involve a large chemistry effort. In addition, ADME studies to assess drug-like activity are brought into the progressions scheme along with some very early safety studies. The aim of this phase of the program is to identify a drug candidate molecule for progression to human studies. An expanded discovery and development team is involved with assessment of safety and pharmacokinetics data as well as preparation of the Investigational New Drug (IND) report to government agencies such as the Food and Drug Administration (FDA) to seek permission to test the drug in humans. Once this is approved, this team also will be involved in assessing human clinical data and also the filing of patents and synthesis of molecules to secure intellectual property and furnish possible back-up compounds.

It can be seen from Fig. 11.3 that in the initial discovery phase (screening), the drug-like properties of the molecule are considered; as pointed out in Chapter 7, Pharmacokinetics I: Permeation and Metabolism (see Fig. 7.5), three separate threads of structure-activity relationship must be satisfied for a drug to emerge: (1) activity at the primary target; (2) pharmacokinetic profile; and (3) safety. Therefore, repeated iterations of the discovery process may be required; this was made evident in the development of the first anti-ulcer histamine H_2 receptor antagonists—see Box 11.1. After a therapeutic area, biological and chemical target have been identified, the two major components of a discovery program become relevant, namely the compound libraries to be tested and the nature of the pharmacological assay systems that will be used to test them.

Libraries and molecules as drug sources

There are numerous sources of molecules for potential drug testing. As noted in Chapter 9, In Vivo Pharmacology, molecules may be identified through the side-effects of already known drugs—see Box 9.3. Another rich source of potential drugs are natural products, that is, molecules found in nature that can either be improved through synthetic chemistry (i.e., see Fig. 11.4) or form the basis of synthetic analogs

BOX 11.1

Persistence pays off.

The first effective treatment of peptic ulcer was blockade of histamine H_2 receptors with selective H_2 receptor antagonists. The proof-of-concept molecule is burimamide which competitively blocks H_2 receptors but is not adequately absorbed in vivo. Medicinal chemists at Smith, Kline, and French continued and arrived at metiamide which competitively blocks histamine H_2 receptors and is absorbed in vivo. However, toxicological issues precluded this molecule from continuing further. Persistence was rewarded when chemists synthesized cimetidine, which has appropriate receptor blocking properties, is absorbed in vivo and has a good safety profile.

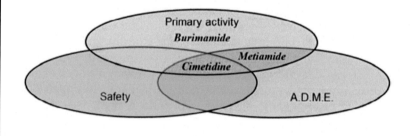

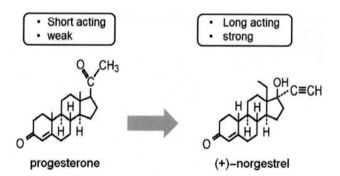

FIGURE 11.4 Improving Nature. While the natural steroid hormone progesterone has many beneficial physiological actions, it is short-acting and relatively weak. In contrast, chemical modification of the natural molecule to (+)-norgestrel yields a strongly efficacious molecule with a long duration of action.

for new drugs. One of the most famous of these is the antimalarial compound quinine from South American tree bark—see Box 11.2. Synthetic modification of a natural product is also seen in penicillin.

Fig. 11.5 shows the natural product drug found in nature (benzylpenicillin from mold) that formed the scaffold for an orally active congener penicillin, namely phenoxypenicillin. Bacteria from soil can produce unique chemicals and some of these can be pharmacologically active—see Box 11.3.

The world of natural products is vast in that only extracts from 5% to 15% of 25,000 species of higher plants, <1% of bacterial, and <5% of fungal sources have been studied for possible therapeutic activity. In addition, the World Health Organization estimates 80% of the world population relies on traditional medicine (natural products). In general, 25% of US prescriptions through the years 1959—80 contain plant extracts or active principles (119 chemical species from 90 plant species) and, of the 67% of 877 new synthetic chemical entities, 16.4% are from pharmacophores derived directly from natural products. On the other hand, natural products can be expensive, structurally complex (not tractable), of unpredictable novelty and intellectual property value, and be high in "stereo complexity," that is, contain fewer nitrogen, halogen, and sulfur atoms and more oxygen rich with many hydrogen donors (consequence of enzymatic biosynthesis) making them less than ideal starting points for new drugs.

Probably the most fertile source of new drug molecules are synthetic libraries of compounds that can be screened in high-throughput test systems. Historically, these have been made up of random samples of chemical space with little regard for drug-like activity. Experience with these has shown that hits can emerge with nondrug-like scaffolds that are difficult to convert to drugs and/or are not tractable. Given this, more recent drug discovery efforts employ molecules in libraries that are specifically designed from drug-like chemical scaffolds. For example, virtual rules for library compounds have been defined that can be used to prescreen new members of screening libraries—see Box 11.2. Virtual in silico methods can be used to filter new drug candidate libraries. For example, Box 11.4 shows how application of the Lipinski rules of five, Veber rules, and other virtual filters can be applied to libraries to remove nondrug-like molecules, in this case molecules that will not permeate cells (Boxe 11.5).

In terms of the identity of library members, it has been estimated that chemical space is enormous (number of molecular weight molecules $< 600 \approx 10^{62}$) and that, given this, to randomly find a hit molecule with nanomolar activity would require screening 21 million compounds. It is known that hits are found with much smaller libraries suggesting that there are pockets of "drug-like" molecular structures where the

BOX 11.2

Drugs from natural products.

There are many drugs derived from natural plant, fungal, marine, and bacterial sources. One of the most famous is quinine from the bark of *Cinchona officinais* used by the Quechua peoples of Bolivia, Peru, and Ecuador to treat shivering due to malaria. The fame of the treatment came after a bout of malaria contracted by the Countess of Chincon was successfully treated by her bathing in the bitter water (due to the presence of quinine) beneath the tree. In honor of the curative effects on the countess, the tree was named cinchona. The Jesuit Brother Bernabe Cobo (1582–1657) brought the bark of the "fever tree" to Europe where it entered apothecaries and became a famed medicine. So important did this medicine become, Peru and surrounding countries outlawed the export of cinchona seeds and saplings in the 19th century to maintain a monopoly. From quinine came the present-day treatments for malaria—chloroquine and mefloquine.

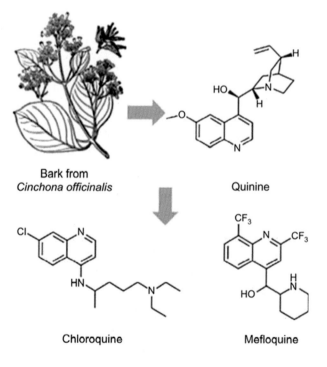

Bark from
Cinchona officinalis

Quinine

Chloroquine

Mefloquine

Natural product   Synthetic

Benzylpenicillin   Phenoxypenicillin
(discovered 1928 in mold)   (orally active synthetic)

FIGURE 11.5   Penicillin was discovered by Alexander Fleming in 1928. Upon a return from a holiday, Fleming noted that Petri dishes containing Staphylococcus bacteria had mold growing and that around the mold no bacteria thrived. This led to the characterization of what he referred to as "mold juice" as penicillin. Chemical modification of the penicillin originally discovered (benzylpenicillin) to phenoxypenicillin converts the antibiotic to an orally active drug.

probability of finding drugs is greater. Support for this notion also comes from the identification of so-called "privileged" structures that re-occur in drug chemical space repeatedly—see Fig. 11.6. These ideas also lead to the notion that once a structure has been identified then the class may be explored further to find "follower" drugs. This idea is based on the fact that no drug has all of the features required and that existing drugs can always be improved. Thus, further structural exploration within a known drug structural motif may lead to an improved drug—see Box 11.6. In addition, approved drugs can be studied in humans without causing harm and this may lead to other activities of the drug for other diseases; this is referred to as drug re-purposing.

Pharmacological assay design

The other major component of a discovery program is the detection system in place to sift through the compound libraries. Historically, binding screens have been used because they are robust and amenable to robotic assays that can handle a large number of compounds in a short time; technology at that time did not allow the same to be done with functional assays. However, the pharmacological functional effects of compounds are the relevant property for drug activity and there are many advantages to functional screening over screening with binding. For instance, many allosteric compounds would not have been detected with binding and only seen with function—see the example with the HIV-1 entry inhibitor aplaviroc (Box 11.7). In general, binding assays

BOX 11.3

Special soil: antibiotics from the Earth around us.

Soil can contain complex natural products not found anywhere but in certain locations. For example *Rapamycin*, an immune suppressant for transplant patients and treatment of certain cancers, inhibits kinase mTORC1 to decrease cell proliferation. It is isolated and active from the soil bacteria *Streptomyces hygroscopicus* found only in the soil of Easter Island. The molecule is named for the source Rapa Nui (Easter Island). Similarly, the anticancer drug *doxorubicin*, which intercalates into DNA causing DNA damage and death of the cancer cells, is isolated from the bacteria *Streptomyces peucetius* found only in the soil around Castle del Monte in Apulia, Italy.

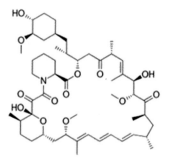

Rapamycin

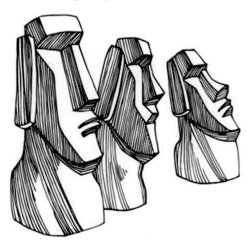

BOX 11.4

"Quality In" yields "Quality Out."

Considering the instances where the drug is only a few synthetic steps away from the original hit in screening, there may be little opportunity to introduce "drug-like" activity into the molecule. Experience with generic legacy libraries where drug-like activity was not considered has resulted in the conscious stocking of screening libraries with molecules that already have drug-like character. To this end, virtual criteria in the form of rules roughly based on current virtual criteria, such as the "rule of five" to guide the inclusion of new compounds in libraries have been defined. One such set of rules are shown [2] with an example of the minimal difference between the screening hit responsible for the drug Zofenopril.

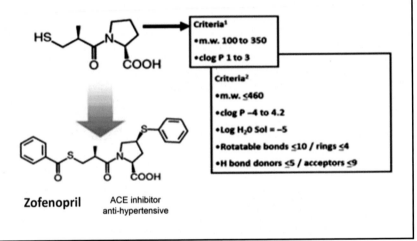

Criteria[1]
• m.w. 100 to 350
• clog P 1 to 3

Criteria[2]
• m.w. ≤460
• clog P −4 to 4.2
• Log H_2O Sol = −5
• Rotatable bonds ≤10 / rings ≤4
• H bond donors ≤5 / acceptors ≤9

Zofenopril   ACE inhibitor
anti-hypertensive

measure different protein species than do functional assays (see Box 11.8) and can be misleading due to the fact that the functional receptor species producing pharmacological response are the ones relevant to therapy.

The most direct means to determine the physiological effect of a potential drug is to test it in a functional assay. These can be natural cellular systems, isolated organ systems, in vivo animal systems, or recombinant cellular systems. The last category has been criticized for the fact that recombinant systems can yield abnormal and unphysiological

BOX 11.5

Virtual screening for drug-like properties.

Many aspects of drug-like properties can be quantified through physico-chemical indices and these, in turn, can be calculated in silico. Criteria such as the "Lipinski Rule of Five" can be used to filter libraries and remove molecules with predicted poor drug-like properties that serve only to waste valuable drug development resources—see Chapter 7, Pharmacokinetics I: Permeation and Metabolism. The figure shows the application of the Rule of five and three other virtual criteria of drug-like properties to the permeation of molecules through lipid bilayers. It can be seen that the application of the in-silico screening techniques to remove nondrug-like molecules greatly enhanced the library in terms of permeation. Specifically, while testing the entire library for permeation yielded the expected normal distribution of permeation criteria (blue bars), removal of molecules from the library that did not meet virtual drug-like property enriched the remainder to a library with extremely favorable permeation properties (red bars) [3]. Such virtual screening of libraries could be used to conserve development resources in the drug discovery and development process.

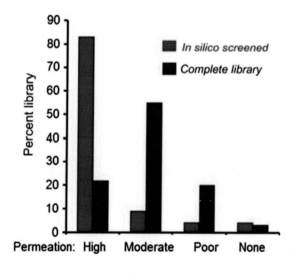

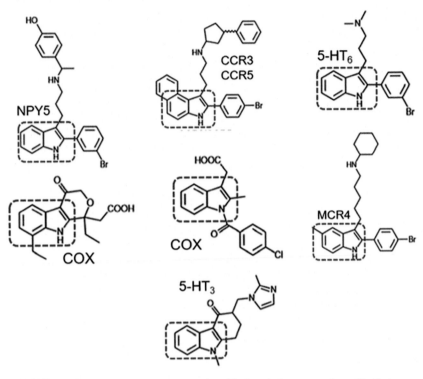

FIGURE 11.6 There are certain "privileged" chemical structural motifs thatappear repeatedly in drugs for a variety of targets. Shown are drugs for seven different targets all containing the indole group.

effects due to aberrations in the stoichiometries of the components. However, this is true only if it is assumed that the effects seen in the in vitro assay will necessarily be seen in the therapeutic in vivo system. From the point of view of having the assay reveal what the molecule can do (not necessarily what it will do), recombinant systems are still valuable to delineate the properties of new drug candidates.

The two variables in recombinant systems are the host cell type and the level of receptor expression. The first variable also includes the cointeracting species with the target which may be associated with a particular cell type or may be cotransfected to produce a desired combination of reactants. The level of receptor expression in a cell leads to functional assays of varying capability (Fig. 11.7). Low levels of receptor expression lead to assays where agonists show partial agonism and this, in turn, allows the separate characterization of changes in agonist affinity (location parameter of the concentration−response curves) and efficacy (maxima of concentration-response curves) for lead optimization—see Fig. 2.10. These data are best to assess the linkage of chemical structure

BOX 11.6

If you do not succeed the first time; follower drugs.

First-in-class drugs are rarely if ever complete in having the ideal therapeutic activity, pharmacokinetic properties and safety profile. Therefore, such first in class drugs can serve as a template for "follower" molecules that retain primary activity but also may have improved properties. Seventy-five first in class drugs screened between 1999 and 2008 spawned 157 follower drugs with improved profiles.

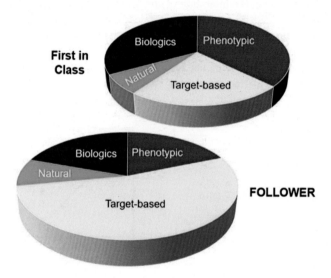

Source: *From D.C. Swinney, J. Anthony, How were new medicines discovered? Nat. Rev. Drug Disc. 10 (2011) 506—519.*

with molecular activity. Higher levels of receptor expression led to more sensitive assays where agonists produce full agonism. While this provides less specific information regards the structure-activity relationship of agonism (changes in potency cannot be identified as due to affinity or efficacy, only a complex function of both properties), the added sensitivity is better for low efficacy agonist detection, that is, screening. Finally, even higher levels of receptor expression can yield constitutively active receptor systems due to the fact that enough receptor exists in the spontaneously active state to cause an elevated basal response due to receptor activity. These types of assays allow the

---

BOX 11.7

Functional versus binding screens.

As noted in Chapter 5, Allosteric Drug Effects, allosteric protein effects can be probe dependent. While this is a caution for known allosteric mechanisms, it can also be an issue with screening unknown chemical targets as well. For example, the target for HIV-1 entry in AIDs therapy is the chemokine CCR5 receptor. Screening with the AIDS virus is not practical therefore discovery programs instituted a surrogate screen incorporating the inhibition of chemokine binding and/or chemokine function. CCR5 has multiple natural ligands including the chemokines CCL3 and CCL5. The allosteric HIV-1 entry inhibitor aplaviroc blocks HIV-1 entry and also the pharmacological effects of CCL3 and CCL5 in functional experiments. However, while aplaviroc blocks $[^{125}I]$-CCL3 binding, it has no effect on $[^{125}I]$-CCL5 binding. Therefore, if an initial HIV-1 entry inhibitor screen had employed $[^{125}I]$-CCL5 binding instead of $[^{125}I]$-CCL3, aplaviroc would never have been found [4].

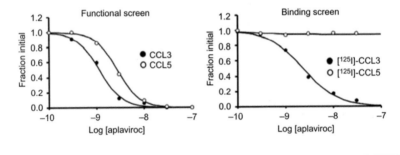

detection and quantification of inverse agonist activity, which may yield information about possible antagonist tolerance or unique signaling. For agonists, the type of functional assay also involves the choice of efficacy to be observed, that is, a cyclic AMP assay will reveal a Gs protein effect but not a β-arrestin effect. The impact of choosing various functional readouts of response is discussed in Chapter 2, Drug Affinity and Efficacy, with regards to the appropriate choices of functional responses for therapy. In terms of screening, although it is optimal to choose a functional assay that gives a therapeutically relevant response, it may not be essential. This is because most drug targets are protein in nature

BOX 11.8

Binding and function are different.

The notion that binding assays and functional assays measure the same drug behavior is false. (Panel A) shows the different receptor species measured in binding assays (top—protein species associated with the agonist and/or antagonist species) while the bottom panels show the activated receptor species measured in functional assays. Another notion is that binding assays are simpler than functional assays and this too may not be the case. (Panel B) shows the receptor species operative in an allosteric system [5]. It can be seen that there are many parameters of interaction that are not independently verifiable; this leads to the use of more simple partial models in practical binding experiments as approximations of the complex complete systems.

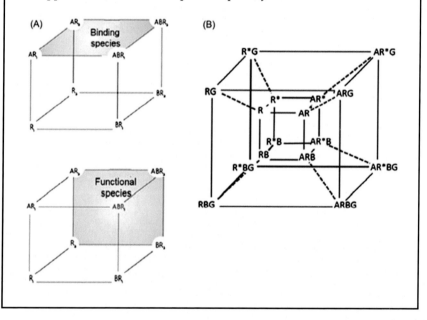

and binding to proteins is not a passive process, that is, if a molecule binds to a protein there is a high probability it will change the energy and conformation of the protein and that this will be detected by most assays that monitor the drug target. On the other hand, there are extremely biased ligands that predominantly produce a selected signal and it would be possible that such compounds would not be detected, if the incorrect screening assay were chosen.

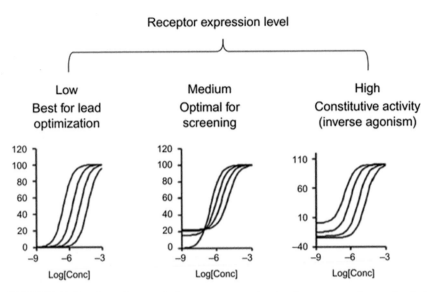

FIGURE 11.7 Through control of receptor expression levels, assays can be constructed to optimally measure agonist affinity and efficacy (low receptor expression), provide a sensitive screening assay for detection of low levels of agonism (medium receptor expression) or measurement of negative efficacy as inverse agonism (constitutively active system with very high receptor expression).

Identification and validation of drug targets

The next step in the discovery process is the identification of biological drug targets. The conventional method of doing this is through the identification of some unique failure in natural physiology that can be compensated for by activating or blocking a physiological target. For example, it was known that the activation of the histamine H_2 receptor by the autocoid histamine caused the release of acid in the stomach and that this prevented ulcers from healing. Professor Sir James Black instituted a discovery program at Smith, Kline, and French to have medicinal chemists modify the natural autocoid histamine to reduce efficacy and increase affinity of histamine; these efforts led to the identification of the histamine H_2 receptor antagonists that bind to the receptor to prevent activation by histamine and subsequent acid release. The inhibition of acid release allows ulcers to heal. A variant of this approach is the detection and exploitation of special functions of physiological components. For instance, the immune system contains several types of cells whose function it is to detect and destroy diseased cells. Augmentation of these "killer" cells is a viable target in many diseases, such as cancer—see Box 11.9.

BOX 11.9

Unlocking nature's gateway to the immune system with antibodies.

T cells of the immune system (often called natural killer cells) are designed to recognize antibodies on the surface of foreign cells and destroy them. A natural fail safe in the immune system is the checkpoint system whereby bodies on the surface of the host cells that are not a threat and the T cell (PD-1 and PD-L1) recognize each other and the lethal cascade is halted. However, if cancer cells adopt this checkpoint system, they can cloak themselves as normal healthy cells and escape the vigilance of T cells. A strategy to allow the immune system to recognize cancer cells for the threat they are is to prevent the interaction of the checkpoint proteins from canceling the immune response. Thus, antibodies that bind to PD-L1 sites to prevent them from binding to the checkpoint PD-1 site on the T cell prevent the cancellation of the immune response and lead to the elimination of the cancer cell.

Checkpoint Prevents T Cell Destruction of Cancer Cell

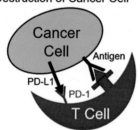

Ab-Blockade of Checkpoint Allows T Cell to Destroy Cancer Cell

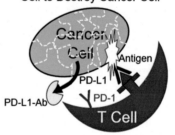

Another mechanism that can be used is the application of receptor mutation to identify a unique target-based pathophysiology. For example, the identification of the D32 CCR5 mutation of the CCR5 chemokine receptor (causing prohibition of receptor expression on the cell surface) and the linking of that effect to a unique resistance to AIDs led to the identification of the target mediating HIV-1 viral entry into cells—see Box 11.10.

Another approach to finding new drug targets is through "reverse pharmacology." Specifically, it is known that biological targets such as receptors can spontaneously form active states that can then couple to signaling proteins and produce detectable signals. Usually, the setpoint for this type of activity is very low such that very little spontaneous

BOX 11.10

Nature's mistake identifies a key cause of AIDS.

HIV-1 infects cells to produce the lethal disease AIDS (Acquired Immuno Deficiency Syndrome). For several years, the target for HIV-1 infection of cells was not known but research finally unveiled the target to be CCR5 (C-C chemokine receptor type 5). A key factor in absolutely confirming the essential role of CCR5 in HIV-1 infection was the discovery that certain individuals possess a gene that produces only a mutant version of the receptor called D32 CCR5. This mutation produces a receptor devoid of a 32 amino acid segment that prevents the transport of the receptor to the cell surface. Thus, the absence of CCR5 on the cell surface prevents HIV-1 binding.

CCR5   Δ32 CCR5

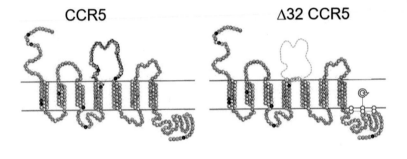

physiologic activity is observed. However, if the expression of biological target is elevated, then a significant level of spontaneous active state receptor will be produced in the system and an elevated basal response will be observed. Under these circumstances, an unstable system results whereby an elevated level of spontaneously activated receptor target is present in the system and any binding of molecules to alter this state will result in a demonstrable change in the basal receptor response. As discussed in the chapters on the mechanisms of efficacy, binding of a molecule to a biological target will necessarily change the interaction of that target with signaling proteins. Therefore, if a ligand binds to the orphan receptor, then the basal activity produced by that orphan receptor may be increased or decreased, depending on the outcome of the receptor conformation stabilized by the binding reaction. What this means (identification of a molecule binding to the orphan receptor) in practical terms is that a tool is created that can then be used to assess the relevance of the orphan receptor—see Box 11.11. In this sense, orphan screening can be thought of as a way to identify new drug

BOX 11.11

Receptors stand up to be counted: constitutive orphan screening.

Orphan receptors have no known ligand that can be used as a probe for screening but binding to receptors in a constitutively active receptor system can demonstrate either positive or inverse agonism. The figure below shows the effects of peptides binding to the calcitonin receptor in constitutively active systems of varying levels of receptor expression. It can be seen that ligands binding to this receptor alter the basal activity.

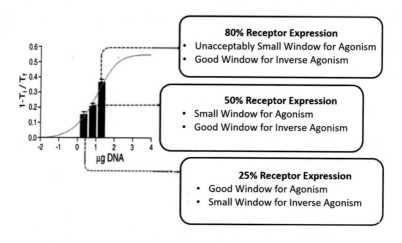

80% Receptor Expression
- Unacceptably Small Window for Agonism
- Good Window for Inverse Agonism

50% Receptor Expression
- Small Window for Agonism
- Good Window for Inverse Agonism

25% Receptor Expression
- Good Window for Agonism
- Small Window for Inverse Agonism

Source: Data from G. Chen, C. Jayawickreme, J. Way, S. Armour, K. Queen, C. Watson, D. Ingar, W.-J. Chen, T. Kenakin, Constitutive receptor systems for drug discovery, J. Pharmacol. Toxicol. Meth. 42 (1999) 199–206.

targets. If the molecule found for the orphan receptor produces a favorable physiological response, then it might qualify as a good new drug target.

There are other obvious indications for biologic targets. For example, a deficit or surfeit of a natural biological target can be corrected by changing the availability of the natural substrate. Thus, therapeutic effect could be achieved by replacement of a protein that is deficient or abnormal, the addition of one to augment an existing pathway, and addition of one to introduce a novel function. Protein replacement and correction historically has been developed for the treatment of hemophilia. Thus, an absence of coagulation factor VIII (FVIII) leads to Hemophilia A and a lack of coagulation factor XI (FIX) leads to Hemophilia B. Current proteins for hemophilia include AL prolix (recombinant factor IX Fc-fusion for hemophilia), Beloctate (recombinant factor VIII-Gc fusion for hemophilia A), Adynovate (recombinant factor VIII PEGylated for hemophilia A), and Idelvion (recombinant factor IX albumin fusion for hemophilia B). Other examples of protein replacement are aflibercept (VEGF Fc-fusion for macular degeneration), tbo-filgrastim (G-CSF growth factor for neutropenia), peginterferon beta-1a (PEGylated IFNb-1b for multiple sclerosis), etanercept-szzs (TNFR-Fc-fusion for arthritis), glucarpidase (enzyme for kidney failure), taliglucerase alfa (β-glucoerebrosidase for Gauchet Syndrome), ocriplasmin (enzyme for symptomatic vitreomacular adhesion), and sebelipase alfa (lysosomal acid lipase for lysosomal acid lipase deficiency). The converse to protein replacement is selective protein elimination as in the removal of the cancer protein BRD4 with PROTACs technology (see Box 4.4).

Not all drug targets are single entities. Complex targets made up of a combination of components can produce unique phenotypes in cells. For instance, the amylin / adrenomedullin system consists of multigene target of calcitonin receptors and proteins called RAMP (Receptor Activity Modifying Protein) to produce unique phenotypes—see Box 11.12. The formation of receptor dimers in the cell membrane is a similar application of complex target pharmacology. Some receptors naturally function as dimers such as Class C GPCRs (i.e., $GABA_{B1}$-$GABA_{B2}$), taste receptors (TR3) with TR1 and/or TR2, and mGlu2 Receptors. There is evidence for hetero-dimerization in native tissues for a_{2A}-adrenoceptor + morphine m receptor, b-adrenoceptors, and thyroid stimulating hormone receptors, and the chemokine receptors CCR2, CCR5, CXCR4.

In addition to outright activation or blockade of pharmacological targets, nuance in target function can be obtained through allosteric modulation. For instance, activation of muscarinic receptors can produce serious toxic effects, which precludes the use of direct muscarinic agonists in therapy. However, there are data to show that mild potentiation of muscarinic receptor in the brain through allosteric modulation (positive allosteric modulators) can increase cognition to be a useful therapy. Thus, the manner in which the target is pharmacologically manipulated allows the target to be prosecuted for therapeutic activity. A related application of pharmacology to therapy is the palliative treatment of disease. For example, in asthma allergic sensitization, the failure of neuronal and hormonal balance in airway

BOX 11.12

Phantom genes: it takes two to Tango.

Unique "receptors" are made from complexes of a single receptor and single transverse membrane-spanning proteins called RAMP proteins (Receptor Activity Modifying Proteins). For instance, the human calcitonin receptor is more sensitive to human calcitonin than the hormone amylin (see panel A). However, in some physiological systems (i.e., the nucleus accumbens of the brain), there is an amylin "receptor" that has a unique phenotype whereby the hormone amylin is more potent than human calcitonin. This target has been of interest for the treatment of diabetes and considerable efforts were made to clone the amylin receptor from the gene. All of these efforts failed because there is no amylin gene. Rather, the phenotype comes from a complex of two proteins expressed by the calcitonin receptor gene and the gene for RAMP3—see panel B.

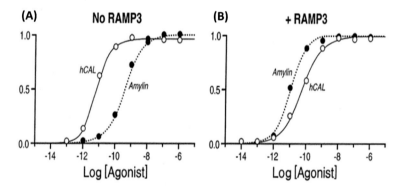

Source: From S.L. Armour, S. Foord, T. Kenakin, W.-J. Chen, Pharmacological characterization of receptor-activity-modifying proteins (RAMPs) and the human calcitonin receptor. J. Pharmacol. Toxicol. Meth. 42 (1999) 217–224.

smooth muscle, and hyperreactivity of smooth muscle leads to a multisystem breakdown resulting in hypercontracted bronchial smooth muscle (bronchospasm). Historically, these systems were controlled, not be addressing the cause of the bronchial hyperreactivity but rather in producing a system override by relaxation of the constricted airways through b-adrenoceptor agonist-induce bronchodilation. While not specifically producing a cure, this treatment saves lives—see

Fig. 11.1. Finally, the role of serendipity should be mentioned in the drug discovery process; through a favorable confluence of conditions, researchers have been presented drug profiles that have proven to be remarkably valuable—see Box 11.13.

Once a drug target has been identified, it is important to validate it as a true mediator of the disease. An example of the process of target validation can be found in the determination of the chemokine receptor CCR5 as being the key entry point for HIV-1 in AIDS.

1. Cells require presence of chemokine receptors for HIV infection.

BOX 11.13

Happy pharmacologic accidents.

Scientific lore favors the concept that logic and reason coupled with hard work leads to great discoveries and this largely is the case. However, serendipity has played a role in the history of pharmacologic drug discovery as well. For instance, returning from a holiday in 1928, Dr. Alexander Fleming entered his laboratory to find mold growing on a Petri dish of Staphylococcus bacteria. However, he then made the perspicacious observation that the mold appeared to be preventing the bacteria around it from growing. This led to the discovery of penicillin as a major antibiotic responsible for saving countless lives. Similarly, Robert Furchgott, who in spite of being Chairman of Pharmacology at the SUNY University Department of Pharmacology, always found time to do experiments in his laboratory once a week. Studying the effects of acetylcholine in vascular smooth muscle, Furchgott noticed that when his technician experimented, acetylcholine-produced contraction; when he experimented, it produced relaxation. The difference was that Furchgott did not clean the interior of the artery with a cotton swab (a common practice to remove extraneous material) and his technician did. Cleaning the vascular preparation stripped the fragile layer of endothelial cells, which are critical for vascular patency and vasorelaxation. Furchgott determined that loss of the endothelial layer led to elimination of acetylcholine-mediated release of EDRF (Endothelial Derived Relaxation Factor, later to be identified as nitric oxide), a critical mediator of vascular function. This became one of the most important discoveries in cardiovascular pharmacology and led to Furchgott receiving the Nobel Prize in Medicine, along with Louis Ignarro, in 1998.

continued

BOX 11.13 *(cont'd)*

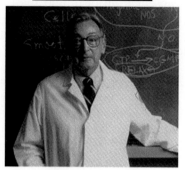

Robert Furchgott
(discovery of EDRF)

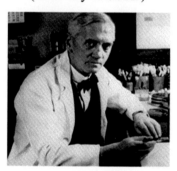

Alexander Fleming
(discovery of penicillin)

2. Ligands for CCR5 are potent inhibitors of HIV infection in vitro.
3. CCR5 mouse knockout healthy and more resistant to some inflammations.
4. Allelic variants of the CCR5 promoter leads to accelerated progression of AIDS.
5. Individuals homozygous for the D32 CCR5 allele are highly resistant to HIV infection and otherwise apparently healthy—see Box 11.10.

The technology of gene knockout has been an important part of the target validation process. However, it should be noted that this is primarily done in mice and there can be differences between mouse and human target proteins that could lead to divergence of activity.

Moreover, gene knockouts are done in adult systems where the animal has had the target operative from birth; this is different in some cases from the target being absent from birth and these differences can lead to differences in the predictions of knockouts.

Target validation can also be achieved through tool compounds (molecules that do not have full drug profiles but nevertheless have a primary activity that can be exploited to determine the possible importance of a target in a disease process). For instance, preliminary data show that the NPY5 receptor is involved in feeding and thus could be considered to be a possible target for obesity. However, testing of tool NPY5 antagonists injected directly into rat brain indicated that no changes in feeding were produced thereby negating this receptor as a therapeutic possibility.

High-throughput screening

- The next step in the process is to sift through the library with an appropriate screening assay; the main prerequisites for this assay are sensitivity (high) and low variability (robust). There are four basic formats for drug screening: the first relate to agonists and antagonists.
- Agonist screens: basal response is stable and low and there is a high range for increased response (agonism). The screen is run with no chemical context (no other molecule is present in the assay). Increased response is the desired effect—see Fig. 11.8A. Potential active molecules are subjected to a dose—response test to determine the curve for activity.
- Antagonist screens: same requirements for basal and maximal effects as agonist screens. The screen is run with a chemical context, usually an agonist to detect inhibition at a concentration that produces between 50% and 80% maximal response. Decreased agonist response is the desired effects—Fig. 11.8B. Potential active molecules are subjected to an IC_{50} type of analysis where a concentration-range of the putative antagonist is tested against a constant submaximal response of the agonist.

Historically, the compounds that produced the greatest apparent agonist response in an agonist screen were progressed to secondary assays; in this process, no examination of the quality of efficacy was made. A preferable strategy is to test all compounds showing any efficacy in the screening assay in another functional assay measuring another signaling pathway mediated by the same receptor (Fig. 11.9). Comparison of the responses in the two functional assays then yields an array of biased

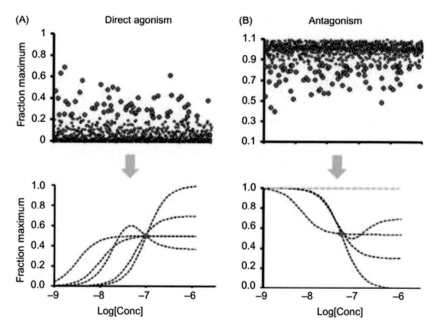

FIGURE 11.8 Screening for agonists (panel A) and antagonists (panel B). (A) A sensitive functional assay is exposed to test compounds and increases in functional response (red-filled circles) are regarded as possible agonist responses. These are then tested in a concentration–response mode to hopefully unveil as dose–response relationship. (B) A functional preparation is preequilibrated with a submaximal concentration of agonist (producing between 50% and 80% maximal response) and then exposed to test compounds. Responses that fall below control levels (red-filled circles) are regarded as possible antagonists which are then tested in a concentration–response model to determine possible IC_{50} values.

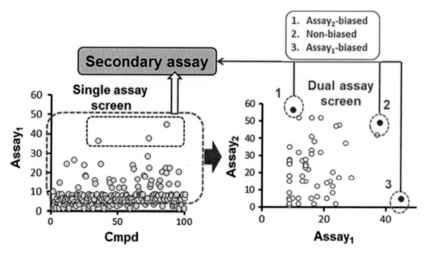

FIGURE 11.9 Choosing screening hits for progression to secondary assays. Historically, the most active screening hits in an agonist were progressed for secondary testing. Testing of a larger array of hits in the initial screen in another functional assay uncovers biased agonists which, when progressed, yield a better likelihood of producing unique phenotypic agonist response in the secondary assay.

agonists, which can then be selected to progress to the secondary (in vivo) assay. This process ensures that agonists of differing quality of efficacy are progressed with the greater potential to unveil unique phenotypic activity in the secondary assay(s).

- *Constitutively active screens*: The receptor levels (or level of reacting signaling proteins) are high enough to cause the functional assay to have an elevated basal response due to spontaneously active receptors. No chemical context is needed in this assay making it amenable to the screening of orphan receptors for which no natural ligands are known.

The basal response and effect of hits are shown in Fig. 11.10. The basal response in a constitutively active receptor system consists of an unstable array of active state receptors coupled to signaling proteins and spontaneously producing an elevated basal signal. Such a system is therefore a mixture of active and inactive receptor conformations. If any ligand binding to this collection of conformations has a preferential affinity for any of the states, it will stabilize that state at the expense of others and through Le Chatelier's principle, bias the entire system toward that state. If the state is an active receptor, then agonism will result (red-filled circles); if an inactive state is stabilized, the basal constitutive activity will be decreased and inverse agonism will result (blue filled circles).

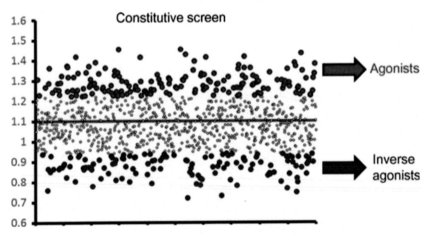

FIGURE 11.10   The basal response in a constitutively active receptor system consists of a collection of active and inactive receptor states. Ligands stabilizing the active state will produce positive agonism (red-filled circles) and those stabilizing the inactive state will produce inverse agonism (blue filled circles).

Allosteric screen: this assay detects molecules that modify an existing submaximal agonist response. The assay has a chemical context of a low-level activation of the receptor by the natural agonist. This screen can detect positive allosteric modulators (PAMs) with an increased response and negative allosteric modulators (NAMs) with decreased response.

In an allosteric screen, the receptor is preequilibrated with the endogenous agonist to produce a submaximal activation (usually between 25% and 35% maximal response). Prospective allosteric molecules that bind to the receptor then may increase or decrease the pre-existing agonist response to detect PAMs or NAMs, respectively. Fig. 11.11 shows output from an allosteric screen detecting PAMs. One feature of allosteric screens is they are inherently more variable with respect to basal response (due to the fact that ligand effects are superimposed on a biologically generated agonist response by a low level of agonist); this can lead to a higher than usual level of false positives. In addition to a more rigorous requirement for testing in an allosteric program, there is a possibility that animal ortholog receptors for the drug activity may not be available due to the absence of the allosteric binding site on the animal receptor. While adherence of orthosteric binding sites between humans and animals is often encountered (due to the similarity of the molecules binding to those sites in the form of common neurotransmitters and hormones), the same adherence may not extend to subsidiary sites on the protein mediating allosteric activity—see Box 11.14.

In general, modern high-throughput screening is more than an informed "numbers game" in that the libraries contain drug-like molecules that may be biased toward privileged structures. Recently the technology

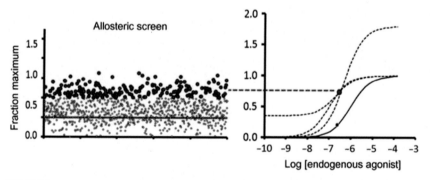

FIGURE 11.11 Receptors are preequilibrated with the endogenous agonist to produce a submaximal activation in an allosteric screen. Shown are potential PAMs or PAM-agonists which increase the agonist response (red-filled circles).

BOX 11.14

Allosteric site variation in ortholog ATP P2X7 receptors.

In the development of drugs, it is important to have animal models to confirm putative therapeutic activity in humans. For orthosteric ligands where the binding sites for identical transmitters in humans and animals show extensive correspondence, receptor activity often transfers from animal to human tissue. For allosteric ligands, there may not be the same teleological pressure to conserve protein binding sites and more variation between animal and human receptors can be seen. The P2X7 receptor is a ligand-gated cation channel gated by ATP which is important in the release of the pro-inflammatory cytokine interleukin-1b from immune cells. It can be seen from the figure that Cmpd-22, an allosteric antagonist of ATP for the human receptor (3 μM essentially completely blocks the effects of ATP) is inactive at the Guinea Pig P2X7 receptor [6]. This raises issues for the testing of Cmpd-22-mediated antiinflammatory activity in guinea pigs.

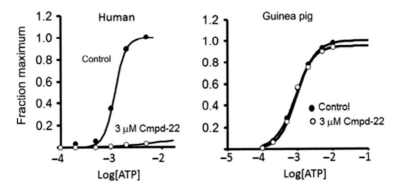

Source: *Data from J. Arrowsmith, Trial watch: phase II failures: 2008–2010, Nat. Rev. Drug Discov. 10 (2011) 328–329. [1].*

employed for DNA-encoded libraries has greatly facilitated the screening of millions of compounds in a short amount of time—see Box 11.15.

Fragment-based screening also has proven to be a great advance to the discovery of new molecules. This approach is based on the concept that extraneous chemical groups on molecules preclude binding of the whole molecular scaffold, thus losing the information inherent in the substructures of the molecule that otherwise could have fit into the

---

BOX 11.15

Finding a needle in a haystack: DNA-encoded libraries.

A limitation of screening very large numbers of compounds is the separation and identification of bound molecules ("hits") from inactive molecules. Historically, separate samples of each test molecule are physically separated by testing in a separate location (binding well); for millions of compounds this leads to logistical problems. DNA-encoded library technology (DEL) enables the mixing of molecules in a single tube; the problem of identifying which molecule is a hit is solved by linking of each molecule with a unique DNA sequence barcode that can identify the molecule identification of the hit molecule. Thus, the various mixtures of "hits" can be processed together in the same tube through polymerase chain reaction (PCR) to amplify the single DNA chain for each hit and then sequenced with next-generation sequencing (NGS) to identify the barcode, which then leads to identification of the hit molecule. Unbound molecules are washed away and bound molecules identified through DEL technology. Literally billions of molecules, each encoded with a unique DNA sequence, can be tested together since each can be identified through PCR and NGS to identify which molecule bound to the target.

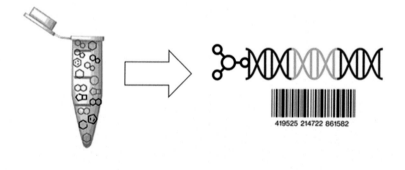

---

binding site of the target. With this approach molecules are reduced to their substructure components and screened for binding activity; the substructure components that do bind then can be assembled to form a complete molecule that fits the target binding site—see Box 11.16.

Drug screening also has greatly benefited from the determination of receptor structure. The elucidation of drug-binding sites can greatly assist in the design of molecules that better engage the target. For GPCRs, historically these have been considered intractable protein

BOX 11.16

The whole is greater than the sum of its parts: fragment-based screening.

Large chemical structures that bind to complex protein binding pockets have a close complement interaction. Molecules that partly bind into these pockets may fail to completely engage the binding pocket due to interference from the parts of the molecule that do not correspond to the binding pocket. Thus, in a screening assay, there may be several molecules that "partly" bind to the pocket but do not show up as hits due to the weak interaction. Fragment-based screening decomposes complex chemical structures into smaller pieces, which might fit into parts of the binding pocket without interference. If these fragments can be identified, then they may form the basis of a complex structure that completely fits into the binding site. A historical short-coming of this approach has been the technical inability to detect weak fragment binding but advances have been made in this regard and fragment-based screening is now a viable approach to finding new drugs.

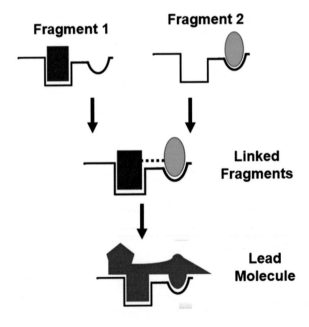

structures for the determination of an X-ray structure suitable for binding analyses. This is because, these targets are known to be extremely malleable with respect to tertiary conformation with changes in free energy. However, unique biochemical manipulations of these difficult targets have resulted in methods to "freeze" conformations long enough to allow X-ray structures to be determined. These new technologies have revolutionized the application of protein structure to the development of molecular binding models to receptors—see Box 11.17.

Since 2006, the application of receptor protein crystal structures to discovery has risen exponentially.

Another technological advancement made in screening is the development of docking and virtual screening techniques. In this endeavor, virtual libraries of millions of molecules are electronically docked into binding sites on receptor structure images to yield optimal binding poses that can then be verified experimentally. A successful example of the application of virtual screening is the de-orphanization of the proton-sensing receptor GPR68 and the discovery of the positive allosteric modulator ogerin—see Box 11.18. Finally, as stated earlier, the fact that receptors can spontaneously form active states to produce constitutively active systems can be applied to detect ligand binding for agonists and antagonists.

These techniques are target-based in that they begin with the definition of a biological target protein for the binding of molecules. An alternative to this approach is phenotypic screening where the screening system is actually a complex collection of targets. Thus, while the goal of a target-based screen is a drug-like molecule with primary activity that can be absorbed, distribute to the therapeutic tissue, remain there long enough to produce effect and cause no harm, the goal of a therapeutic screen does not require drug-like character in that the endpoint is not necessarily a drug entity but rather a new mode of altering pathophysiology. Molecules are tested in a complex multitarget system that have a "phenotype" (complex set of properties that can be modified by drug action). Phenotypic screens assess a much wider sample of readouts than do target-based systems, i.e., they yield multiparametric data (generated by multiplexed staining and image analysis) that can be analyzed for nuanced assessment of effects on a system. Large collections of parameters (classifiers) are accumulated that mathematically reduce sensitive phenotype clustering (using machine learning algorithms). Thus, additional outcomes can be determined from a phenotypic screen. Chemically unattractive scaffolds are not excluded from the hit collection since removing such compounds would lose value in terms of providing probes for exploring new modes of action, i.e., accessing different biology may require

BOX 11.17

The receptor becomes more than a concept.

On October 10, 2012, Drs Brian Kobilka and Robert Lefkowitz won the 2012 Nobel Prize in Chemistry "for studies in G-protein-coupled receptors" (GPCRs). The vision for this work was stated early on by Lefkowitz: "At such time as purified receptor preparations are available, detailed physicochemical characterization will become possible. Such studies should lead to an intimate understanding of 'the b-adrenergic receptor'" (R.J. Lefkowitz, Life Sci. 18 (1976) 461−472). After the cloning of the first gene for the hamster b_2-adrenoceptor, they prophetically stated that "our proposed model for the structure of the b-adrenergic receptor and its interaction with pharmacologically important ligands should, together with the biochemical and genetic studies now possible, provide a rational basis for a new approach to the development of more selective drugs" (Dixon et al., Nature, 321 (1986) 75−79). There were still considerable obstacles in the path to the determining receptor structure including obtaining adequate protein production and issues with purification, protein stability and homogeneity. However, as put by Kobilka: "while the challenges facing GPCR structural biologists are formidable, I believe structures will begin to appear within the next several years. The problems are solvable." The result was successful and culminated in the award of the Nobel Prize for Chemistry for the determination of the structure of the b_2-adrenocepto (B.K. Kobilka, Biochim. Biophys. Acta 1768 (2007) 794−807; Cherezov et al., Science 318 (2007) 1258−1265; Rasmussen et al., Nature 469 (2011) 175−180).

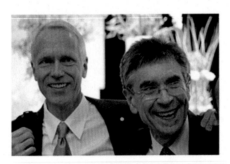

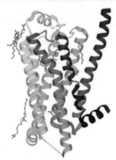

BOX 11.18

Billions of possibilities: virtual screening.

Yeast-based screens with the orphan receptor GPR68 were used to identify the benzodiazepine drug lorazepam as a nonselective GPR68 positive allosteric modulator. Sequence alignment of GPR68, GPR4, GPR65, and GPR132 to CXCR4 and docking of lorazepam and compound libraries to five distinct binding sites on 3307 GPR68 homology models allowed ranking of lorazepam versus decoy molecules. 3.1 million molecules were then docked into the sites (3.3 trillion docking complexes) to optimize the optimal lorazepam binding mode. The outcome was the discovery of ogerin, a positive allosteric modulator of the proton sensor protein GPR68.

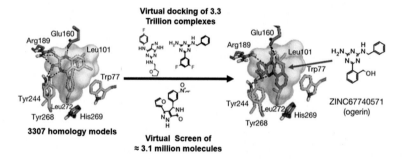

Source: Huang et al., Allosteric ligands for the pharmacologically dark receptors GPR68 and GPR65, Nature 527 (2015) 477.

different chemical matter. This can yield new information about mode of action of molecules or a new cellular mechanism in disease.

Decision gates for phenotypic screens versus target-based screens will be different as potency will not be paramount; unique patterns of activity will be more important. Gain of signal is preferable to a loss of signal as the latter can be due to toxic effects and thus be a false positive. Optimal systems consist of highly disease-relevant assays stimulated by disease-relevant stimuli with assay readouts as close to the desired clinical outcome as possible, i.e., assay systems should have a clear link to the disease (i.e., patient-derived cells) and the assay readout should be as proximal as possible to the clinical endpoint and disease pathophysiology (systems that do not require an endogenous stimulus are preferred)—see Box 11.19.

BOX 11.19

Can complex systems unveil new therapeutic mechanisms? Phenotypic screening.

Phenotypic screens seek to find activity (preferably gain of function) in primary cells that emanates from human donors (preferably more than one donor). Successful molecular series must pass key counter screens and validation assays and hopefully the mode of action of hit molecules will be differentiated from the known mode of action of other compounds. Ideally, evidence of structure-activity relationships (>10-fold difference in activity with changes in molecular scaffold structure) with no obvious chemical groups known to cause toxicity will emerge and these will be profiled against targets with known safety issues, i.e., there is a divergent structure-activity relationship for efficacy and cytotoxicity.

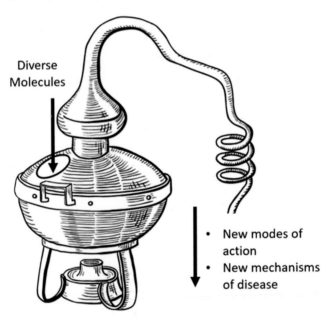

Diverse Molecules

- New modes of action
- New mechanisms of disease

Source: *Vincent et al. Hit triage and validation in phenotypic screening: considerations and strategies, Cell Chem. Biol. 27 (2020) 1332−1346.*

Summary

- Four essential properties of drugs must be known to allow prediction of possible therapeutic effect: affinity, efficacy, orthosteric versus allosteric interaction, and kinetics of drug offset from the target.
- With regards to drug "efficacy", it should be recognized that drugs have many efficacies and it is important to detect and quantify all of them to prepare for complex profiles seen in vivo.
- There are fundamental differences between programs aimed at improving existing drugs and producing first in class drugs.
- Whereas target-based discovery is aimed at finding new drug entities, systems-based discovery is focused on identifying new mechanisms, and cellular pathways in disease that can be utilized in drug therapy.
- The fact that final drug candidates are often similar to the screening starting point scaffolds, the use of drug-like molecules in screening libraries is now commonplace.
- Two types of assay are detection assays (screening)—these must be sensitive, robust and selective and "lead optimization assays," which must return correct pharmacology for the molecule and data to advance structure activity studies and determine mechanism of action.
- Target validation is an essential part of the drug discovery process but is now extended to "pathway validation" in light of the discovery of biased signaling.
- Technology (i.e., fragment-based screening, constitutive screening, virtual screening, structure-assisted screening, and DNA-encoded libraries) has greatly expanded the four types of screening (agonists, antagonists, allosteric modulators, and constitutive screening).

References

[1] J. Arrowsmith, Trial watch: phase II failures: 2008–2010, Nat. Rev. Drug Discov. 10 (5) (2011) 328–329. Available from: https://doi.org/10.1038/nrd3439.

[2] M.M. Hann, T.I. Oprea, Pursuing the leadlikeness concept in pharmaceutical research, Curr. Opin. Chem. Biol. 8 (3) (2004) 255–263. Available from: https://doi.org/10.1016/j.cbpa.2004.04.003.

[3] D.E. Clark, P.D.J. Grootenhuis, Predicting passive transport in silico—history, hype, hope, Curr. Top. Med. Chem. 3 (11) (2003) 1193–1203. Available from: https://doi.org/10.2174/1568026033451970.

[4] C. Watson, S. Jenkinson, W. Kazmierski, T. Kenakin, The CCR5 receptor-based mechanism of action of 873140, a potent allosteric noncompetitive HIV entry inhibitor, Mol. Pharmacol. 67 (4) (2005) 1268–1282. Available from: https://doi.org/10.1124/mol.104.008565.

[5] T.P. Kenakin, Cellular assays as portals to seven-transmembrane receptor-based drug discovery, Nat. Rev. Drug Discov. 8 (8) (2009) 617−626. Available from: https://doi.org/10.1038/nrd2838.

[6] A.D. Michel, S.W. Ng, S. Roman, W.C. Clay, D.K. Dean, D.S. Walter, Mechanism of action of species-selective P2X 7 receptor antagonists, Br. J. Pharmacol. 156 (8) (2009) 1312−1325. Available from: https://doi.org/10.1111/j.1476-5381.2009.00135.x.

The science of finding drug molecules II: demonstrating target engagement and therapeutic value

Lead optimization

The mechanism of action of new drugs is usually determined by the verisimilitude of the complex patterns they produce in pharmacologic assays to the theoretical models of drug action derived from mass action models and pharmacologic experience. The best models for this purpose are mathematical models that furnish rules of behavior governing drug effects under a range of physiological conditions. The importance of these rules is that they furnish two critical elements to the lead optimization process: (1) they allow us to make predictions of what the drug will do under different physiologic conditions, which can then be tested and (2) they furnish checkpoints to test adherence to the model(s) and eliminate happenstance as a reason for the similarity of the experimentally observed effects and predictions of the models. As put by the astrophysicist Stephen Hawking... "what is it that breathes fire into the equations and makes a universe for them to describe?" (Stephen Hawking, 1991). What Hawking meant was that, once a set of rules for future behavior is established by mathematical description of a model, then a "universe" of behaviors can be predicted.

The lead optimization process of linking the experimental observations with the mechanism of action of the drug then begins with the experiment, the building of the model, using the model to make a prediction of the new behavior of the system, and designing a new experiment to compare the prediction to the new data—Fig. 12.1. The importance of the internal checks cannot be overemphasized. Thus dextral displacement of agonist concentration-response curves with no diminution of maxima is a hallmark of simple competitive antagonism but the displacements must be such that the slope of regression of the logarithm of the dose ratios-1 upon the logarithm of the antagonist concentration producing the dose-ratio must furnish a linear regression with a slope of unity. Failure to satisfy this internal check would constitute doubt on the conclusion that the molecule is a true simple competitive antagonist. Of course, it is not possible to definitively prove

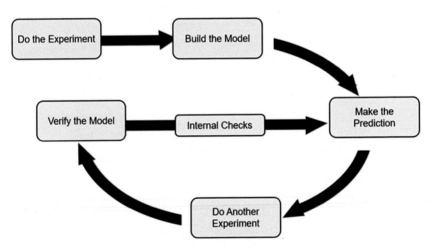

FIGURE 12.1 Comparison of experimental data to models to delineate mechanism of action. After data is collected from an experiment, a model is devised (mathematical with equations and rules). The model then can be used to predict a behavior of the system under different circumstances and then another experiment is done to see if the prediction holds. If the prediction does not hold, the model is modified and the cycle is repeated. Also, the model will usually have rules as to how the data will be presented and if these internal checks are not verified, this negates the model.

the mechanism of the drug through such a procedure as there may be a prediction and an experiment that would unveil differences. However, the iteration can be often enough to yield a level of confidence that, with adherence of observed effect to model prediction, a correct model can be identified.

Historically, pharmacologic models were derived from the mass action model first published in 1864 [1,2] that states;

$$A + B \rightleftharpoons A' + B' \qquad (12.1)$$

This model is deceptively simple but it does state that matter cannot be created or destroyed. Combinations of the mass action model form the basis for all linkage receptor models ranging from enzymes, G protein coupled receptors, ion channels and allosteric proteins—Fig. 12.2.

Models can be classified according to their relative complexity and also how verifiable the parameters that go into the model are. This latter factor is important since a complex model requiring a large number of parameters that cannot independently be verified cannot be used to fit data effectively. The verisimilitude of models to data is the main criterion for assessment of the model as a descriptor of system but it should be recognized that it cannot be certain that a given mathematical fit is the correct one; this is consistent with but not proof of veracity—Box 12.1.

1. Mass Action : Enzymes

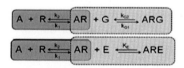

2. Series Mass Action : GPCRs

3. Parallel Mass Action : Ion Channels, Allosteric Proteins

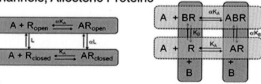

FIGURE 12.2 The Mass action law as a building block for pharmacologic models. Mass action equations in series model GPCR behavior and the operational model for receptor function. Mass action equations in parallel model ion channels and allosteric receptor systems.

BOX 12.1

How good is good enough?

'Nothing can be proven to be correct...only incorrect...'

'If apparently correct you just may not have designed the right experiment that would have proven it to be incorrect...'*

Karl Popper 1902-1994

*why we always must disprove the null hypothesis

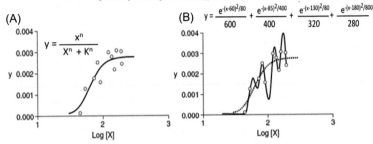

(A) $y = \dfrac{x^n}{X^n + K^n}$

(B) $y = \dfrac{e^{-(x-60)^2/80}}{600} + \dfrac{e^{-(x-85)^2/400}}{400} + \dfrac{e^{-(x-130)^2/80}}{320} + \dfrac{e^{-(x-180)^2/800}}{280}$

The similarity of mathematical models to data patterns is assessed by how well the predicted curve approximates the data curve, that is, a low sum of squares of the differences between real and calculated values. This raises the question; how good must the fit be to be considered the ultimate fit reflecting true behavior of the system? As stated by Karl Popper (1902–94), one of the most influential philosophers of science of the 20th century, there never is a limit that definitively denotes true veracity. For example, in the concentration-response curves shown below, the data points can be fit with the Hill equation in panel A. However, there is always a better equation that might reduce the sum of squares, such as the equation for the curve in panel B. At some point, the researcher must take on the responsibility of assessing "this is the model I choose" and move on.

There are two important and equal components to the model fitting process: (1) the quality of the mathematical model, and (2) the quality of the representation of drug effect, that is, the quality of the pharmacologic assay. In the previous chapter, assays were discussed in terms of how well they detect signals, specifically low-level signals, such as might come from a screening assay. With these types of assays, sensitivity is the prime consideration and it may not be expected that the signal accurately reflects the equilibrium kinetics of the drug-receptor interaction, that is, it basically furnishes a binary, "yes-no" output. Such detection assays must be sensitive, robust, and selective. This is not the case for assays used in the lead optimization stage of a project where the data is used to determine the mechanism of action of the drug. These assays will be used to assess the verisimilitude of the data to the model to furnish the mechanism of action of the drug and also to guide medicinal chemistry efforts to modify activity. This being the case, the assay must truly reflect the pharmacology of a drug as it interacts with the receptor. In addition, a range of predictions of the model should be employed in the assessment. Fig. 12.3 shows the effect of a test partial

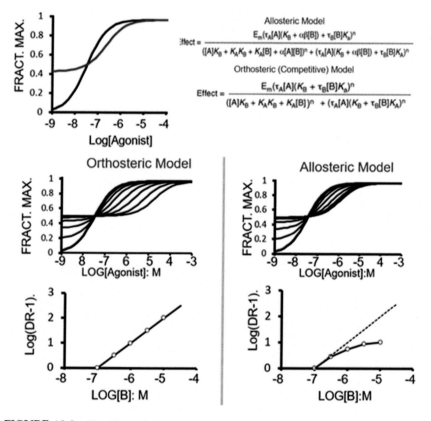

FIGURE 12.3 The effect of a partial agonist on the response to a full agonist is shown by the curve in red in the top left panel. However, this single pattern is predicted by an orthosteric or an allosteric partial agonist. These mechanisms can be distinguished by testing a range of partial agonist concentrations and observing the pattern of dextral displacement of the full agonist curve. Orthosteric effects predict a straight line for Log(Dr-1) (the Schild regression) whereas an allosteric mechanism shows saturable behavior resulting in a curved relationship.

agonist on the concentration-response curve of a full agonist. It can be seen that a profile of elevated-basal response and dextral displacement of the agonist concentration-curve result. This pattern can be produced by an orthosteric partial agonist or an allosteric partial agonist and it is not possible to discern, which of these is true from the two curves shown. However, orthosteric and allosteric mechanisms are different and it may be possible to unveil the mechanism by observing the effects of a range of concentrations of the test partial agonist. Specifically, allosteric effects are saturable as the allosteric effect comes to limiting value due to the saturation of binding to the allosteric site. In contrast, orthosteric effects are competitive and continue depending upon the relative concentrations of the two competing ligands (agonist and partial agonist). As shown in Fig. 12.3, differentiation between an allosteric versus orthosteric mechanism is straightforward upon observation of the full range of effect of the experimental ligand.

Not all assays are capable of demonstrating the full range of thermodynamic effects produced by a ligand on a target receptor. For instance, the measurement of calcium transient response from a hemi-equilibrium assay reflects only the first few seconds of response as the agonist binds to the receptor. Therefore any action where concomitant sustained responses must be measured cannot be studied with the calcium assay. Antagonists that selectively stabilize the inactive receptor state produce a reversal of elevated basal responses due to constitutive receptor activity revealing the property of inverse agonism. The property of inverse agonism may be a harbinger of antagonist tolerance in some systems so it is a valuable property of the antagonist to be detected. Fig. 12.4 shows two assays monitoring ghrelin receptor activation of Gq protein. The equilibrium IP1 assay accurately reflects the elevated basal response due to receptor overexpression and, importantly, the reversal of this elevated basal by the inverse agonist. In contrast, the calcium transient assay does not demonstrate a sustained elevated basal response and thus cannot reveal the inverse agonist activity of SPA. This reveals the importance of using the right assay to demonstrate the drug effect.

Not only does the quality of the assay affect the lead optimization process, but also the type of data that is used. In general, highly transformed data (the result of multiple readouts of activity) should not be used as different structure-activity trends may cause the cancellation of *bona fide* effects of changes in the molecular structure. Box 12.2 shows what can happen when the transform for potency (pEC_{50}) is used for SAR instead of estimates of affinity and efficacy; the canceling affinity and efficacy effects of structural changes cause the transform (EC_{50}) to not reveal any changes in activity whereas the determination of affinity and efficacy show a rich structure-activity relationship.

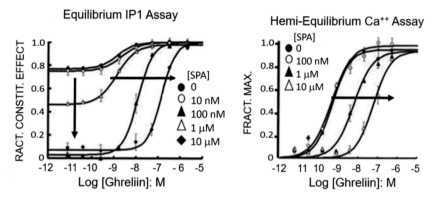

FIGURE 12.4 Concentration-response curves to the agonist ghrelin activating Gq protein in ghrelin-receptor transfected HEK293-GSHR1a cells. Curves shown in the absence (control, filled circles) and presence of the inverse agonist SPA. [D-Arg1, D-Phe5, DTrp7, 9, Leu11]-substance P (10 nM, open circles), (100 nM, filled triangles), (1 μM, open triangles), and (10 μM, filled diamonds). The equilibrium IP1 assay is constitutively active (elevated-basal response) and displays the inverse agonist activity of SPA. The hemi-equilibrium calcium assay cannot sustain an elevated-basal response and thus does not reveal inverse agonism. Source: *Redrawn from Bdioui S, Verdi J, Pierre N, Trinquet E, Roux T, Kenakin T. (2018) Equilibrium assays are required to accurately characterize the activity profiles of drugs modulating Gq-protein-coupled receptors. Mol. Pharmacol. 94: 992—1006.*

Models allow the fitting of complex concentration-response data to multicomponent systems. Historically, early models were designed to yield linear transforms as these were amenable to analysis without computers (when rulers ruled the world). Linear models hold the advantages of being simple and predictable with simple statistical tests to assess quality (linearity, elevation, and slope). Thus transforms of equations to describe enzyme activation (Lineweaver-Burke plots—see Fig. 6.1) and simple competitive receptor antagonism (Schild regressions—see Fig. 4.6) were applied to numerous pharmacologic analyses. While this can simplify analysis, transforming to a linear model can also skew data and provide heteroscedasticity in the estimation of error. Linear models also can be misleading as in the oversimplistic linearization of receptor binding data with Scatchard or Hanes plots. On the other hand, the fact that linearized models are overly sensitive to variations in data can be used to discover in-equilibrium as in binding studies that utilize too much protein in the assay. While this may not be apparent in the raw data, a Scatchard analysis greatly amplifies the error and makes it evident. However, as a means of deriving meaningful drug parameters, linear transforms have fallen by the wayside now that computers can analyze raw data.

Once a molecule has been identified as a possible drug candidate studies must be done to see if it really does fulfill the therapeutic need

---

BOX 12.2

Complex transforms of drug activity can be misleading

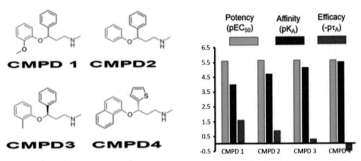

CMPD 1   CMPD2

CMPD3   CMPD4

Pharmacologic activity data drives medicinal chemistry structure-activity relationships (SAR); this is the core of the lead optimization process. The data used to guide this process can be important in that the wrong type of data may miss valuable trends that could guide chemists. For example, the potency of an agonist is descriptive data for the molar concentration of the agonist producing 50% maximal effect (usually expressed as $-\text{Log}(EC_{50} = pEC_{50})$. However, the pEC_{50} is a transform of the molecular scales of affinity and efficacy ($pEC_{50} = pK_A - \text{Log}(\tau_A + 1)$ where K_A is the equilibrium dissociation constant of the agonist receptor complex and τ_A is the efficacy of the agonist from the operational model). There is a danger in using transformed data in that opposing trends may cancel each other and thus make it appear no change has taken place. For example, shown are four bronchodilators with essentially equal potencies. Chemists would have no guidance as to the effects of the structural changes. However, when the respective affinities and efficacies of the compounds are analyzed, it can be seen that there is a rich SAR with increasing affinity and decreasing efficacy; this provides chemists with data to subsequently modify agonist activity. The changes in structure modify the molecular properties controlling agonist binding and activation but the transformed data (pEC_{50}) did not reveal this.

---

in alleviating and/or curing the disease. Presumably the target chosen for the drug has been validated for treatment of the disease but it still may not be clear if the drug has the complete set of characteristics to satisfy the pathophysiological deficit. This, in fact, may be one of the reasons that, despite all best intensions and planning, over 50% of new drug candidates fail in the clinic due to lack of therapeutic efficacy.

There are two possible reasons for this; (1) the elements of the pathology of disease were not adequately known and (2) the complete range of efficacies (or lack of efficacies) of the candidate molecule were not known.

One possible reason for late candidate failure in a therapeutic setting is that the complexity of the disease and the pleiotropic nature of drug efficacy (drugs can have many efficacies) cause a mismatch and inadequate treatment results. Another reason may be that a particular collection of efficacies may be required for effective treatment. For example, 16 β-adrenoceptor blockers have been tested in clinical trials for congestive heart failure with varying results. If the single property of β-adrenoceptor blockade were the sole criterion for successful treatment, then all of these should have shown efficacy. In fact, of the 16 β-blockers tested, 13 showed moderate activity, 2 (bisoprolol, metoprolol) showed better activity, and carvedilol showed superior activity. One hypothesis for this difference is that carvedilol has a galaxy of activities that satisfied the pathological need (i.e., blockade of β-adrenoceptors and α_1-adrenoceptors, antioxidant activity, antiendothelin effects, and antiproliferative properties) to give a superior profile in this disease [3].

In addition, target-based strategies assume that the principal factor in the disease has been identified and that treatment of that single factor will produce a therapeutic effect. However, disease often is a multicomponent array of system that go awry and it may be that fixing a single target may be inadequate—see Box 12.3.

Target engagement

At some point, it is useful to convincingly demonstrate that the lead molecule directly engages the drug target, that is, functional effects in a cell containing the targets sometimes can be ambiguous. There are two general approaches to doing this: (1) Physical interaction and (2) functional response. In terms of showing a physical interaction between the drug candidate and the target, biochemical binding can be employed in the form either of showing a physical complex of a radioligand congener of the molecule through saturation binding or physical displacement of a surrogate radioligand bound to the target by the candidate molecule. Binding can be a one-way experiment in there are several possibilities that the direct physical interaction of a candidate molecule may not be made evident through binding. For instance, if the candidate is an allosteric modulator binding to a different locus on the target than the tracer radioligand, then no effect may be seen.

A more comprehensive approach can take with isothermal titration calorimetry. This technique takes advantage of the fact that two bodies

BOX 12.3

Sometimes there is no "magic bullet"

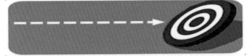

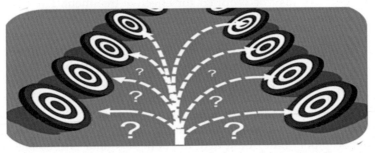

Disease can be a complex system failure where several components of a physiological system need adjustment. In these cases, it may not be possible to alleviate the disease with a single drug aimed at a single target. For instance, there are drugs for several classes approved for the treatment of Alzheimer's disease (Acetylcholinesterase, BACE-1, GSK-3b, MAO-B, metal chelation; Zhang et al. (2019) Eur. J. Med Chem 176:228). Pharmacological treatment of disease is put into perspective by Nobel Laureate Sir James Black:

"... angiogenesis, apoptosis, inflammation, commitment of marrow stem cells, and immune responses. The cellular reactions subsumed in these processes are switch-like in their behavior.... biochemically we are learning that in all these processes many chemical regulators seem to be involved. From the literature on synergistic interactions, a control model can be built in which no single agent is effective. If a number of chemical messengers each bring information from a different source and each deliver only a subthreshold stimulus but together mutually potentiate each other, then the desired information-rich switching can be achieved with minimum risk of miscuing."

Sir James Black (1986)

Nobel Lectures

binding to each other either release energy (exothermic reaction) or consume energy (endothermic reaction). The important point is that a change in the energy of the system is observed upon binding. Thus two chambers are set at equal temperatures with one being the reference chamber and one housing the binding reaction. A very sensitive thermocouple links the two chambers and can detect minute differences in their temperature. As the binding reaction progresses, the thermocouple registers the differences to yield a surrogate of the binding curve. Fig. 12.5 shows the binding of guggulsterone-E to DNA; it is noteworthy that this technique can be applied to a wide variety of ligand/target pairs, not only protein-receptor receptor binding. A variant of this thermodynamic approach is through Cellular Thermal Shift Assay (CETSA). This technique depends upon the concept that the melting point of proteins (temperature at which the protein becomes disordered and melts) is higher when proteins have an additional factor causing order, that is, binding of ligand. Therefore the melting point of the protein will be higher in the presence of a ligand that specifically binds to the protein,

Another method of determining physical interaction is through Free Solution Analysis (FSA)—see Fig. 12.6. With this procedure, a binding reaction is carried out in a capillary tube filled with physiological solution; another tube with solution is compared as a reference. A compensated interferometer detects solution changes through fringe pattern phase shift and Fourier Transform and image data constructs FSA

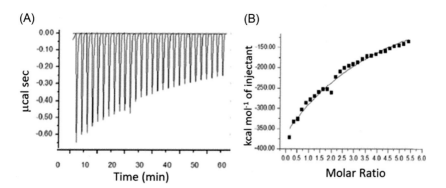

FIGURE 12.5 Application of isothermal calorimetry to demonstrate the binding of guggulsterone-E (5 μM) binding to ctDNA (0.2 mM). Panel A: Heat burst curve showing differences in thermo-cell heat exchange between the reference and binding chamber. Panel B: Normalized heat signals versus molar ratio. Source: *From Ikhlas S, Ahmad M. (2018) Binding studies of guggulsterone-E to calf thymus DNA by multi-spectroscopic, calorimetric and molecular docking studies. Spectrochimica Acta Part A: Mol Biomol Spectrosc. 190: 402–408.*

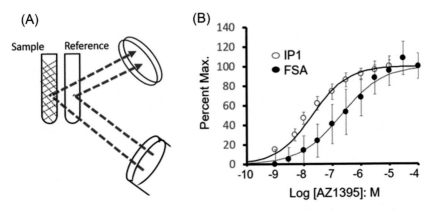

FIGURE 12.6   The measurement of binding through changes in refractive index and dielectric constants in a capillary-bound solution. This technique measures the extent of immobilization of the ligand and the target in the sample cell. Panel B shows the effects of AZ1395 on GPR39; Cell response is measured through IP1 metabolism and direct interaction of AZ1995 with GPR39 shown with FSA. FSA, Free solution analysis. Source: *Redrawn from Fjellstrom et al. (2015) Novel Zn2 + modulated GPR39 receptor agonists do not drive acute insulin secretion in rodents. PlosOne December.*

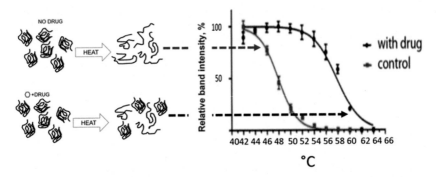

FIGURE 12.7   Application of the cellular thermal shift assay (CETSA) to verify binding of a ligand to a protein. Source: *Redrawn from Martinez Molina D, Jafari R, Ignatushchenko M, Seki T. Larsson EA, Dan C, Sreekumar L, Cao Nordlund P. Monitoring drug target engagement in cells and tissues using the cellular thermal shift assay. Science 341: 84—87.*

signals discerns the difference. Binding induced solvation, conformational, and electronic structure all alter refractive index and dielectric constants and the extent of this modification quantifies the extent of interaction of the ligand and the target.

A new technology to demonstrate target engagement is through CETSA (Fig. 12.7). In this technique proteins are denatured by increased temperature and the temperature at which denaturation occurs is inversely proportional to how structured the protein is. Binding ligands to proteins increase their structure; thus the melting point (temperature at which denaturation occurs) of a protein increases when a ligand is bound. This thermal shift can be used to identify ligand binding.

Another way of demonstrating target engagement is through changes in the functional response of a system with ligand binding. Label-free technology is invaluable in this regard since it can detect perturbation of cell function in a target-agnostic manner, that is, no need to know what target the ligand interacts with. One technique, such as dynamic mass redistribution, utilizes the movement of bodies 150 nM into the cell cytosol; when these are detected, this can be associated with interventions. Another approach is with the "CellKey" system whereby electrical impedance through a cell monolayer is measured; activation of metabolic processes in the cell by any means causes the impedance to change and this ligand interaction can be detected. An early version of these label-free techniques is microphysiometry where minute changes in pH in the medium surrounding cells are detected. As with impedance, alteration of cellular function changes the level of secretion of $H+$ into the medium from the cell and these are detected as changes in pH by the microphysiometer.

Fig. 12.8 shows how this can be applied to the detection of target engagement. Addition of a ligand (calcitonin) to a host HEK cell produces no change in pH. However, when the same cell contains the calcitonin receptor through expression, then addition of calcitonin produces a response. This is presumptive evidence that the calcitonin engages the calcitonin receptor as a target.

A method to delineate, which target a given molecule interacts with is through multiple pathway analysis. For instance, the delineation of

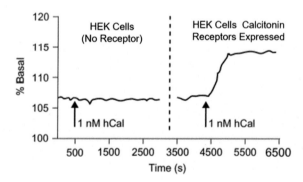

FIGURE 12.8   The label-free assay microphysiometry measures minute changes in $H+$ secretion from cells produced by changes in cell metabolism, (such as those brought about by ligand-receptor interaction). This can be used to measure target engagement. HEK cells produce no microphysiometry response when exposed to human calcitonin. However, when the human calcitonin receptor is transfected into HEK cells, addition calcitonin produces a microphysiometry response (indicative of a change in cell metabolism) thereby suggesting an engagement of calcitonin with the receptor.

the target for the diaryl sulfonylurea compound MCC950/Cytokine Release Inhibitory Drug 3 CRID3 is achieved through the monitoring of two pathways yielding the levels of IL-1β and IL-6 from cells. As shown in Fig. 12.9, while CRID3 reduces levels of IL-1β (the desired effect) it does not change levels of IL-6. In contrast, nonspecific inhibitors of IL-1β also reduce levels of IL-6. These data suggest that CRID3 is a selective inhibitor of the NLPR3 inflammasome (the desired target).

Biosensors have become extremely important in the delineation of target activation. Specifically, these are molecules that signal when a component from a given receptor is activated, that is, there are biosensors for various G proteins such as Gs, Gi, and Gq. Therefore if a biosensor signal is observed when an experimental molecule is exposed to the cell, this is presumptive evidence that a receptor interacting with that signaling pathway has been activated. Ligand-receptor interactions often lead to alterations in protein-protein interactions (i.e., receptor/ G protein) and biosensors can indicate receptor activation. These are two-subunit systems for intracellular detection of protein-protein interactions (Large BiT (LgBiT; 18 kDa) + Small BiT (SmBiT; 11 amino acid peptide)) expressed as fusions of proteins of interest. The technology of such systems has been radically improved and spectral resolution and a

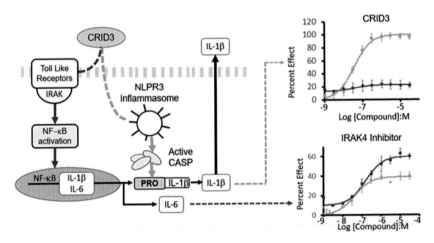

FIGURE 12.9 Determination of the target for CRID3. CRID3 reduces IL-8β but this can be observed through numerous pathways; the objective of these experiments is to determine if CRID3 targets the NLPR3 inflammasome. CRID3 reduces IL-1β but this can also occur through inhibition Toll-like receptors (an unwanted effect). Exploring multiple signaling pathways indicates that inhibitors of IRAK4 (an unwanted effect) depresses IL-1β levels and also reduces IL-6. This was not observed with CRID3, thereby indicating that the IRAK4 pathway is not involved in CRID3 activity. *Source: Data from Vincent F, Nueda A, Lee J, Schenone M, Prunotto M, Mercola M (2022) Phenotypic drug discovery: recent successes, lessons learned and new directions. Nature Rev Drug Disc 21: 899–914.*

greater dynamic range over current BRET technologies have been demonstrated. The small size of the NanoBiT complementation partners minimizes interference with normal protein function and the bright signal: improved sensitivity accommodates low, native expression levels. These experiments can now be done in real time in living cells, Fig. 12.10 shows dopamine receptor activation by dopamine and blockade of the response by sulpiride.

Finally, target engagement can be refined to detect not only what target a drug binds to but also what components of that target's capability to produce a response are activated. It is known that many receptors are pleiotropic with respect to the coupling proteins they interact with, and with the discovery of biased signaling, it cannot be assumed that all agonists activate the same links to the receptor or which of the links is therapeutically important. Knockouts of specific signaling proteins can be useful in this regard. Fig. 12.11 shows how parathyroid hormone (PTH) builds bone in a normal mouse but not in β-arrestin knockout mouse. This indicates that the $_{\beta}$-arrestin component of PTH signaling is the therapeutically relevant component of the agonism.

These techniques demonstrate target engagement in in vitro experiments but it is important to see that these same engagements occur in vivo. There are three components to this stage: (1) presence of the drug in the receptor compartment, (2) some indication that the drug engages the target in vivo, and (3) some indication that the engagement results in a therapeutically relevant response. Data for the first element (presence) results from pharmacokinetic studies. The second element involves an in vitro indication that the drug and target engage, or at least that the drug is in the vicinity of the target. There are two types of data to indicate this.

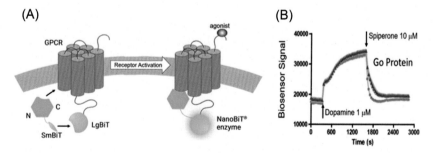

FIGURE 12.10 Biosensor for Go and the dopamine receptor. (A) Schematic shows how activation of the receptor recruits G protein binding and brings the large bit and small bit of the fluorescent biosensor in close proximity to give a signal. (B) Activation of the receptor by dopamine and blockade of response by sulpiride. Source: *Redrawn from Machleidt T et al. (2015) NanoBRET-A novel BRET platform for the analysis of protein − protein interactions. ACS Chem. Biol. 10:1797−1804.*

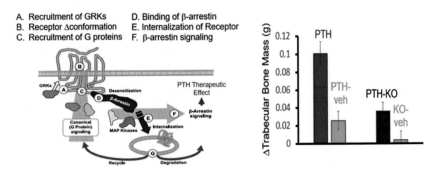

FIGURE 12.11 Identification of therapeutically relevant signaling pathway for para-thyroid hormone (PTH) bone building effects of osteoporosis. Panel on the left shows the variety of signaling mechanisms triggered by PTH receptor activation. Panel on the right shows PTH-induced increase in trabecular bone mouse in normal mice after PTH treat-ment (red column) and in β-arrestin knockout mice (blue column). *Source: Data redrawn from Ferrari SL et al. (2005) Bone response to intermittent parathyroid hormone is altered in mice null for β-Arrestin2. Endocrinol 146:1854−1862.*

The first is the observation of a biomarker (see Fig. 9.6). While the appearance of a biomarker after in vivo drug treatment is not direct evi-dence of target engagement, it does indicate that the drug enters the body and has some physiological effect. The second is a more direct indicator of target engagement and this can be attained through imag-ing. Specifically, this can be obtained with positron emission tomogra-phy (PET) where a very low amount of a radioactive substance (radionuclide or radioactive tracer) is used to determine the presence of the tracer in various tissues. There are two settings for PET scanning to denote drug presence: (1) utilize a radioactive congener of the molecule itself or (2) use the molecule to displace an externally administered radionuclide. Fig. 12.12 shows PET scans of various organs after admin-istration of a ^{18}F- analog of the antifungal fluconazole. The color spec-trum is used to quantify the amount of tracer in the tissue.

Showing, the presence of the drug in the correct location and target engagement still does not ensure a productive therapeutic effect, that is, drug effectiveness. However, the demonstration of presence in the correct therapeutic drug compartment and interaction with the therapeutic target is strong presumptive evidence favorable therapeutic effect. An example showing presumptive evidence of effectiveness is shown in Fig. 12.13 where a positive allosteric modulator of the mGLUR5 receptor is injected into mice. PET (displacement of a PET tracer for mGLUR5) indicates binding to the correct brain region (striatum) and, through separate in vivo behavioral studies, antipsychotic behavior is produced in a close approximation of the same concentration range. These studies link in vivo presence, target engagement, and effectiveness for this molecule.

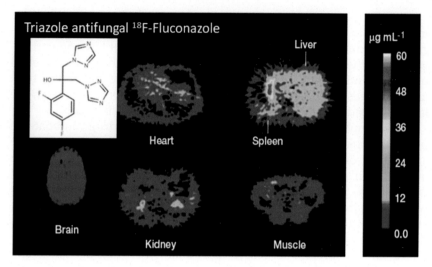

FIGURE 12.12 Positron emission tomography (PET) scans of ^{18}F-fluconazole. Color code denotes that fluconazole concentrates in the spleen. Source: *From Rudin M, Weissleder R. (2003) Molecular imaging in drug discovery and development. Nature Rev. Drug Disc. 2:123−131.*

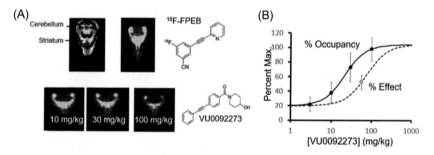

FIGURE 12.13 Displacement of a PET imaging tracer for mGLU5 receptors showing binding of a positive allosteric modulator (VU0092273) in the cerebellum. (A) Concentration dependent decrease in tracer binding. (B) Percent displacement of tracer from data in panel A (solid line, filled circles) and percent effect of VU0092273 on reversal of amphetamine-induced hyperlocomotion (indicative of antipsychotic activity). *PET,* Positron emission tomography. Source: *(A) From Rook JM et al. (2015) Relationship between in vivo receptor occupancy and efficacy of metabotropic glutamate receptor subtype 5 allosteric modulators with different in vitro binding profiles. Neuropsychopharmacol 40: 755−765. (B) Data for hyperlocomotion from Noetzel MJ et al. (2012) Functional impact of allosteric agonist activity of selective positive allosteric modulators of metabotropic glutamate receptor subtype 5 in regulating central nervous system. Mol Pharmacol. 81: 120−133.*

The foregoing discussion illustrates techniques for showing the engagement of a molecule with a target for a single target disease and how this may be sufficient for associating the target binding with therapeutic effect. However, sometimes, multiple targets are required to be modified in some diseases (i.e., schizophrenia, depression) and drugs may need to practice "polypharmacology" and engage multiple targets—see Box 12.4. A variant of this idea are drugs that have no particular target other than the whole cell. For example, antibodies with lethal payloads (anticancer drugs, radioactive tracers) can be targeted to bind to cancer cells that then absorb them in the cytosol. Once absorbed, the lethal payload becomes free to kill the tumor cell—see Box 12.5.

Once a molecule has been identified as a potential drug candidate its pharmacologic characteristics should be completely characterized. There are two reasons for this; the first is to prepare researchers for what the molecule will do in much more complex in vivo systems and the second is to identify profiles that, should the first molecule fail, the follow-up will not share. There are basically three types of pharmacologically active molecular patterns; agonism, antagonism, and allosteric modulation and checklists for the possible variations of these should be completed in the process of characterization. After the detection and

---

BOX 12.4

Some diseases may require "magic shotguns"

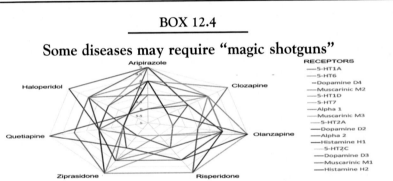

An attractive feature of the target-based discovery strategy is the relative simplicity of need to concentrate on only one target and optimize drug activity for that single target. Unfortunately, that is not always an optimal strategy for the treatment of some complex CNS disorders, such as schizophrenia and depression. For example, a review of atypical antipsychotic drugs indicates that the most successful antipsychotics have multiple activities at multiple receptors suggesting that this type of pan receptor activity is the discerning feature determining effective therapy. The radar plot shows the pKi (-log affinity) for 7 atypical antipsychotic drugs for 12 receptors. Data from Roth BL, Sheffler DJ, Kroeze WK (2004) Magic shotguns versus magic bullets: selectively nonselective drugs for mood disorders and schizophrenia Nature Rev Drug Disc 3: 353–359.

BOX 12.5
_____

Providing cancer with a lethal Trojan horse

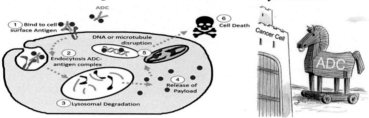

There are cases where there is no particular molecular target for the drug other than to achieve a given end result; such a case is the killing of cancer cells. Antibody drug complexes (ADC's) are antibodies targeted to cancer cells that carry with a lethal payload (often an anticancer drug or radioactive killer molecule). As cells bind and absorb these antibodies, the antibody becomes consumed by the cell proteolysis system and the poisonous payload is released within the cell to cause cell death.

---

collection of prospective active molecules from a screen, dose-response relationships for these molecules must be established and each pharmacologically characterized.

For *agonists*, the following effects should be determined:

- Agonist potency (pEC$_{50}$) and preferably affinity (K_A) and efficacy (τ); for full agonists, determine Log(τ/K_A)—see Chapter 3, Predicting Agonist Effect
- Agonist external cell (receptor) selectivity: relative potency (and or Log (τ/K_A) values) of the molecule on primary versus secondary receptors
- Agonist internal selectivity (bias): the number of signaling pathways that are activated by the agonist and the relative activity (in the form of $\Delta\Delta$Log(τ/K_A) values) of the molecule for each pathway (signaling bias).

For *antagonists*, the following must be determined:

- Antagonist potency (affinity): pK_B value for the primary receptor
- Antagonist selectivity: pK_B values for other relevant receptors
- Efficacy: positive efficacy (leading to weak agonism in sensitive tissues) or negative efficacy (leading to inverse agonism in constitutively active systems and possible antagonist tolerance with chronic use)

- Target residence time: the rate of offset of the antagonism determines how well it will block the receptor in vivo.

For *allosteric modulators*, the following must be determined:

- The maximal degree of sensitization (magnitudes of α and β-see chapter: Allosteric Drug Effects) for the natural agonist
- The binding potency, which for PAMs will be related to α in the form of K_B/α.
- Binding potency for NAMs as pK_B value
- Probe dependence: for multiple natural agonists, α/β values for each separate agonist
- Determination of possible induced bias on natural signaling (determine α and β values for selective signaling pathways).

The lead optimization process consists of synthetic chemistry applied to a chemically tractable scaffold to modify activity to optimize a defined index of drug activity. For example, Fig. 12.14 shows a series of pK_B values for receptor antagonists; in this case, increased potency is the goal. It can be seen that the first 10 compounds had an approximate mean pK_B value of 4.4. Progress is gauged by molecules that exceed the 95% confidence limits of the values of the previous molecules. As seen in Fig. 12.14, the 11th molecule in the series has a pK_B of 5.2, which exceeds the 95% limits of the previous set of molecules. This defines a step forward for future structural manipulation; it can be seen that the 95% limits of the molecules in the second iteration are exceeded by molecule 18 ($pK_B = 6.25$). The third iteration produced a molecule with $pK_B = 7.0$ (exceeds a previous 95% c. l. of previous molecules) and

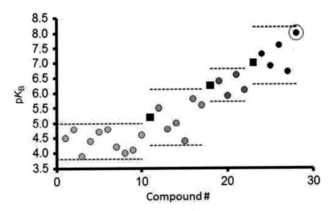

FIGURE 12.14 pK_B values for 28 potential antagonist candidates in chronological progression. The filled squares represent compounds that break out of the 95% confidence limits of the previous compounds and yield a higher pK_B than previous compounds (represent a way forward).

continued work produced a goal compound of $pK_B = 8.0$. Frequently, there are multiple goals, such as target potency and also target selectivity and the structure-activity relationships for these two goals may be independent. This leads to a more complex iterative process of synthesis toward the candidate molecule.

Drug development

The more criteria there are for drug candidacy, the more complex this process becomes; increased criteria come from building drug-like activity (adequate ADME properties) and safety into the scaffold. 12.15 shows a typical inflection point in the lead optimization process that was encountered for the final drug maraviroc, an HIV-1 entry inhibitor. It can be seen from this figure, that various R groups led to molecules that had good permeation but poor hepatic stability and vice versa (Fig. 12.15).

The introduction of drug-like activity recruits the various assays quantifying permeation, and stability into the process by the overall scheme

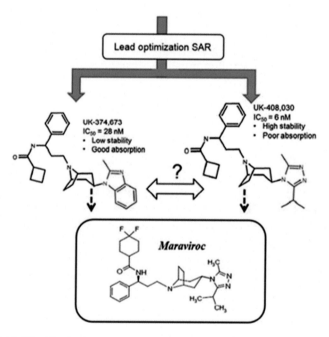

FIGURE 12.15 The lead optimization process. From the initial screening hit for the HIV-1 entry inhibitor maraviroc, two scaffolds showed divergent activity on permeation and hepatic stability. Such bifurcations in activity are common in the lead optimization process and judgments as to the utility of various chemical moieties must be made.

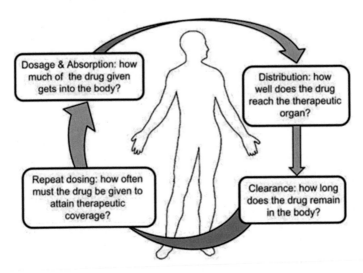

FIGURE 12.16   ADME studies aim to answer four questions regarding the in vivo therapeutic use of the new drug candidate.

for drug discovery as outlined in Fig. 11.2. The pharmacokinetic profile of a new drug candidate basically seeks to answer four questions of a dosage given in vivo: (1) how much will be absorbed into the body? (2) where will it distribute in the body? (3) how long with the drug remain in the body? and (4) how often must the drug be administered to attain a therapeutic steady-state concentration in the bloodstream (Fig. 12.16)?

The dramatic improvement in the quality of assays for predicting ADME properties is largely responsible for the elimination of pharmacokinetics as the roadblock it once was in drug development—see Box 12.6.

If a substantial correlation exists between LogP (or LogD) values, then theoretically modification of the LogP may eliminate unwanted activity in the target molecule. For instance, the β-adrenoceptor blockade scaffold shown in Fig. 12.17 shows a correlation of LogP with inhibitory activity for Cyp3A4, (which could lead to a drug-drug interaction). If a region of the molecule could be found that did not interfere with β-adrenoceptor activity, then reduction of the LogP may eliminate the Cyp3A4 activity; this is suggested by the addition of the hydroxyl group, which could reduce the Ki for Cyp3A4 activity 30-fold.

Clinical testing

The endpoint of discovery and development studies to furnish a bona fide drug candidate that can be used to cure or alleviate the

BOX 12.6

The power of PK assays

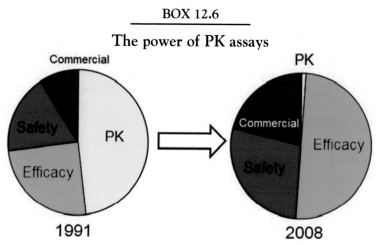

In 1991 lack of adequate pharmacokinetic properties accounted for 49% of new drug candidate failures. By the year 2000 this was reduced to 12% and by 2008 to nearly insignificant levels (1%). Thus at present, there is little reason to suppose that a new molecule will fail because of inadequate ADME properties. The reason for this impressive improvement is the availability of new inexpensive and facile in vitro assays to measure permeation into cells, effects on transport and efflux processes and stability of molecules. This latter factor stems from the availability of hepatic enzyme preparations (in the form of microsomes, S9 and hepatocytes) from animal species and humans. With these tools, the correct predictive species can be identified to link PK effects from animals to humans.

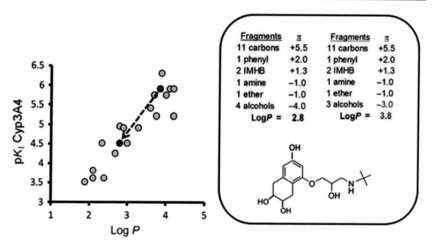

Fragments	π		Fragments	π
11 carbons	+5.5		11 carbons	+5.5
1 phenyl	+2.0		1 phenyl	+2.0
2 IMHB	+1.3		2 IMHB	+1.3
1 amine	−1.0		1 amine	−1.0
1 ether	−1.0		1 ether	−1.0
4 alcohols	−4.0		3 alcohols	−3.0
LogP =	2.8		LogP =	3.8

FIGURE 12.17 Addition of the hydroxyl group to the β-adrenoceptor scaffold would reduce LogP by 1 log unit and possibly reduce Cyp3A4 activity 30-fold.

symptoms of disease. The type of therapeutic environment for the drug is important and may modify the criteria for candidate progression. If the treatment has a clear endpoint (i.e., removal of an infection), the treatment is of short duration or the disease is intractable, and lethal then certain concessions on safety may be allowed. Ultimately it becomes a balance of the least harm done; administering a drug that may have some toxicity versus denial of a life-saving treatment. Modern views on this balance take into account new technology to assess this risk: four considerations are [4]:

1. What is the safety margin? This can depend on the nature of the dose-limiting adverse event, the intended patient population, the therapeutic indication being sought, the competitive environment and present standard of care.
2. Is the toxicity reversible? Irreversible toxicity is unacceptable
3. Is there a biomarker? Without the ability to monitor toxicity, it could become irreversible.
4. What is the mechanism? This could speak to the question is the toxicity species specific?

The next step is to design a statistically robust clinical trial to assess the effects of the drug in humans and the first step for that is to determine a starting dose. Clearly, if this is too high (and thus enters into concentrations that could cause toxicity) then harm can be done. Alternatively, if the dose is too low, then large amounts of resources could be wasted as the study progresses through periods where nothing is observed.

Once clinical trials are anticipated then human safety must be considered as well as pharmacokinetics. Starting doses for human trials incorporate animal data in the norm of no observed adverse effect levels (NOAELs); Fig. 12.18A shows the NOAELs for a drug in four animal species and how this can be correlated with clearance; assuming the clearance in these four species is similar to clearance in humans, this may predict a NOAEL in humans. There are several methods to predict the starting dose for human clinical studies; Fig. 12.18B shows a retrospective on predicted starting doses for nine drugs that have undergone clinical trials compared to the actual dose range of the clinical trial. As can be seen, all but one of the predictions fell within the actual range tested.

Once the parameters of the proposed clinical trial have been established, permission to do the trial must be obtained; this is permission for an IND (Investigational New Drug Application). Specifically, this is a request for a Phase I study (safety in healthy volunteers), Phase II (safety and efficacy in small patient population), and Phase III (pivotal safety and efficacy in diverse patient population) trials. The IND must contain information about the design of clinical trial(s) and descriptions preclinical pharmacology, safety, ADME, and toxicology, a compendium of

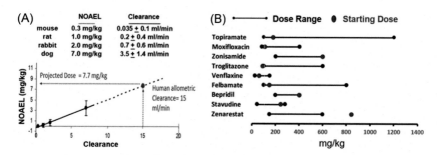

FIGURE 12.18 Determination of first-time dose in humans for clinical testing. A NOAEL (No Observed Adverse Effect Level) is determined in animal species to gauze the safety profile of a candidate. Insofar as these values can be linked to in vivo concentrations, one approach to making predictions is to correlate the clearance of the drug in each species with the NOAEL. In panel A, the NOAEL of a drug is correlated with clearance in each species to produce a regression that could predict the NOAEL in humans. Panel B shows the predicted first-time starting dose in humans (red dot) for nine drugs and the real starting and ending doses of the trials for those drugs. In all cases, except for Zenarestat, the prediction fell within the actual experimental range. Source: *Data redrawn from Mahmood I, Green MD, Fisher JE. (2003) Selection of the first-time dose in humans: comparison of different approaches based on interspecies scaling of clearance. J Clin Pharmacol 43:692–697.*

chemistry and manufacturing controls, and description of proposed use of clinical trials material in humans. Should an IND be successful, then an new drug approval (NDA) is requested. Clinical trials should have social value, scientific validity, fair subject selection with respect for human subjects, and informed consent, offer a favorable risk-benefit ratio, and be subject to independent review. In terms of cost, effort and time, **Phase 0** trials are the lowest. These employ 1/100 of the active dose for any effect and are mainly done to obtain PK data that is, negative data, such as the compound is not absorbed. They rely on radiolabeled substance and track location and amount of drug in the body through PET imaging. They are of short duration (7 days to 1 month), done at low cost ($1M–2M) and have a low number of subjects (as low as 10). Phase 0 trials are mainly done for cancer drugs (i.e., does the compound enter the tumor?). The next level is the **Phase I** trial. These trials are run mainly to assess safety and are the first time where drug is tried in humans. A secondary aim of Phase I trials is to assess Pharmacokinetics and Pharmacodynamics. These trials usually are run in healthy subjects although critically ill patients may be given the option after considering risk/benefit ratio. They usually are open label, have between 10 and 100 subjects and may take several months to 1 year (at a cost of approximately $10 M). Should a drug not show safety issues and appear to be absorbed adequately, then the process progresses to **Phase II** trials. This is where the safety and effectiveness of the drug in targeted disease groups are examined. These trials often utilize biomarkers (definitive or surrogate). Definitive biomarkers show therapeutic outcomes; for example, in a study of hypertension, a definitive biomarker would be incidence of stroke. For a cancer study, a definitive biomarker would be mortality. Surrogate biomarkers are indirect; for hypertension a surrogate would be cholesterol level, for cancer tumor size, levels of p53, or TGF-α. Phase I trials are aimed at the determination of effective dosing regimen, frequency and duration of effect. They contain between 50 and 500 subjects, may be several months to 1–2 years in length and have a cost of >$20 M. At this point many drugs fail, that is, success rate of Phases I/II ≈ 30%. In a phase II trial, if the new drug is designed to test if it is better than existing treatment then the trial design must include data to show that the existing treatment provided benefit (over placebo); if this is not done then the trial is invalid. This is because if the trial does not demonstrate existing treatment is effective, then the FDA assumes the sponsors did not know how to design a proper trial. The next step toward drug approval are **Phase III** trials (at least 2 are required); these trials are designed to confirm the efficacy of a drug in a large patient group. These trials (conducted in several locations (multisite trial) to determine effect of ethnic responses) set the dosage, treatment frequency, duration and target patient groups for the drug. They involve several hundreds to thousands of patients, can be 3–5 years in duration and cost approximately $50 M to $100 M. In Phase III trials, if a drug does not show overall improvement over existing treatment, changes may be made to analyze certain subgroups in efforts to determine if effects are greater in one group over another. This process could define parameters for understanding the safety and effectiveness of the drug.

Data from Phase III trials are subject to extensive and detailed statistical analysis. Such analyses are designed to detect two types of error. The first is a Type I error (denoted α, a false positive). If this error occurs, then the trial would wrongly conclude that a difference exists when in fact there is no real difference. This would put a useless medicine on the market. The criteria for Type I errors are usually $\alpha < 5\%$ (95% certainty). A second type or error is a Type II error (β, false negative); these are more serious as they would wrongly conclude there is no difference when in fact there is a difference. The outcome of this would be to keep a good medicine away from patients. The criteria for Type II errors are usually $\beta = 0.05 - 0.2$ (80%–95% certainty).

In general, statistical analyses determine four main questions:

1. Central Tendency: What is the true value?
2. Variability: How accurate is the estimate?
3. Difference: Did the intervention produce a real difference?
4. Verisimilitude to Models: Are we entitled to apply a complex model to the data?

An important tool in statistical procedures is the manipulation of the power of the analysis. Power analysis takes into consideration the level of difference researchers wants to determine (denoted δ) and the level of risk they wish to take that they are wrong (90%, 95%?). Given this, the analysis yields the number of replicates (n) required to meet those criteria. An example of how power analysis is used is should in Fig. 12.19. Several replicates of a value measured experimentally will yield a bell-shaped curve of the frequencies of the values versus the values. The peak of the curve will show the mean value and the width of the curve will show the relative similarity of values to the mean. Thus a wide curve represents a wide distribution of values from considerably lower to considerably higher than the mean, that is, a high level of uncertainty. As the number of replicates increases, the curve becomes less wide and there is less difference between individual values and the mean, that is, less uncertainty. In a clinical trial, there is usually a value to improve whether it be a dosage or therapeutic readout and a data sample yield a bell-shaped curve of those values around a mean. As the new drug is tested, a new population of values will be generated with a new distribution; the difference in the means is the δ value and is the main criterion for quality of improvement. The respective areas under each curve are a measure of the distribution and the convergence of the control and experimental curves may produce a commonality whereby there is no difference between the treatments; these are the shaded areas in

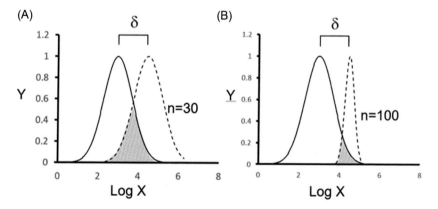

FIGURE 12.19 Distributions of repeated estimates of the potency of a standard therapy (lefthand curve) and a new therapy. When 30 subjects were tested for the new therapy, there was a difference in the mean potency (designated as δ) but it can be seen that there is approximately a 30% crossover of values between the standard and the new therapy (shaded area). If more subjects are added to the estimate for the experimental therapy, the distribution narrows and it can be seen so too does the area shared by the two curves, that is, there is increased confidence in the estimate of difference between the two means.

Fig. 12.19. The larger the common area, the less confidence there can be that δ is significant, that is, the mean values are different. In panel 12.19 A, the common area for a sample of 30 patients is approximately 25% of the area of the control curve; this translates into a 75% level of confidence that the values are actually different. In Fig. 12.19B, a sample of 100 patients necessarily improves the accuracy of the mean value (curve is less wide) and shows that the common area is now about 5%; this leads to an increased confidence value that the mean values are different to a level of 95%. It can be seen that power analysis demonstrates that increasing the number of replicates increases the confidence in difference estimates and will also allow for greater discernment of small differences.

Another powerful statistical tool is hypothesis testing. This is a procedure that allows the comparison of data between the two models to discern, which one of them best fits the data. The models are usually chosen to be of varying complexity, that is, one is a "simple" model and the other a "complex" model. Fig. 12.20 shows an example of this procedure. A set of data is shown, which could be simply a random array of replicates or a *bona fide* dose-response curve. Thus the data is fit to the simple model (the mean of the replicates) (Fig. 12.20A) and a complex model (a four parameter logistic function defining a sigmoidal curve) (Fig. 12.20B). How well the models fit is assessed through a sum of squares, which is the sum of the squares of the differences between each value and the value calculated by the model:

$$SSq = \sum (x - x_m)^2 \tag{12.2}$$

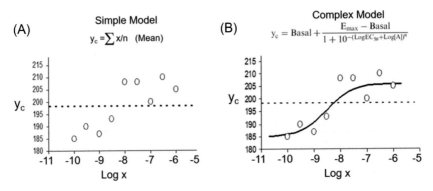

FIGURE 12.20 An array of ordinate values (responses to a drug) is shown in panel A. There is no supposed pattern to this dataset and it can be assumed to be a representation of a mean potency (simple model). Panel B shows the same dataset fit to a formal pattern (4 parameter logistic function) thereby assuming a dose-response relationship (complex model). Hypothesis testing calculates whether the complex model (and better fit) can legitimately be applied to the dataset.

The better fit is denoted by the lower SSq value. A statistical value denoted F is then calculated by comparing the SSq values for the fits to the simple (SSq_s) and the complex (SSq_c) models:

$$F = \frac{(SSq_s - SSq_c)/(df_s - df_c)}{(SSq_c)/df_c} \tag{12.3}$$

Each SSq value has an associate parameter called the degrees of freedom (df). This value denotes any possible constraint on the value imposed by the model. In the case above, the simple model (mean value) has no constraint so the degrees of freedom are equal to the number of values; in the example in Fig. 12.20A $n = 10$ so $df = 10$. In the case of the complex model, however, the outcome has four constraints, namely, the values of basal. E_{max}, slope n and EC_{50}, therefore the df for the complex model is n-4; example in Fig. 12.20B $n = 10$, $df = 6$. The object of calculating F is not to determine the better fit. The complex model will always be a better fit ($SSq_c = 5.34$ while $SSq_s = 31.19$) but there is a penalty to fitting a very complex model with arbitrary parameters set to control the fit. This begs the question "what gives us the right to impose the constraints of basal, E_{max} n and EC_{50} on the dataset?" and that doubt is reflected in the reduced df. The values of SSq and df are compared in a statistical F table, which penalizes such constraints in the form of artificially reducing the SSq needed to get a large value of F. If the experimental value of F is larger than the F in the table (chosen for a given level of confidence), then this states that we have the right to assume the complex model is a better fit. For the example shown in Fig. 12.20 the calculated value of F is 9.1; for a $p < 0.05$ (95% confidence) value of F from a two-tailed F table (column for df_c and row df_s) is 7.87. Since the experimental F is greater than the F from the table, this means that with 95% certainty, the dataset represents a dose-response curve and not a random array. Hypothesis testing is used extensively to compare various models in experimental and clinical pharmacology.

There is a final phase of "testing" called **Phase IV** where, once the drug is approved, continued surveillance is maintained to check for untoward effects. This is done to take advantage of the enormous increase in data received once the drug is approved. Whereas 3000–5000 patients provide data for Phase III studies, this increases to millions after drug approval. Thus very low incidence of toxicity would be detected at this stage that would not have been detected in Phase III (note the example of Vioxx given in chapter 10). Phase IV trials are also called postmarketing approval trials and are designed to monitor side effects of drugs in uncontrolled real-life situations. The main focus is on detecting rare side effects, cost effectiveness, and monitoring the patient's quality of life. In addition, Phase IV trials can furnish data to give additional indications for the drug. They also provide pharmacoeconomic data obtained to convince health care payers that new drug offers significant benefit over existing therapy (time to recovery, quality of life).

Possibly the most significant hurdle for a new drug candidate to overcome is the transition from activity in phase 1 and 2 clinical trials to phase 3 trial activity in patients. The former trials are considered "efficacy" trials where the main objective is to demonstrate that the drug has some effect and is also safe. Efforts are taken at this stage to reduce noise in the baseline activity of the patient population so that even small effects can be detected (see Fig. 12.21). Accordingly, the patient population is restricted to providing a uniform baseline and homogeneous sample for drug testing. In contrast, in phase 3 trials (considered "effectiveness" trials) the patient population is heterogeneous and the baseline can be extremely noisy. Under these circumstances, a modest drug effect may well be lost in the level of baseline noise and thus go unnoticed [5]. This would translate to a loss of effectiveness of the drug in the therapeutic situation.

In general, an enormous dataset is evaluated to determine whether a new molecule has the efficacy, drug-like properties and safety profile

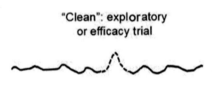

"Clean": exploratory or efficacy trial

Efficacy trial
- Narrow patient selection
- Clear definition of concomitant medication
- Monitor patient adherence
- Intergroup difference easily detected

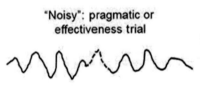

"Noisy": pragmatic or effectiveness trial

Effectiveness trial
- More heterogeneous population
- Treatment resembles everyday clinical practice
- Signal may be lost in noise

FIGURE 12.21 Effect of a modest drug effect (broken line) amongst the low variability in an efficacy trial (phase 1 and 2) versus the much higher variability and noise level in an effectiveness trial (phase 3). Source: Redrawn from H.-C. Eichler, E. Abadie, A. Breckenridge, B. Flamion, L.L. Gustafsson, H. Leufkens, et al., Bridging the efficacy—effectiveness gap: a regulator's perspective on addressing variability of drug response. Nat. Rev. Drug Discov. 10 (2011) 495—506.

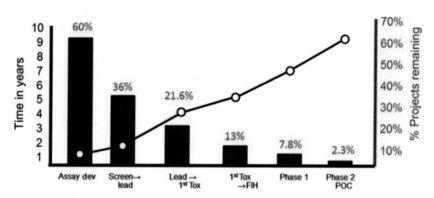

FIGURE 12.22 Graph showing the percentage of projects remaining after various phases of a discovery/development project (blue bars) and the number of years spent in that particular phase (line with open circles).

required to be used therapeutically in humans. As seen in Fig. 11.3, the process of drug discovery spans the time taken from identification of the therapeutic need, biological target, assessment of which chemical intervention may be appropriate to address the need, consideration of other factors, such as market, cost, and tractability, through the detection of a hit (screening) to the chemical optimization of the hit to a tractable lead. The milestone at this point is the choice of drug candidate, which then progresses into testing in humans (phase 1, 2, and 3 clinical trial). Fig. 12.22 shows a typical chronology for this process; it should be noted that the therapeutic area can modify these estimates as discussed previously in this chapter with the extended time required for central nervous system drugs. An important theme in this process is one of "fail fast-fail early," a way of stating that it is in the best interests of the discovery program if compounds that will fail in late stages of the process be identified early on so as not to waste precious resources for other better compounds. Approximately, 64% of projects fail before they reach the lead optimization stage. This may be because no molecules could be found in screening that fulfill criteria or that the molecules found did not possess the chemical tractability to allow synthetic manipulation to alter activity.

Summary

- Fitting data to quantitative pharmacologic models (defined by mathematical equations) allows the differentiation of pharmacologic mechanisms (defining behaviors) and random coincidence of patterns of response

- The fact that the models have mathematical equations defining the behavior of the model under a variety of conditions allows prediction of drug effect under different circumstances (i.e., in vivo).
- The two main approaches to demonstrating target engagement of ligands with a defined target are: (1) demonstration of physical interaction, and (2) demonstration of effect after ligand-target cobinding
- Development changes in chemical scaffolds can be, and often are, introduced early on in the drug development process in attempts to optimize drug-like activity.
- The data from clinical trials are aimed at identifying two types of statistical error: Type 1 error where an ineffective drug candidate is approved for therapy, and Type 2 error where an effective therapy is deemed inactive and patients are deprived of a useful new medicine.
- While Phase I and II trials are designed to determine safety, pharmacokinetics and effect, Phase III trials are aimed at determining therapeutic effect in patients. The difference is that the patient selection in Phase I and II trials is designed to be uniform (to determine possible low-level effects), the patient baseline response in Phase III trials is high and low-level responses are often not identified. Thus many drugs fail in Phase III trials.

References

[1] C.M. Guldberg, P. Waage. Studies concerning affinity. C. M. Forhandlinger: Videnskabs-Selskabet i Christiana 1864; 35.
[2] C.M. Guldberg, P. Waage, Concerning chemical affinity, Erdmann's J. Pr. Chem. 127 (1879) 69–114.
[3] M. Metra, L. Dei Cas, A. di Lenarda, P. Poole-Wilson, Beta-blockers in heart failure: are pharmacological differences clinically important? Heart Fail. Rev. 9 (2004) 123–130.
[4] J.A. Kramer, J.E. Sagartz, D.L. Morris, The application of discovery toxicology and pathology towards the design of safer pharmaceutical lead candidates, Nat. Rev. Drug. Disc 6 (2007) 636–649.
[5] H.-C. Eichler, E. Abadie, A. Breckenridge, B. Flamion, L.L. Gustafsson, H. Leufkens. Bridging the efficacy–effectiveness gap: a regulator's perspective on addressing variability of drug response. Nat. Rev. Drug Discov. 10 (2011) 495–506.

A

Derivations and proofs

Successive saturable functions leads to amplification of signals

For Chapter 1

In a cell, biochemical reactions function in series, whereby the product of one reaction becomes the substrate for the next, etc. In these types of systems, the sensitivity of the complete system to an initial substrate will always be higher than the sensitivity of any one step in the system. Thus, the K_{eq} for a series of reactions will always be of lower magnitude than the K_{eq} for any one step.

Cellular stimulus–response coupling is represented by a series arrangement of saturable functions of the form:

$$\text{Output}_1 = \frac{[\text{Input}_1]}{[\text{Input}_1] + K_1} \tag{A.1}$$

Under these circumstances, the midpoint (sensitivity) of the function defined by Eq. (A.1) is K_1. A series arrangement leads to the output from one function becoming the input for the next, thus, the output from a second function in the series is:

$$\text{Output}_2 = \frac{[\text{Output}_1]}{[\text{Output}_1] + K_2} \tag{A.2}$$

Substituting for output$_1$ from Eq. (A.1), the equation for output$_2$ is:

$$\text{Output}_2 = \frac{[\text{Input}_1]}{[\text{Input}_1] + (1 + K_2) + K_1 K_2} \tag{A.3}$$

Rearranging to isolate input$_1$ yields:

$$\text{Output}_2 = \frac{[\text{Input}_1]}{[\text{Input}_1] + \frac{K_1 K_2}{(1 + K_2)}} \tag{A.4}$$

The sensitivity for $output_2$ (denoted $K_{observed}$), in terms of $input_1$, is given by:

$$K_{observed} = \frac{K_1 K_2}{(1 + K_2)} \tag{A.5}$$

It can be seen from Eq. (A.5) that for all nonzero values of K_2, $(1 + K_2)$ > K_2, $K_{observed}$ will always be $<K_1$. Thus, the equilibrium constant for the series of reactions is always less than the equilibrium constant for a single reaction. This means that series saturable functions always amplify initial signals.

The potency of a full agonist depends on both affinity and efficacy

For Chapter 2

Denoting the affinity of a molecule as K_A and the efficacy as τ (see Chapter 3, Predicting Agonist Effect, for details on this parameter), the response to an agonist is given by (see Chapter 3, Predicting Agonist Effect, for explanation of this equation and Eq. (A.3) for derivation):

$$Response = \frac{E_m \cdot [A] \cdot \tau}{[A](1 + \tau) + K_A} \tag{A.6}$$

where E_m is the maximal response of the system. It can be seen that as $[A] \to \infty$, the maximal response (Max) is given by:

$$Max = \frac{E_m \cdot \tau}{(1 + \tau)} \tag{A.7}$$

Defining the EC_{50} as the point where response is half maximal E_m defines the following equality:

$$0.5 = \frac{[EC_{50}](1 + \tau)}{[EC_{50}](1 + \tau) + K_A} \tag{A.8}$$

Under these circumstances, the equation for EC_{50} for a partial agonist reduces to:

$$EC_{50} = \frac{K_A}{(1 + \tau)} \tag{A.9}$$

It can be seen from Eq. (A.9) that EC_{50} is a function of both affinity (K_A) and efficacy (τ).

Derivation of the Black−Leff operational model

For Chapter 3

Beginning with a form of the Michaelis−Menten equation for enzymes:

$$\text{Response} = \frac{[A]E_m}{[A] + \nu} \tag{A.10}$$

where the concentration of agonist is [A], E_m is the maximal response of the system, and ν is a fitting parameter for the hyperbolic function, then the concentration of drug [A] can be expressed as:

$$[A] = \frac{\text{Response} \cdot \nu}{E_m[A] - \text{Response}} \tag{A.11}$$

Mass action defines the concentration of agonist-receptor complex as:

$$[AR] = \frac{[A] \cdot [R_t]}{[A] + K_A} \tag{A.12}$$

where $[R_t]$ is the receptor density and K_A is the equilibrium dissociation constant of the agonist-receptor complex. A second function for [A] can then be derived:

$$[A] = \frac{[AR] \cdot K_A}{[R_t] - [AR]} \tag{A.13}$$

Equating Eqs. (A.11) and (A.13) and rearranging yields:

$$\text{Response} = \frac{[AR] \cdot E_m \cdot K_A}{[A](K_A - \nu) + [R_t]\nu} \tag{A.14}$$

If $K_A < \nu$ then negative and/or infinite values for response are allowed (no physiological counterpart to such behavior exists). Therefore, this allows only a linear relationship between agonist concentration and response (where $K_A = \nu$) or a hyperbolic one ($K_A > \nu$). Very few cases of truly linear relationships between agonist concentration and tissue response can be found; therefore, the default for the relationship is a hyperbolic one.

A hyperbolic relationship between response and the amount of agonist-receptor complex, response is defined as:

$$\frac{\text{Response}}{E_{max}} = \frac{[AR]}{[AR] + K_E} \tag{A.15}$$

where K_E is the fitting parameter for the hyperbolic response. K_E has a pharmacological meaning in that it is the concentration of the [AR] complex that produces half the maximal response and it defines the ease with which the agonist produces response (i.e., it is a transduction constant). The more efficient the process from production of [AR] to response the smaller is K_E. Combining Eqs. (A.14) and (A.15) yields the primary equation for the operational model:

$$\text{Response} = \frac{[A] \cdot [R_t] \cdot E_m}{[A]([R_t] + K_E) + K_A \cdot K_E} \tag{A.16}$$

A constant is defined that characterizes the propensity of a given system and a given agonist to yield response as the ratio $[R_t]/K_E$. This is denoted by τ. Substituting for τ yields the working equation for the operational model (Eq. 3.3):

$$\text{Response} = \frac{[A] \cdot \tau \cdot E_m}{[A](\tau + 1) + K_A} \tag{A.17}$$

Derivation of variable slope Black–Leff operational model

For Chapter 3

If the stimulus-response coupling mechanism has inherent cooperativity, then a model with variable slope must be defined. The method for doing this involves re-expressing the receptor occupancy and/or activation expression (defined by the particular molecular model of receptor function) in terms of the operational model with a Hill coefficient not equal to unity. The operational model utilizes the concentration of response-producing receptor as the substrate for a Michaelis–Menten type of reaction, given as:

$$\text{Response} = \frac{[\text{Activated Receptor}]E_m}{[\text{Activated Receptor}] + K_E} \tag{A.18}$$

where K_E is the concentration of activated receptor species that produces half-maximal response in the cell and E_{max} is the maximal capability of response production by the cell. Cooperativity expressed at the level of the cell can be expressed as a form of Eq. (A.18) shown as:

$$\text{Response} = \frac{[\text{Activated Receptor}]^n E_m}{[\text{Activated Receptor}]^n + K_{E^n}} \tag{A.19}$$

where n is the slope of the concentration-response curve. The quantity of activated receptor is given by $\rho_{AR} \times [R_t]$, where ρ_{AR} is the fraction of total receptor in the activated form and $[R_t]$ is the total receptor density of the preparation. Substituting into Eq. (A.19) and defining $\tau = [R_t]/K_E$ yields:

$$\text{Response} = \frac{\rho_{AR^n} \tau^n E_m}{\rho_{AR^n} \tau^n + 1} \tag{A.20}$$

The fractional receptor species ρ_{AR} is generally given by:

$$\rho_{AR^n} = \frac{[\text{Active Receptor Species}]^n}{[\text{Total Receptor Species}]^n} \qquad (A.21)$$

where the active receptor species are the ones producing response and the total receptor species is given by the receptor conservation equation for the particular system (ρ_{AR} = numerator/denominator). It follows that:

$$\text{Response} = \frac{(\text{Active Receptor})^n \tau^n E_m}{(\text{Active Receptor})^n \tau^n + (\text{Total Receptor})^n} \qquad (A.22)$$

Therefore, the operational model for agonism can be rewritten for variable slope by passing the stimulus equation through a forcing function to yield (see Fig. 3.5):

$$\text{Response} = \frac{\tau^n \cdot [A]^n \cdot E_m}{([A]+K_A)^n + \tau^n(A)^n} \qquad (A.23)$$

Derivation of the Gaddum equation for competitive antagonism

For Chapter 4

Analogous to competitive displacement binding, agonist [A] and antagonist [B] compete for receptor (R) occupancy:

$$A + R \xrightleftharpoons{K_a} AR \qquad (A.24)$$

where K_a and K_b are the respective ligand-receptor association constants.
The following equilibrium constants are defined:

$$[R] = \frac{[AR]}{[A]K_a} \qquad (A.25)$$

$$[BR] = K_b[B][R] = \frac{K_b[B][AR]}{[A]K_a} \qquad (A.26)$$

$$\text{Total receptor concentration } [R_{tot}] = [R] + [AR] + [BR] \qquad (A.27)$$

Leading to the expression for the response-producing species [AR]/[R_{tot}] (denoted as ρ):

$$\rho = \frac{[A]K_a}{[A]K_a + [B]K_b + 1} \qquad (A.28)$$

Converting to equilibrium dissociation constants ($K_A = 1/K_a$) and redefining $[A]/K_A = C_A$ and $[B]/K_B = C_B$ leads to the Gaddum equation (Eq. 4.1):

$$\rho = \frac{C_A}{C_A + C_B + 1} \tag{A.29}$$

Correction of IC$_{50}$ to pK$_B$ for competitive antagonists

As shown by Leff and Dougall (Chapter 4, Drug Antagonism Orthosteric Drug Effects; Ref. [3]) mass action equations can be used to derive the relationship between the concentration of antagonist that produces a 50% inhibition of a response to an agonist (antagonist concentration is referred to as the IC$_{50}$) and the equilibrium dissociation constant of the antagonist-receptor complex (K_B). The response in the absence of an antagonist can be fit to a logistic curve of the form:

$$\text{Response} = \frac{E_m[A]^n}{[A]^n + [EC_{50}]^n} \tag{A.30}$$

where the concentration of agonist is [A], E_m is the maximal response to the agonist, n is the Hill coefficient of the dose-response curve, and [EC$_{50}$] is the molar concentration of agonist producing 50% maximal response to the agonist.

In the presence of a competitive antagonist, the EC$_{50}$ of the agonist dose-response curve will shift to the right by a factor equal to the dose ratio; this is given by the Schild equation as ($[B]/K_B + 1$) where the concentration of the antagonist is [B] and K_B is the equilibrium dissociation constant of the antagonist-receptor complex:

$$\text{Response} = \frac{E_m[A']^n}{[A']^n + ([EC_{50}](1+[B]/K_B))^n} \tag{A.31}$$

The concentration of antagonist producing a 50% diminution of the agonist response to concentration [A] is defined as the IC$_{50}$ for the antagonist. Therefore:

$$\frac{0.5E_{max}[A]^n}{[A]^n + [EC_{50}]^n} = \frac{E_m[A']^n}{[A']^n + ([EC_{50}](1+[IC_{50}]/K_B))^n} \tag{A.32}$$

After rearrangement (Eq. 4.5):

$$K_B = \frac{[IC_{50}]}{((2+([A]/[EC_{50}])^n)^{1/n}) - 1} \tag{A.33}$$

Derivation of the equation for noncompetitive antagonism

For Chapter 4

It is assumed that the noncompetitive antagonist reduces the fraction of available receptor population. Assuming the noncompetitive antagonist removes a fraction ρ_B from the receptor population, the fraction of agonist remaining after binding of B (ρ_{AB}) is given by:

$$\rho_{AB} = \frac{[A](1 - \rho_B)}{[A] + K_A} \tag{A.34}$$

Expressing ρ_B from mass action:

$$(1 - \rho_B) = ([B]/K_B + 1) - 1 \tag{A.35}$$

Eq. (A.35) can be rewritten for any slope value n:

$$\rho_{AB} = \frac{[A]^n}{([A] + K_A)^n ([B]/K_B + 1)^n} \tag{A.36}$$

Substituting in Eq. (A.20) yields (Eq. 4.6):

$$\text{Response} = \frac{[A]^n \tau^n E_m}{[A]^n \tau^n + (([A] + K_A)([B]/K_B + 1))^n} \tag{A.37}$$

Derivation of the equation for allosteric modulation

For Chapter 5

The equilibrium equations for the receptor species are:

$$[AR] = [ABR]/\alpha[B]K_b \tag{A.38}$$

$$[BR] = [ABR]/\alpha[A]K_a \tag{A.39}$$

$$[R] = [ABR]/\alpha[A]K_a[B]K_b \tag{A.40}$$

The receptor conservation equation for total receptor $[R_{tot}]$ is:

$$[R_{tot}] = [R] + [AR] + [BR] + [ABR] \tag{A.41}$$

The potential response-producing species are [A] and [ABR]; therefore, the fraction of receptors that may produce response is given by:

$$\rho_{A/B/AB} = \frac{[A]/K_A + \alpha[A]/K_A[B]/K_B}{[A]/K_A(1 + \alpha[B]/K_B) + [B]/K_B + 1} \tag{A.42}$$

multiplying by $K_A K_B$ yields

$$\rho_{A/B/AB} = \frac{[A]K_B + \alpha[A][B]}{[A]K_B + \alpha[A][B] + [B]K_A + K_A K_B} \tag{A.43}$$

From Eq. (A.20):

$$\text{Response} = \frac{(\tau_A[A](K_B + \alpha[A][B]))^n E_m}{(\tau_A[A](K_B + \alpha[A][B]))^n + ([A]K_B + \alpha[A][B] + [B]K_A + K_A K_B)^n} \tag{A.44}$$

Defining τ_B as $= \beta\tau_A$ gives (Eq. 5.2):

$$\text{Response} = \frac{(\tau_A[A](K_B + \alpha\beta[B]))^n E_m}{(\tau_A[A](K_B + \alpha\beta[B]))^n + ([A]K_B + K_A K_B + K_A[B] + \alpha[A][B])^n} \tag{A.45}$$

Derivation of the equation for allosteric modulation with direct agonism

In this case, the modulator occupied receptor can also produce response due to direct efficacy. Therefore, the potential response-producing species are [A], [BR] and [ABR]; therefore, the fraction of receptors that may produce response is given by:

$$\rho_{A/B/AB} = \frac{[A]/K_A + [B]/K_B + \alpha[A]/K_A[B]/K_B}{[A]/K_A(1 + \alpha[B]/K_B) + [B]/K_B + 1} \tag{A.46}$$

$$\rho_{A/B/AB} = \frac{[A]K_B + [B]/K_A + \alpha[A][B]}{[A]K_B + \alpha[A][B] + [B]K_A + K_A K_B} \tag{A.47}$$

From Eq. (A.20)

$$\text{Response} = \frac{(\tau_A[A](K_B + \alpha[A][B]) + \tau_B[B]K_A)^n E_m}{(\tau_A[A](K_B + \alpha[A][B]) + \tau_B[B]K_A)^n + ([A]K_B + \alpha[A][B] + [B]K_A + K_A K_B)^n} \tag{A.48}$$

Defining τ_B as $= \beta\tau_A$ gives (Eq. 5.3):

$$\text{Response} = \frac{(\tau_A[A](K_B + \alpha\beta[B]) + \tau_B[B]K_A)^n E_m}{(\tau_A[A](K_B + \alpha\beta[B]) + \tau_B[B]K_A)^n + ([A]K_B + K_A K_B + K_A[B] + \alpha[A][B])^n} \tag{A.49}$$

Derivation of the Michaelis—Menten equation for enzymes

For Chapter 6

The reaction scheme for Michaelis—Menten kinetics is:

$$E + S \underset{k_{-1}}{\overset{k_1}{\rightleftharpoons}} ES \overset{k_2}{\longrightarrow} E + P \tag{A.50}$$

The substrate binds reversibly to the enzyme to form a complex ES, which either dissociates or progresses to enzyme plus a product P. The product P is assumed to have no affinity for the enzyme and thus dissociates. The second half of the reaction describes an irreversible formation of product plus regeneration of the active enzyme. From the reaction scheme Eq. (A.50) comes an expression for the velocity v for the enzyme reaction:

$$v = k_2[ES] \tag{A.51}$$

The assumption here is that the overall reaction velocity is limited by the formation of the product. At this point, the assumption is made that the amount of ES complex is nearly constant, such that the rate of formation of ES (controlled by rate constant k_1) is equal to the rates of dissociation going forward (k_2) and backward (k_{-1}):

$$k_1[E][S] = k_{-1}[ES] + k_2[ES] \tag{A.52}$$

which rearranges to:

$$\frac{K_1[E][S]}{(k_{-1} + k_2)} = [ES] \tag{A.53}$$

A rate constant K_m (the Michaelis–Menten constant) is defined:

$$\frac{(k_{-1} + k_2)}{k_1} = K_M \tag{A.54}$$

which allows Eq. (A.53) to be written:

$$\frac{[E][S]}{K_M} = [ES] \tag{A.55}$$

The total enzyme concentration $[E_0]$ is given by the conservation equation:

$$[E_0] = [E] + [ES] \tag{A.56}$$

Solving for [E] and substituting into Eq. (A.55) yields:

$$\frac{([E_0] - [ES]) + [S]}{K_M} = [ES] \tag{A.57}$$

Rearrangement of Eq. (A.57) and solving for [ES] yields:

$$\frac{[E_0][S]}{[S] + K_M} = [ES] \tag{A.58}$$

Substituting Eq. (A.58) into Eq. (A.51) yields:

$$v = k_2 \frac{[E_0][S]}{[S] + K_M} \tag{A.59}$$

Defining a maximal rate of enzyme reaction V_{max}, which occurs when $[S] \gg [E]$ (also defined as $[A] \to \infty$) yields:

$$V_{max} = k_2[E_0] \qquad (A.60)$$

Substituting Eq. (A.60) into Eq. (A.59) yields the Michaelis–Menten equation:

$$v = \frac{V_{max}[S]}{K_M + [S]} \qquad (A.61)$$

Index